Psychosocial Occupational Therapy
practice in a pluralistic arena

Psychosocial Occupational Therapy
practice in a pluralistic arena

Roann Barris, MS, EdD, OTR
Assistant Professor

Gary Kielhofner, MA, DrPH, OTR, FAOTA
Assistant Professor and Director of Graduate Studies

Janet Hawkins Watts, MS, OTR
Assistant Professor

Department of Occupational Therapy
Virginia Commonwealth University
Richmond, Virginia

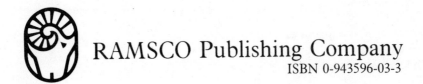

RAMSCO Publishing Company
ISBN 0-943596-03-3

RAMSCO Publishing Company is a subsidiary of RAM Associates LTD, P.O. Box N, Laurel, Maryland 20707.

ISBN 0-94359603-3

Library of Congress Catalogue No. 83-62206

First Printing, August 1983

RAMSCO Order No. 00600

TO:

Patients and clients, whose needs give meaning to the profession

Our fellow therapists, with whom we share the search for professional identity and

Our students, who will continue to shape the profession

Acknowledgments

This book grew out of a shared commitment to a vision for occupational therapy. Its writing represents a true collaboration in that, although each of the authors had primary responsibility for various sections, all contributed to the final content and shaping of every chapter.

While the three authors cooperated in the writing, many others contributed to the book's development. From the beginning stages of conceptualization to the final revisions, we sought input and feedback from our colleagues. The following individuals read the manuscript and offered helpful criticism and commentary: Cathy Andberg, Bette Bonder, Tara Broderick, Tina Brollier, Bob Jenkins, Kathy Kaplan, John Morgan, Ann Neville, Burke Rochford, Joan Rogers, Mark Rosenthal, Cheryl Salz, and Gerald Sharrott. Several students contributed effort and time to the preparation of the manuscript—Beverly Billau, Jamie Cook, Laura Hardee, and Gail Leininger. Our undergraduate and graduate students were our testing grounds and preliminary critics, good naturedly using early chapter drafts instead of a text.

To Sally Cubie goes our special appreciation for her insightful and prompt feedback every time she received another bulky package of drafts in the mail.

Our department head, Patti Maurer, was supportive, diplomatic, and encouraging throughout the period during which we worked on this book.

We are indebted to our family members, who tolerated our frantic efforts and who have foregone our attention and time. Our warm thanks to Allen, Kimberly, Nancy, and Robbie, who graciously supported and endured our work on this volume.

No book comes into existence without an editor and publisher. Our special thanks to Bob Malone for his faith in us and his unwavering and expert support of the text throughout each stage of its development.

Table of Contents

Introduction

Psychosocial occupational therapists practice in a pluralistic arena with a diverse group of professionals who represent a variety of perspectives on psychosocial disorder. Like a large weaving, these different ideologies intermix in varying configurations. One particular school of thought, like a single thread, can become lost in the overall pattern. Those who work in psychosocial practice, however, must be able to both discriminate individual strands, while still recognizing the larger pattern.

The occupational therapist must know the language of and share concepts with several disciplines and frames of reference, while at the same time offering a unique and focused contribution to the health care of psychosocially dysfunctional people. This complex task can be exacerbated when there is a lack of consensus about what the field's unique role is or whether such a role even exists. While many occupational therapists do experience ambiguity over the nature of their service, this need not be the case. Occupational therapy has a rich and long history that readily yields a vision of therapists' roles and functions in a pluralistic psychosocial arena. One purpose of this book is to identify the role and mission of occupational therapy, beginning two centuries ago as moral treatment and continuing today in the use of occupation as a psychosocial health determinant. These principles and practices are unique and contribute substantially to the care of psychosocially dysfunctional people.

We began this book by reflecting on and drawing from our clinical experiences in psychosocial occupational therapy. The following examples represent some of the experiences that led us to compose this volume.

In my work at a county facility for the long-term treatment of chronic patients, I initially tried to fit into the established occupational therapy role. This involved leading or co-leading task groups that used short-term craft projects to develop long-term interests, attitudes, and skills. However, the activities often seemed, to patients, irrelevant or unconnected to their lives. These patients were willing to work on life skills and activities they chose, but they rejected arbitrary choices of such activities as a collage and its apparent irrelevance to their daily life. In fact, I was just as uncomfortable with this arbitrary use of activity as they were and began to search for an approach to developing life skills that would use activities in a meaningful way for these patients. In changing these groups, I had to "reeducate" others (including those in my department) in the hospital about the role of occupational therapy. To do this, however, required a framework that would make sense out of what I thought we should be doing. Here, I was stuck—or rather, thrown back to the traditional occupational therapy approach of taking pieces of theory and ideas from a variety of sources. I emerged with an explanation of occupational therapy that resembled one of the collages more than it articulated a cohesive occupational therapy role.

*   *   *

In my job at a mental health center, working with many other disciplines and no other occupational therapists, I was offered the opportunity to co-lead a group of depressed middle-aged ladies with a highly respected and experienced social worker. After I sat in on a few sessions, the focus on verbal supportive therapy and the use of movement experiences to express feelings became apparent. Although I viewed this as a very exciting opportunity to work with a highly trained therapist, her approach seemed incompatible with my training and experience as an occupational therapist. I realized that the social worker had a different view of these persons' problems from mine. Further, the focus on verbal exchange and emotive expression through movement conflicted with my identity as a therapist who used meaningful activity to develop skills and self-confidence. While I wanted to articulate this situation, I lacked the training to analyze the relationship of different treatment approaches to that of occupational therapy. After two uncomfortable months of trying to figure out how to use my skills in that group, I simply expressed my error in agreeing to co-lead the group.

*   *   *

My first patient as an affiliating student was a young man hospitalized with a label of adjustment reaction of adolescence. This person occasionally in private used women's cosmetics, and concern emerged over the formation of his sexual identity. Most of the treatment team, led by a psychoanalytic psychiatrist, zeroed in on this problem. As an occupational therapist, I did not feel particularly interested in nor prepared to address a problem of sexual identity. On the other hand, I had observed that this young man (who was obese) was inactive, had very few interests, hobbies, or skills, and was isolated from the social recreational activities of his peers. My therapy addressed these problems, but I always felt on the periphery of what most of the team considered the main problem, his sexual identity. In team meetings it seemed that what I had to say about him or his treatment was brushed aside or considered nice but not necessary for his care.

*   *   *

At one point in my practice I was engaged in research with a number of social scientists. I was eager to demonstrate to these anthropologists and sociologists my genuine concern for and ability to address my retarded clients' problems. Thus, it was disconcerting for me when one sociologist pointed out that I had undeniably, because of my perceptions of the tremendous deficits of one man with Down's syndrome, overlooked much of his very real competence. I suddenly became aware that the very situation which cast him as the retarded client and myself as the therapist presented problems that thwarted my goals of recognizing and enhancing his competence. Soon I found myself stepping outside my clinical role and examining my interactions with clients from the perspective of a social scientist asking about the role relationships, the communication processes, and the respective views of each other that my client and I took. Assuming the perspectives of the social scientist not only gave me fresh insight, but made me a better clinician.

*   *   *

In working with numerous other disciplines providing day treatment services to chronic clients in the community, I experienced pride and confidence in my practical orientation as an occupational therapist. However, I was soon dismayed to find other disciplines had begun to adopt that same practical orientation, altering their own traditional treatment approaches to suit the needs of clients in the community. While I felt that my own professional contribution and expertise were being overtaken by other disciplines, I also felt abandoned by many occupational therapists in the field who eschewed the practical orientation and the use of everyday activities as therapy. To top it off I felt insecure in my ability to articulate to other disciplines the exact nature and uniqueness of my practical expertise and the knowledge base that supported it.

Each of these examples reflects one underlying theme: the importance of awareness, knowledge, and critical thinking about different bodies of knowledge. In some cases, as in the first example, therapists find themselves puzzled in the attempt to incorporate several incompletely understood bodies of knowledge into a personal perspective. Other situations involve the interface of people who hold different perspectives based on various bodies of knowledge. Sometimes this interface is harmonious, as in the example where a social science perspective deepens clinical sensitivity. At other times the interface is conflicting, as when people define problems differently or when their views of their respective roles lead to disagreement. In either instance, professionals should appreciate and understand others' perspectives. At the same time, those with a clear identity and commitment to their own professional perspective can more effectively contribute to the function of the team and to patient care. The function of a team is, after all, to bring together people who represent differing ideas and abilities for the purpose of providing optimal health care.

Those who lack clarity and conviction about their professional role identity more often blend into the setting, becoming ancillary to others with stronger perspectives. They tend to follow rather than to direct and develop the goals and activities of the settings in which they practice. This was borne out in a nationwide study of psychosocial occupational therapists.* Therapists who reported that they used activities for psychodynamic reasons (e.g., patients working with clay in order to ventilate anger) generally did so at the request of psychiatrists and psychologists. Such occupational therapy was seen as an extension of psychodynamic approaches championed by other professionals rather than as a unique service. Indeed, several of the therapists in this survey spontaneously volunteered their feelings of insecurity regarding knowledge or the use of theory in psychosocial occupational therapy. Without a strong identity, they were lost in the pattern of ideas and actions represented in the psychosocial arena.

Occupational therapists must both appreciate pluralistic viewpoints and have knowledge and expertise in their own field. Thus, in formulating this book, we were guided by two practical questions: What knowledge comprises the special expertise of the occupational therapist? and What basic knowledge must the occupational therapist have to competently interact with other professionals and to selectively incorporate ideas and approaches into treatment? These two questions led to the development of two major sections in the text. Part One presents eleven bodies of knowledge that are prominent in the thinking of mental health professionals. Part Two is devoted to a detailed description of the occupational therapy body of knowledge and its implementation. Occupational therapy knowledge is covered in greater detail because it is the expertise (or "know how") of the occupational therapist, whereas the other perspectives are covered so that therapists can *know about* them.

Our renderings in Part One of these bodies of knowledge are more absolute than what one typically encounters. However, our goal is to demonstrate a way to identify the many separate lines of thought that contribute to the ultimate configurations of ideas and actions in practice settings.

---

*Barris, R. *Toward an image of one's own: Sources of variation in the occupational therapist's role.* Unpublished doctoral dissertation, Teachers College, Columbia University, 1983.

To facilitate comprehension of each perspective and to enhance critical comparison and evaluation of these bodies of knowledge, all chapters follow the same format. Each chapter begins with a discussion of the *history and purpose* of the body of knowledge. In this section, the following themes are generally covered: (a) how the knowledge emerged and what forces or influences led to its formation, (b) major writers or leaders who developed the ideas and concepts, (c) what fields or professions generally use the knowledge, and (d) particular features that make this body of knowledge interesting, noteworthy, and/or problematic.

The second section of each chapter, *view of order*, examines how the body of knowledge explains the well working of humans. The concept of health approximates what is meant by order, but it presupposes a particular perspective. For instance, some of the bodies of knowledge represented in Part One are not primarily concerned with health and illness. Thus, while they may not address health per se, they do present concepts about how human behavior is organized and influenced. The term *order* was chosen because it is broad enough to encompass many perspectives.

Each chapter then discusses *disorder*, or how the body of knowledge views psychosocial problems. Perhaps here more than in any other section the chapters portray the real differences in bodies of knowledge. How a body of knowledge defines a problem or disorder determines how it will attempt resolution. This is the topic of the discussion that follows next, *action implications*. Here, treatment techniques, a call for social organizational change, or whatever action is prescribed by the body of knowledge is identified.

Two final sections of each chapter provide a perspective for critical evaluation. The *criticisms and limitations* section presents and interprets claims that have been made in the literature pertaining to the weaknesses or limitations of each body of knowledge. The *commentary* section addresses the body of knowledge from the perspective of occupational therapy, discussing its relevance and compatibility. This section offers an assessment of how the body of knowledge should be regarded by occupational therapists.

Needless to say, this chapter format worked more readily for some bodies of knowledge than for others. However, using this structure to organize the presentation of each body of knowledge served to highlight some of the gaps and inconsistencies as well as the strengths of each perspective. The themes of order, disorder, and action implications are of critical concern to any person working in the area of psychosocial dysfunction, and they must be properly balanced in any view. Thus, when a body of knowledge focuses on action without a clear formulation of order and disorder, or when disorder is concentrated on so heavily that order is relatively ignored, the body of knowledge can be said to be incomplete or lacking. Therefore, while our categories are imposed from without on each body of knowledge, this imposition facilitates critical analysis and evaluation.

The second part of the text consists of a comprehensive discussion of occupational therapy that follows the format of the chapters in Part One. However, each section on order, disorder, and so forth is expanded into a full chapter. Our intent in Part Two was not so much to unravel as to interrelate occupational therapy themes so that they could be seen as a whole. The action implications section is greatly expanded to constitute a comprehensive description of practice. It outlines principles of practice and the occupational therapy process, and it discusses assessment and the roles and functions of occupational therapy in remediating psychosocial dysfunction.

The perspective offered as the unique occupational therapy contribution to the psychosocial arena also reflects the authors' convictions about the unique orientation of occupational therapy in general. Thus, it should *not* be construed that the occupational therapy ideas forwarded in this text are essentially different from the approach that should be taken by occupational therapists in physical dysfunction. It is the patient population which leads to differences in practice in the areas of physical and psychosocial dysfunction, not a difference in the body of knowledge that defines the roles and functions of occupational therapy.

The choice of certain words always presents a dilemma for writers; some of our choices bear mentioning. First, every effort was made to eliminate sexist terminology throughout this volume. The terms "patients" and "clients" are both used throughout the text. Their use often reflects the context or setting being discussed. Thus, the term *client* was used in discussions of nontraditional situations, especially community mental health. *Patient* was used in discussions of more traditional medical circumstances. In addition, we used the term most often associated with the body of knowledge under discussion.

The term *psychosocial dysfunction* is used throughout the volume to refer to persons with (a) identified emotional disturbances, (b) mental retardation, and (c) developmental disabilities or physical problems that have precipitated a psychological or social disturbance. In reality these categories overlap. All have in common a disturbance to psychological and interpersonal well-being. More specific terms such as mental retardation, schizophrenia, and the like were used when a particular topic pertained only to that subgroup of those with psychosocial dysfunction. Finally, we sought to avoid such terms as "mental retardates" and "the mentally ill," since such language does not acknowledge the human identity of these persons.

Each chapter contains a glossary and summary table as review and study guides. They also provide a ready means of comparison of different bodies of knowledge. Reference lists provide additional readings for the interested person. Our choice of references in Part One was based on the goal of using authoritative and representative works and is therefore not exhaustive. In Part Two we did attempt to provide complete excursion of relevant occupational therapy references.

Part One

Bodies Of Knowledge In Psychosocial Practice

1
The Medical Model

Any discussion of the medical model must begin with the qualification that no universally accepted version of the medical model exists.[2] This chapter presents the medical model in its classical and purest form, leaving out proposed extensions, alterations, and reformulations.

The medical model is strictly in the possession of medicine, though aspects of it have been used in other paramedical or allied health disciplines. It is both an ideology and a collection of knowledge, which cannot be effectively separated. The ideological component of the medical model includes a set of beliefs about the physician's role as a healer with authority over patients. The knowledge component is a reductionist, biochemical body of information that explains disease as an interruption of normal physiological processes and yields procedures to eliminate disease through manipulation or alteration of somatic structures and processes. The medical model can thus be defined as the beliefs and knowledge that define physicians as authoritative healers and that enable them to cure, ameliorate, or arrest disease through recognition and alteration of its manifestation in bodily states.

HISTORY AND PURPOSE

The current medical model can be partially traced to the medical systems of the ancient Greeks.[5] Hippocrates is viewed as the progenitor of modern medicine, and while his writings presage the medical model, they reflect a broader viewpoint. The Hippocratic view of medicine is based on the ideas embodied in two Grecian gods.

Hygeia, the goddess of health, represented the concepts that health is a state of harmony with nature and one's environment and that disease results from violation of natural laws that govern this harmony. Hygeia was a teacher of wisdom who represented living in an orderly and harmonious fashion as a protection against the ravages of disease. The god, Asclepius, embodied the healer—one who cures with medicinal plants and surgery. The Asclepian authority of the physician derives from this divine healer.[19] Whereas Hygeia disseminated practical knowledge to the populace to guide their actions, Asclepius wielded esoteric knowledge as part of his healing art. He ministered to a passive and compliant recipient of the healing action. Because he was the knowing healer, his authority over the patient was absolute.

Hippocrates took a democratic view of the relative importance of these two modes of medical practice, stressing the role of the physician as both a teacher and a healer.[5] In that sense, Hippocratic medicine is broader than the current medical model, which exclusively embraces the Asclepian mode. Hippocrates does portend one important element of the medical model, namely, its commitment to science. He called for the liberalization of scientific medicine from theological (i.e., mystical and demonic) beliefs.

The history of Western medicine is one of steady growth of scientific knowledge concerning disease and its management.[5] The powers of observation, analytic thought, and experimentation catapulted medicine into one of the most successful enterprises known to human civilizations. This was made possible by the confinement of medical knowledge to the domain of reductionistic cause-and-effect perspectives and to biological phenomena. That is, medical knowledge is concentrated on underlying biochemical constituents of the human body and their cause-and-effect relationships, with a relative lack of concern for more complex biological phenomena, psychosocial phenomena, and connections between mind and body.

At the time when medicine began to increase its scientific base, reductionist thought in the physical sciences was reaching maturity. Scientists had made great strides in understanding the physical world through careful examination of the building blocks of nature and their interrelationships.[4] They sought to understand the universe as a great clockwork of interacting parts. Both the separation of mind from body and this "mechanistic" viewpoint of reductionist science led medicine to adopt the view of the body as a machine and led physicians to adopt the view that their task was to repair breakdowns in the machine (i.e., disease).[4] In practice, physicians using the medical model came to treat the body as separate from psychological and social processes and tended to see the latter as insignificant.

The most central aspect of the medical model is the concept of disease. Foucault[8] documents the long history of medical thought that culminates in the physician's ability to separate the person who is experiencing an illness from the underlying disease that "resides within" the person. This abstraction is at the core of all medical thought and practice.

Historically, the medical model has been the nearly exclusive domain of physicians; in turn, physicians have largely chosen to approach their practice within the framework of the medical model. Psychiatry, however, represents a rather unusual case. Psychiatry's relationship to mainstream medicine has been and remains a matter of concern among physicians. Some believe that psychiatry is a branch of medicine that has collected a variety of perspectives, knowledge, and skills that extend beyond the traditional purview of medicine. They view this as a necessary response to patients' psychosocial problems. Others disagree, arguing that the medical model alone defines both the physician's role and domain of concern. Proponents of the latter viewpoint would support a narrowing of psychiatric practice to concentrate on those psychosocial problems that are true biological diseases, leaving to other health professionals psychosocial problems that have no biological components.

VIEW OF ORDER

The theory base of the medical model includes three major themes: (1) a reductionist cause-and-effect framework, (2) a concern with the biochemical level of structures and processes, and (3) a homeostatic or normative view of order. These are interrelated in the theoretical explanation of health (order). Because the medical model has traditionally been concerned primarily with disorder, the approach to defining order has been to proceed "inductively by enumeration of examples [of disease] and then health is the absence of all of those states" (p. 75).[3] The problem of what constitutes order in the human system is generally not a major issue in the medical model, simply because the prime focus of concern is disorder.

Reductionism and the cause-and-effect conceptualizations of the medical model are derived from the intellectual models of early physical sciences.[4,17] The basic tenets of reductionism are that any phenomenon is ultimately reducible, and thus explicable, in terms of its most elementary constituents and their cause-and-effect relationships.[1,4] In physical science, reductionist strategies were the searches for the building blocks of the inanimate world. They led to such discoveries as the atom—at one time considered the building block of physical phenomena. In the biological sciences and in medicine, the search led to the discovery of the cell and later its molecular constituents, their chemical components, and so forth. Always, reductionism progresses deeper into the system in the search for more and more elemental parts. The goal of reductionist thought is that ultimately all phenomena at a macro level (e.g., bodily functions directly observable to anyone) will be explained in terms of the finite cause-and-effect relations between the most elementary or microlevel components of the body. Thus, tissue can be understood in terms of its cellular makeup, cells in terms of their molecular structures, molecules in terms of their chemical constituents, and so forth.

As a function of its reductionist strategy, the medical model has less concern for macro events (i.e., the body functioning as a whole, as an instrument of the mind, and as an embodiment of someone who has a social position). Rather, the medical model considers psychosocial factors as either inconsequential or as irrelevant to its domain of concern and concentrates on the underlying biological and chemical level. Thus, order primarily refers to integrity of the biochemical constituents of the body.[2,7]

The medical model has also viewed order as homeostasis, a central concept in medical thinking. The classic concept of homeostasis[1] is the notion that living systems try to maintain certain predetermined states. Any substantial movement from a homeostatic state is disturbance to the order of the system. Examples of homeostatic processes in the body are blood pressure and temperature. When conditions change from what is typical for the organism, it seeks to return them to that previous state. Thus, the concept of order in the medical model refers primarily to the maintenance of those bodily states that are considered to be normal.

VIEW OF DISORDER

In the medical model, disorder is disease. As noted earlier, one of the central features of the emergence of the medical model was the ability of the physician to see a disease *in* the person. Thus, disorder is viewed as a correlate to a foreign and disruptive entity dwelling within someone. As Laing and Esterson[11] describe it:

When a psychiatrist diagnoses schizophrenia, he means that the patient's experience and behavior are disturbed *because* there is something the matter with the patient that causes the disturbed behavior he observed. He calls this something schizophrenia, and he then must ask what causes schizophrenia. (p. ii)

In addition, disease is viewed as disrupting the homeostatic order of biological processes. Disease forces certain functions out of bounds, beyond normative limits. Thus, disease represents an attack on an otherwise static order within the system.

In the purest sense, the medical model view of psychosocial problems is that "mental disorders are in fact organic diseases" (p. 911).[2] This extreme position does not represent all of current psychiatric thought, but it is most consistent with the medical model views of nonpsychiatric physicians. Further, such a characterization of the medical model differentiates it from more psychological concepts often used by psychiatrists, such as psychoanalytic thought.

In the strict sense, the medical model is an *organic* model of mental illness. Physiological disturbances must be present if psychosocial problems are to be considered true diseases.[14] Importantly, for the medical model to yield typical medical treatment, there must be physiological dimensions, if not causes, of the psychosocial disorder. True diseases must have a biological component, as is clear from the following assessment of the medical model view of disorder:

> The dominant model of disease today is biomedical, with molecular biology its basic scientific discipline. It assumes disease to be fully accounted for by deviations from the norm of measurable biological (somatic) variables. It leaves no room within its framework for the social, psychological, and behavioral dimensions of illness. The biomedical model not only requires that disease be dealt with as an entity independent of social behavior, it also demands that behavioral aberrations be explained on the basis of disordered somatic (biochemical or neurophysiological) processes. Thus, the biomedical model embraces both reductionism, the philosophic view that complex phenomena are ultimately derived from a single primary principle, and mind-body dualism, the doctrine that separates the mental from the somatic. (p. 130)[6]

While this view is not accepted by all physicians, those of opposing viewpoints might be said to be operating outside the medical model in their practice and thought. Therefore, biological disturbance *must* accompany psychosocial problems in order to confer upon them disease status.[2,14] Further, problems without any clear organic correlates are problems with living, which fall outside the domain of medicine.[19] This is a somewhat controversial position, but it is most closely in line with traditional concepts of the medical model.

Biological factors, however, need not be the sole cause or manifestation of psychiatric diseases. Although this allows that other causes of psychosocial disorder (e.g., environmental or experiential factors) may well exist and probably do contribute to many psychiatric problems, the medical model seeks to explain *only* the biological components or causes of psychosocial problems.[14]

The medical model categorizes psychiatric diseases as neuropsychiatric, medicopsychiatric, and functional psychiatric.[14] Neuropsychiatric diseases emanate from nervous system disorders (e.g., epilepsy or brain tumor) and medicopsychiatric from other medical conditions (e.g., vitamin deficiency). The functional category refers to problems where organic factors are suspected but not yet proven. Excluded from any of these categories are problems with living, such as situational depressions, social deviances, and adjustment reactions. This particular system of classification differs from the *Diagnostic and Statistical Manual of Mental Disorders III* of the American Psychiatric Association, which avows no particular theoretical leanings, and is not offered as a medical model approach to psychiatric illness. It draws in eclectic fashion from the perspectives of many health disciplines, including occupational therapy. There is obviously a difference between the practical and often multifaceted collections of perspectives used by psychiatrists and the pure medical model.

ACTION IMPLICATIONS

Strictly speaking, action which is derived from the medical model is somatic in nature and guided by the germ theory of disease. According to germ theory, disease has an identifiable cause. Control of disease is best accomplished by attacking the causative agent or focusing treatment on that part of the body affected by disease.[5] The primary emphasis is on discovery of a drug or procedure that would attack the disease or alter or excise the diseased component. This requires that the physician begin with careful data to arrive at a correct diagnosis—the diagnosis is the crux of medical treatment. The following passage aptly describes the action process of the medical model:

> The view of medical practice in effect at the beginning of this century—which we may label the "traditional view"—assumed the existence of a set of discrete entities called diseases and a set of other entities called therapies or therapeutic agents. These two sets were thought to be related in an imperfect 1:1 correspondence. The task of the physician was to classify signs and symptoms to determine which of the disease entities were present in his patient. When successful, this process of diagnosis suggested the corresponding therapy which the physician was to apply. (p. 83)[3]

Identifying the disease ordinarily means that the physician will have some degree of ability to predict and control the course of illness. The diagnosis is critical in the medical model, because it predicts the course of treatment and the path of the disease.[15] If treatment is successful, it then confirms the physician's initial diagnosis.

However, only in the case of a limited number of diseases does medicine reach this ideal of sufficient knowledge in order to make efficacious use of the diagnosis.[15] There is a continuum from those diseases for which there is rather certain knowledge of etiology, course, and treatment, to those about which little or nothing is known. Psychosocial problems fall at the latter end of the continuum.

The primary somatic therapies of the medical model are chemotherapy, electroconvulsive therapy, diet management, and surgery.[14] A variety of chemotherapies are used for psychosocial disturbances, or to control or manage other biological problems that are concomitants of the psychosocial problem (e.g., the control of epilepsy). The major use of drugs in psychosocial practice is for the management of psychiatric symptomatology. These psychotropic drugs may be divided into antipsychotics, antidepressants, and minor tranquilizers.[10]

Antipsychotics include several families of related chemical compounds. They are used to reduce the extreme symptomatology of psychotic patients. These drugs routinely have a variety of side effects ranging from the fairly innocuous, such as a dry mouth, to serious and some possibly irreversible complications, such as seizure and tardive dyskinesia.

Antidepressant drugs also include several families of chemicals. These drugs palliate symptoms of clinical depression with fewer side effects than the antipsychotic drugs. Minor tranquilizers are a family of drugs generally used to alleviate the symptom of anxiety, and they are more often given to non-hospitalized patients.[10] Their major side effect is sedation.

In all cases, the drugs, within their major categorizations, may act variously with different patients. Optimal dosage is also a matter of great variation among patients. Thus, medication with psychotropic drugs ordinarily involves a trial-and-error period during which both the desired results and side effects are monitored in order to achieve correct prescription. However, since the variety of antipsychotics is great but effects are generally similar, the choice of drugs is largely based on physician familiarity and preference.

Psychosurgery for psychiatric symptoms (e.g., the classic lobotomy) is much less frequent today. The most likely situation for surgery is removal of an actual brain defect such as a tumor or correction of a somatic problem such as epilepsy. Other somatic therapies such as electroconvulsive therapy and megavitamin therapy tend to vary in their use with the particular clinical conviction of the physician and with diagnoses. Certain psychosocial problems (e.g., mental retardation from phenylketonuria) have been successfully prevented through somatic therapy.

Often, treatment cannot be directed at underlying causes (which may not be known) and instead focuses on managing problems concurrent with the psychosocial disturbance or with managing symptoms without affecting the underlying problem.[14] This means that medical model treatment may be curative, compensatory, syndromatic, or symptomatic.[15] In curative treatment, causative agents are attacked and the condition is reversed. Compensatory treatment aims to minimize further problems and maintain function, while syndromatic treatment manages major problems related to the disease without cure. Finally, symptomatic treatment simply alleviates some problems without altering basic causes or effects of the disease. Only a very small percent of medical treatment is curative.[14]

An interesting aspect of psychiatrists' practice is that while they employ elements of the medical model (e.g., Asclepian authority and diagnostic procedures), treatment often includes a variety of approaches (e.g., behavior modification and psychotherapy) informed by bodies of knowledge other than the medical model. These are loosely viewed as compatible with the medical model.[14]

CRITICISMS AND LIMITATIONS

Engel[6,7] argues that the medical model leaves only two alternatives for reconciling the relationship between disease and behavior: (1) a reductionistic alternative, which is to say that all odd or disordered behavior results from or is caused by disease; and (2) an exclusionistic alternative, which says that behavioral disorders that cannot be explained in biochemical terms must be excluded from the category of disease. Engel also argues that the reductionism of the medical model has led to undesirable treatment practices such as overuse of surgery and drugs and inappropriate use of diagnostic procedures. He criticizes the medical model for its lack of concern for factors other than the biomedical.

The value of diagnostic procedures is directly related to the certainty of etiological and therapeutic implications of the diagnosis. This requires that much be known about the disease, its course, its alterability, and the agents that have power to control the disease processes. Many persons have criticized the use of psychiatric diagnostic processes in the medical model, because in psychiatry few diagnoses approach the degree of knowledge and certainty needed for effective delineation of etiology, course (prognosis), and treatment. Goffman[9] notes in this vein that:

> While some psychiatric cases may be neatly handled within the framework established by the medical model there are very evident sources of difficulty, especially in regard to the largest category of patients, those with so-called "functional" psychoses. (p. 352)

Others argue that it will never be correct to apply diagnostic procedures to psychiatric medicine because psychosocial problems are not diseases but rather problems with living.[13,20]

Recognizing that mental illness appears to involve a complex of social factors, psychological factors, biological factors, and their interrelationships points to the need for a model that can address multilevel, complex phenomena. Matching one-to-one therapies for given psychosocial problems with a mechanistic disease-therapy model is simply not possible.[13]

Leifer[13] has launched one of the most critical attacks on the medical model, claiming that it is an ideological rather than a therapeutic tool in the hands of psychiatry. He compares similarities and differences between psychiatry and somatic medicine, noting that the similarities lie more in the background and the conceptual and ideological views held by physicians than in their patients. Criticizing the purely medical model approach to mental disease, he notes that the "important distinction between medical and mental disease is that action to eliminate the former is directed against bodies while action to eliminate the latter is directed against persons" (p.16).[13] Leifer further notes that it is important "whether psychiatric patients are viewed as suffering from diseases or as experiencing some other kinds of problems" (p. 13).[13] He insists that disease should refer to phenomena not regulated by social customs and belonging to organic structure and function of the body. By calling mental illness a disease, the medical model obscures the fact that psychiatrists are agents of social control. Thus, he concludes, while the work of other physicians is primarily a technical matter, the work of psychiatry is patently moral and political in nature. Leifer[13] concludes that conceptual models are metaphors and they reveal only what is congenial to their form, disguising or diverting attention from those things they cannot assimilate. He calls for an expanded biosocial model of mental illness, identifies the need to conduct research into the relationship between the mind and body, and feels that the medical model in psychiatry impedes this process.

Similarly, Szasz sees the medical model as a sham that obscures psychiatry's real role and justifies wholesale segregation and incarceration of socially deviant individuals.[20] Szasz distinguishes between diseases of the body and what he calls "problems with living." The former are properly the purview of medicine while the latter are in the field of human relations and thus constitute a moral rather than a scientific enterprise.

Laing and Esterson emphatically take issue with the assertion that schizophrenia is an entity, clinical or otherwise. They fundamentally disagree with the medical conceptualization of schizophrenia that asserts that "the patient's experience and behavior are disturbed *because* there is something the matter with the patient that causes the disturbed behavior" (p. 11).[11] They criticize the attempt to use the medical model in psychiatry, claiming that it merely represents an attempt to bring psychiatry in line with mainstream biochemical medicine. Attempts to categorize the behavior and experience of persons with psychosocial dysfunction as symptoms are also seen as artificial strategies for making psychiatric practice more medical. Their alternate proposal is that the social intelligibility of schizophrenic thinking and behavior can be understood by examining the family context of the person identified as schizophrenic.

These major criticisms of the medical model pertain to its limited scope (i.e., biochemical, cause-and-effect concepts) and its irrelevance to many psychosocial problems which likely have their etiology and manifestation at the psychological and social levels. Further, there is disagreement with the approach of diagnosing psychosocial patients, both because most psychiatric diagnoses give only limited information about etiology, prognosis, and treatment, and because they presume the existence of biological disease—a phenomenon discounted by some critics.

In sum, the medical model is relevant to psychosocial dysfunction when psychosocial problems have biological concomitants. Chemotherapy is typically of some use in the management of symptoms. In a few categories of psychosocial problems, physicians can have direct impact on underlying causes. Thus, the medical model has a contribution to make, but not one that warrants the predominance of physician authority in the area of psychosocial dysfunction.

COMMENTARY

Earliest occupational therapy (see the discussion of moral treatment, Chapter 12) was an attempt to deal outside the medical model with psychiatric patients. Rogers[18] points out cogently that there are critical differences between occupational therapy's approach to order and disorder and that of the medical model. So called "problems with living" and those psychosocial aspects of mental disability eschewed by the medical model are the primary concern of occupational therapy. Further, occupational therapy seeks primarily to influence health rather than pathology.[16] In that sense, the respective contributions of the medical model and occupational therapy would be complementary in the area of psychosocial problems, if occupational therapy is granted authority for the management of problems that fall primarily in its domain.

Unfortunately, the Asclepian authority of medicine extends beyond the domain of the medical model into areas where other health practitioners might better serve as primary caregivers or managers of psychosocial services. An apt guideline offered by Siegler and Osmond[19] is that the physician's role does not include states of impairment. Psychosocial dysfunction often entails major impairment of function which must be regained through substantial rehabilitative efforts. Occupational therapists should be aware of both the strengths and limitations of the medical model and of the particular ways in which occupational therapy can make primary contributions to the care of those with psychosocial problems.

SUMMARY

History and Purpose	The medical model is both knowledge and ideology which defines and justifies the physician's role as an Asclepian authority.
	It emerges from a commitment to science as practiced by the physical sciences and focuses on the process of identifying and eradicating diseases that dwell within persons.

View of Order	Concern is with cause-and-effect relations in biochemical structures and processes.
	Order is equated with homeostatic or normative states and defined primarily as the absence of disorder.
	Because medicine employs reductionist science, which delves deeper and deeper into the organism, its concern with order is micro (biochemical) rather than macro (the person functioning as a whole).
View of Disorder	Disorder is disease, which is viewed as a foreign entity dwelling in the human body and causing a disturbance of the homeostasis or normative order.
	Disorder is viewed in biochemical terms. Psychosocial problems without biochemical constituents or causes are, strictly speaking, not included in the medical model view of disorder.
Action Implications	Medical treatment is somatic and guided by the germ theory of disease which entails identifying causes and eradicating disease and/or its symptoms through: chemotherapy, diet therapy, electroconvulsive therapy, and surgery.
Criticisms and Limitations	Critics fault the medical model for using Asclepian authority for social control of deviance when the nature of psychosocial problems does not warrant a medical model approach.
	The medical model is also criticized for being too reductionist and narrow in its view of disorder.
	The relevance of the medical model is limited to psychosocial problems with biochemical correlates and causes.
Commentary	Occupational therapy and the medical model can offer complementary action when the authority of the latter is limited to areas of relevance and when occupational therapy's relevance to "problems with living" is acknowledged.

TERMS AND CONCEPTS

antidepressants   drugs used to alleviate depression.

antipsychotics   drugs used to alleviate psychotic symptoms.

Asclepian authority   a term used to refer to the physician's right to be the ultimate authority in medicine and to expect compliance. It connotes the idea of a moral right to authority.

chemotherapy   the use of drugs to manage disease and/or its symptoms.

compensatory treatment   treatment aimed at minimizing further problems and maintaining function.

curative treatment   treatment aimed at attacking the causative agent and reversing the condition.

electroconvulsive therapy   the use of electric shock to alleviate symptoms of certain mental disorders.

epilepsy   a disorder in which those afflicted experience seizures.

etiology   the source or cause of a disease or dysfunction.

homeostatic   a process of maintaining a static state and returning to it after disturbances (examples are rate of heartbeat and blood pressure).

lobotomy   removal of a portion of the brain usually to reduce aggressive behavior.

medicopsychiatric disease   disease emanating from biochemical disturbances other than those in the nervous system.

minor tranquilizers   drugs used to reduce anxiety.

neuropsychiatric disease   disease emanating from disorders in the nervous system.

problems with living   a phrase used to refer to psychosocial problems which appear to have no biological cause, but reflect difficulty adjusting to life situations and life tasks.

psychosurgery   surgery that involves removal of brain tissue or implantation of devices to affect electrochemical functions in the brain.

reductionist   a viewpoint that focuses on the components of phenomena and their cause-and-effect relationships, assuming that the whole can be explained through description of how its parts intermesh.

symptomatic treatment   treatment that alleviates symptoms or problems, but not the underlying disorder or disease.

REFERENCES

1. von Bertalanffy, L. General systems theory and psychiatry. In S.R. Arieti (ed.), *American handbook of psychiatry* (Vol. 3). New York: Basic Books, 1966.
2. Blaney, P. H. Implications of the medical model and its alternatives. *American Journal of Psychiatry*, 1975, *132*, 911–914.
3. Brody, H. The systems view of man: Implications for medicine, science, and ethics. *Perspectives in Biology and Medicine*, 1973, Autumn, 71–92.
4. Capra, F. *The turning point: Science, society, and the rising culture*. New York: Simon & Schuster, 1982.
5. Dubos, R. *The mirage of health*. New York: Harper & Row, 1959.
6. Engel, G. L. The nature of disease and the care of the patient: The challenge of humanism and science in medicine. *Rhode Island Medical Journal*, 1962, *65*, 245–251.
7. Engel, G. L. The need for a new medical model: A challenge for biomedicine. *Science*, 1977, *196*, 129–135.
8. Foucault, M. [*The birth of the clinic*] (A. M. S. Smith, trans.). New York: Pantheon Books, 1973.
9. Goffman, E. *Asylums*. New York: Doubleday, 1962.
10. Kline, N., & Davis, J. M. Psychotropic drugs. *American Journal of Nursing*, 1973, *73*, 54–62.
11. Laing, T. D., & Esterson, A. *Sanity, madness and the family*. Baltimore: Penguin Books, 1970.
12. Lazare, A. Hidden conceptual models in clinical psychiatry. *New England Journal of Medicine*, 1973, *288*, 345–350.
13. Leifer, R. Medical model as ideology. *International Journal of Psychiatry*, 1970, *9*, 13–34.
14. Ludwig, A. M., & Othmer, E. The medical basis of psychiatry. *American Journal of Psychiatry*, 1977, *134*, 1087–1092.
15. Mechanic, D. The doctor's view of disease and the patient. In D. Mechanic (ed.), *Medical sociology* (2nd ed.). New York: Free Press, 1978.
16. Reilly, M. Occupational therapy can be one of the great ideas of 20th

century medicine. *American Journal of Occupational Therapy*, 1962, *16*, 1–9.

17. Riley, J. N. Western medicine's attempt to become more scientific: Examples from the United States and Thailand. *Social Science and Medicine*, 1977, *11*, 549–560.

18. Rogers, J. Order and disorder in medicine and occupational therapy. *American Journal of Occupational Therapy*, 1982, *36*, 29–35.

19. Siegler, M., & Osmond, H. *Models of madness, models of medicine*. New York: Harper & Row, 1974.

20. Szasz, T. *The myth of mental illness*. New York: Delta, 1961.

2
Classical Psychoanalysis

Psychoanalysis was one of the first systematic approaches to understanding and treating mental illness. A distinguishable approach to the treatment of mental illness as early as 1895, it has become identified and merged with the entire domain of general psychology.[3] For the layman as well as for those professionals who are psychoanalytically oriented, classical psychoanalysis is nearly synonymous with the name of Sigmund Freud, who initiated and developed it.

Psychoanalysis underwent significant changes throughout Freud's 40-year period of active theorizing and practice. While many subsequent psychoanalysts have interpreted and extended his writings, this presentation of classical psychoanalysis will include only the original theories of Sigmund Freud and significant elaborations and interpretations that are congruent with Freud's basic theory. Neo-Freudian theories, which tend to dispute major tenets of Freudian thinking, are presented in the next chapter.

HISTORY AND PURPOSE

The development of psychoanalysis was influenced by then current scientific and social trends and reflects Freud's personal and career development, his medical training, and his professional influences. Several notable scientific and social influences and special interests pervade Freud's work.

The Helmholtz school of physiology that emphasized cause and effect sequential thinking and the belief that all science could be reduced to the laws of physics had a strong impact on Freud's works.[1] Freud believed that explaining human psychological functioning in terms of scientific laws was not only possible, but offered the best means of clearly understanding human behavior. The following quote characterizes his views on this issue:

> The hypothesis we have adopted of a psychical apparatus extended in space, expediently put together, developed by the exigencies of life, which gives rise

to the phenomena of consciousness only at one particular point and under certain conditions—this hypothesis has put us in a position to establish psychology on foundations similar to those of any other science, such, for instance, as physics . . . . Our procedure in psycho-analysis is quite similar. We have discovered technical methods of filling up the gaps in the phenomena of our consciousness, and we make use of those methods just as a physicist makes use of experiment. In this manner we infer a number of processes which are themselves "unknowable" and interpolate them in those that are conscious to us. (pp. 53-54)[6]

Other influences reflected in Freud's work include a personal interest in Shakespeare and Goethe, Victorian English values (especially those relative to sexuality), and the flourishing, yet controversial Darwinian theory of evolution.[1,5] Thus, while his theories were original, they reflected both sophisticated intellectual trends of his day as well as other social and cultural influences.

Freud was born in 1856 in an area now called Czechoslovakia. When he was 4, Freud's family moved to Vienna, where he eventually received a medical degree and centered his life and career. In the 1920s he fled from Nazism to England, where he died in 1939.[1,5]

Before settling on the study of psychological phenomena, Freud had a varied medical background. He originally worked as a neurological and neuroanatomical researcher. Then in private practice he worked as a general physician, surgeon, and finally as a psychiatrist at the Vienna General Hospital under Theodor Meynert, a leading brain anatomist. Later, Freud studied at the neurology clinic of Jean-Martin Charcot in Paris, where he developed an interest in hysteria and in the use of hypnosis as a psychiatric treatment. Although Freud eventually found hypnosis to be a limited treatment technique, his interest in it led to more concern with inner, unconscious phenomena. Freud then worked with the Viennese physician Josef Breuer to begin development of what he called a "talking out" technique that is still the primary method of psychoanalysis.[2,5] It is at this point, during Freud's work with Breuer in the study of hysteria and the use of hypnosis, that psychoanalysis has its identifiable origins.

Freud's development of psychoanalytic theories has been identified as reflecting six stages.[1] The first was the period of collaboration with Breuer. Together they described hysterical symptoms as being caused by pent-up emotion related to an unpleasant event stored in the unconscious. Treatment involved helping the patient to recall the memory of this event from the unconscious and express the related emotion, effecting relief and release of undischarged energy. This process was termed "cathartic abreaction." Freud noted that such traumatic events often occurred in childhood and were routinely sexual in nature. This led to his theorizing about childhood sexuality.[1] Freud eventually split with

Breuer over the former's sexual emphasis, and he was ostracized from one of the prominent medical societies for the same reason.

The second stage, around 1900, began with the study of dreams. Freud noted that dreams and symptoms bore strong similarities; both seemed to be distortions formed by the tension between the forces of unconscious childhood wishes seeking expression and the other aspects of mental life exerting a controlling or repressive effect on these wishes. Freud's insights and under-standings came about partly from self-analysis. His most significant thesis was that mental life is primarily characterized by dynamics of conflict between the conscious and unconscious—that is, between what is realistic and logical versus sexual and impulsive. This theory is called the *topographic theory* since it relates to layers of consciousness.[1]

In the third stage, Freud sought an explanation for psychotic behavior. The tension between sexual urges and the more adaptive, logical mental forces seemed inadequate for explaining psychoses. He theorized that tension between investing libidinal energies (sexual drives) in the self versus objects external to the self better explained psychotic behavior.[1] The fourth stage was his attempt at synthesis and reorganization; he tried to organize his concepts as a metapsychology. This was a transitional phase prior to a major theory revision.[1] In the next stage, Freud revised his drive theory to make it a dualistic theory including both libido (sex) and aggression, which are derived respectively from broader biological bases called Eros (love) and Thanatos (the death instinct).[1]

In the sixth and final stage, Freud formed his *structural theory* of the mind's organization, in which the components of mental function were identified by the roles they played in conflict. He divided the psychic apparatus into id, ego, and superego. Mental health and mental illness were viewed as dependent on how well the ego mediated between mental conflicts and external reality factors. Anxiety was identified as a warning signal of mental imbalance, alerting the ego to activate a defensive strategy for self-protection.[1]

The current status of psychoanalysis in the United States is largely influ-enced by policies of the psychoanalytic training institutes affiliated with the American Psychoanalytic Association. With a few exceptions, they limit their admissions to those with a medical degree who have completed a psychiatric training residency. Thus, in-depth psychoanalysis in this country is provided mainly by psychiatrists. However, other mental health disciplines receive training from psychoanalytic organizations not restricted to medical doctors and frequently provide care based on psychoanalytic concepts.[1]

VIEW OF ORDER

Describing the view of order in psychoanalytic theory seems paradoxical since psychoanalytic concepts were developed by Freud largely in response to and from observation of pathological processes. However, some themes that characterize how the human being's mental processes interrelate and unfold can be said to constitute a view of order—though, in the end, psychoanalysis gives the clear impression that order is less probable than disorder in the human being.

The view of order in psychoanalytic thinking reflects linear cause-and-effect thinking, concern with levels of consciousness, the views that causation always comes from lower, more covert levels and that human actions always seek to avoid tension or disequilibrium.

Order is a function of drives that emanate from biological inheritances. These drives are mediated and interrelated at different levels of consciousness though they emanate from lower levels. Conflict is a pivotal feature of all mental processes, and order involves the process of minimizing conflict or tension. Psychoanalysis is a "psychology of conflict" (p. 1),[1] and much as behaviorists consider a person's outward behavior to result from attempts at tension-reduction, psychoanalysts see the operation of the mind to be a product of attempts to reduce or adjust to tensions within the psychic apparatus. These tensions exist between the conscious and the unconscious, internal and external demands, and also result from demands on the organism for growth and development. Many of the themes and principles of psychoanalysis reflect this concern with conflict.

Psychoanalytic Principles

Four major principles of psychoanalytic theory are psychic determinism, the topographic viewpoint, the dynamic viewpoint, and the genetic viewpoint.[1]

Psychic determinism argues that mental events such as feelings and thoughts have specific causes; these are often unconscious and related to earlier life events.

According to the *topographic viewpoint*, mental events are organized into layers of consciousness—the conscious, preconscious, and unconscious. The conscious level is the same consciousness referred to in daily conversation. That content which is easily remembered describes the preconscious. Other psychic material that is inaccessible to the conscious and must be inferred or otherwise recognized is in the unconscious. Conflicts arise from efforts to move psychic material from one level to another or to keep it on one particular level of awareness. A dynamic related to the topographic viewpoint is repression, the process of keeping mental material from conscious awareness to avoid unpleasant events. Another dynamic, resistance, occurs in the analysis when the ego of the patient persistently opposes the perceived threat of the analysis process and the moving of unconscious content to levels of greater awareness.[6] Overcoming this resistance is a significant part of the analyst's work. This topographic theory has been supplanted by Freud's structural theory (i.e., his reference to the id, ego, and superego) as a more useful guide to practice.

The third principle of psychoanalytic theory is the *dynamic viewpoint*. This refers to forces that interact, stimulating the mind to function and change. These forces are libidinal and aggressive drives that emanate from the human biological endowment. Freud referred to these drives as ultimate causes of all human activity. Drives—sometimes called need or tension states—function to motivate the organism to act with the goal of tension reduction; action so motivated or caused brings a sense of relief, gratification, or pleasure.[1]

According to Freud these drives were derived from two basic instincts, Eros (love) and Thanatos (the destructive instinct): "The aim of the first of these basic instincts is to establish ever greater unities and to preserve them thus—in short, to bind together; the aim of the second is, on the contrary, to undo connections and so to destroy things" (p. 5).[6] He described their nature as oppositional, resulting in a process of attraction and repulsion. The psychic energy correlate of Eros is the libido, and the correlate of Thanatos is aggression.

The fourth principle of psychoanalytic theory, referred to as the *genetic viewpoint*, traces "origins of later conflicts, character traits, neurotic symptoms, and psychological structure to the crucial events and wishes of childhood and the fantasies they generated" (p. 12).[1] Freud argued for the pivotal role of childhood development in later personality structure. This theme is seen in the development of object relations (i.e., the emotional connections to persons or things, as opposed to one's self-regard). Freud theorized that the selection of love objects in adulthood as well as other object relations revealed in other interests and activities were dependent on the quality and type of object relationships in early childhood. Thus, childhood development has pervasive effects on all later life.

The stages of psychosexual development and the child's discovery of erotogenic zones (body areas that are sensitive and provide a sense of pleasure) is also understood in terms of the genetic viewpoint. According to Freud, erotogenic zones vary as development progresses. Each is tied to psychological development so that faulty psychological development will be evident by the inappropriate predominance in later life of one of these erotogenic zones. The first zone of importance developmentally is the mouth. This is particularly important as a source of nourishment and satisfaction for the infant. Next the anal zone gains importance, as the growing child learns to control excretory functions. The phallic phase follows. During this phase, Freud described different developmental events for boys and girls as they each work out their relationships to the same- and opposite-sexed parents and resolve the related tensions of jealousy and rivalry. Finally, during the genital phase of puberty, no new erogenous areas are discovered, but the events of previous stages are synthesized, and the child begins to direct his or her attention to the opposite sex.[2,6]

Additional Concepts

In Freud's later *structural theory* of the psychic apparatus, he described the psyche as organized into the id, the ego, and the superego. The id exists as a disorganized collection of instinctual drives and related energy; it is genetically inherited. The ego is a collection of functions characterized by concern with self-preservation through avoiding pain while seeking pleasure. Anxiety is the signal to the ego of impending displeasure and alerts the ego to action. The ego serves as mediator between the id's desires and the superego's demands and reality factors. The superego is the mental structure that functions as the moral agent. It is influenced by parental training and contains ideals for action.[5,6]

Anna Freud elaborated on her father's thinking about defense mechanisms. These mechanisms are evident in everyday life as the ego performs its mediating role. While defenses are part of order, they can be pathological if immature mechanisms from pregenital phases of development are used excessively in adulthood. An example of an immature defense is regression, in which a person returns to a developmentally earlier level of function for the purpose of avoiding discomfort in the present. A mature defense may be the use of humor, in which a person expresses feelings without discomfort to self or others.[5]

Order, as suggested by these concepts, is directly related to the adequacy of ego function in protecting the mind from an upsurge of conflictual material through skillful use of defense mechanisms. The difference between mental health and illness relates to how well the ego manages this task. Order is a delicate balance of forces, easily disrupted, or as one author states, it is a "tenuously stable equilibrium" between id, superego, and reality maintained by "successful repression" (p. 16).[1] Order is manifest as "the capacity to need others, to love, to want to please, and to become like others" (p. 15).[1]

VIEW OF DISORDER

Disorder occurs when psychic forces are in conflict and out of balance, when the person cannot appropriately release tension through defenses, when serious conflicts prevent the normal progression through psychosexual stages of development, and when libidinal drives are misplaced.

Neuroses

The disorder most commonly dealt with in classical psychoanalysis is neurosis.

Neurosis results when a balance (order) between the id, superego, and reality is not maintained. Anxiety, a common symptom of neurosis, acts as a warning signal, enabling the ego to mobilize defensive mechanisms that assist in coping or in maintaining this balance.

Freud noted that neurotics experience the same life demands as others and possess the same general dispositions to deal with these demands but suffer greater discomfort and anxiety. Freud's conclusion was that the difference between neurotics and nonneurotics is the ability of some individuals to deal comfortably and effectively with greater demands than others.[6]

Childhood conflicts are seen as playing a central etiological role in the later emergence of neurotic behavior. All children are viewed as having conflicts, and many have neuroses such as apprehensions, nightmares, and phobias. Children's feelings about their parents are seen as a key to understanding their later psychic configuration. The predominant psychoanalytic dogma is that neuroses are acquired in early childhood before the age of six; however, symptoms may not appear until much later. These childhood neuroses seem to pass, yet may reemerge in adulthood when the delicate balance between drives and defenses is upset.[1,8]

Freud noted that "weakening of the ego" (caused by childhood conflicts) is a precondition to psychopathology and that excessive demands may paralyze the ego's functioning and precipitate a state of disorder (p. 29).[6] Examples of excessive ego demands are the overchallenges presented by new developmental tasks (job, role change, etc.), illness, loss, or disappointment. Any of these could create imbalance in a vulnerable psyche and cause anxiety as old childhood conflicts reemerge and the individual turns to immature responses.

Schizophrenia

Freud's original view of the etiology of schizophrenia was that the libido is withdrawn from external objects and invested in the self.[5] This view is personified by the individual who is withdrawn and preoccupied with delusions, hallucinations, and other idiosyncratic thoughts and sensations.

ACTION IMPLICATIONS

Psychoanalysis as a treatment method developed by Freud and his followers will be discussed in terms of the general therapy process, specific therapeutic techniques, the therapist's and patient's roles, the dynamics of therapy, and the desired outcomes of therapy.

In the general *process of psychoanalysis*, the therapist tries to bring repressed mental content back to conscious awareness for the purpose of helping patients recognize their emotional needs, identify unconscious motivation, and find realistic ways to resolve unconscious conflicts. Therapy directly flows from the psychoanalytic view of neurotic disorder, in that treatment aims at curing the basic neuroses, and practitioners pride themselves in this effort, rather than attempting more superficial symptomatic relief. This requires recalling childhood events and reexperiencing, in the context of the therapeutic encounter, one's immature responses, and finally analyzing these responses and one's resistance to treatment.[5]

The *analytic situation* refers to the patient/therapist relationship that provides the necessary context in which therapy can occur. It literally includes certain patient positioning, such as lying on a couch with the therapist unseen, and setting the expectation that the patient be as honest in reporting mental content as possible. It also involves the therapist's maintaining an "attitude of benign curiosity" (p. 19).[1] This situation creates a relationship in which the patient can freely express mental content with as little influence as possible from other forces and in which the therapeutic regression occurs.

The *analytic process* involves the actual therapy phases and the process of the patient's regression. This process can be divided into phases of initiation and establishment of the analytic situation, transference and its analysis, and termination.[5]

In the first phase, everything patients do and say and the ways they act are observed. The nature of the problem is explored in the interview, while the therapist looks for emerging themes in the patient's content and manner of expression. In the second phase, the patient develops an emotional bond with the therapist and begins to relate to the therapist as though the therapist were another significant person in the patient's life. This relationship, called transference, is analyzed, and understanding of the transference relationship is constantly deepened. In the termination phase, the therapeutic relationship is typically ended with the patient temporarily resuming immature behavior in an effort to prolong the relationship. The therapy process can take several years to complete, with therapy sessions as frequent as four times weekly.

Techniques include the use of free association, analysis of the transference relationship, analysis of resistance, and interpretation. *Free association* involves making the unconscious conscious by having the patient report all thoughts, uncensored and regardless of their seeming insignificance.[5] The information revealed may include content from dreams. *Analysis of the transference relationship* is one of the most integral events of therapy. During this, the therapist helps the patient to distinguish current reality from past events and to align more mature, appropriate responses with the present. *Analysis of the patient's resistance* to therapy also provides further insight into personality configuration and dynamics, such as understanding defenses and resistance. These three sources of information about the patient's mental life provide the raw material from which the therapist attempts *interpretation*. The therapist's comments are carefully timed responses shared when the patient is perceived by the therapist to be ready to personally understand or make use of new viewpoints or links. Freud expressed this in the following way:

> As a rule we put off telling him of a construction or explanation till he himself has so nearly arrived at it that only a single step remains to be taken, though that step is in fact the decisive synthesis. (p. 35)[6]

To do this, the therapist needs to be able to empathize with the patient and to work intuitively, by managing the wealth of information meaningfully on other than a conscious level. The therapist must work introspectively, allowing by silent free association an interpretation to surface, which is then validated by the patient.

In summary, the therapist establishes the analytic situation, remaining relatively passive to allow the free, unhampered expression of thoughts. The therapist focuses thoughts on understanding the transference neurosis, and shares carefully timed responses with the patient. The patient's role is to reveal all, uncensored, to the therapist; to work with dedication, discipline, and earnest effort to solve his or her problems; and to accept the fact that the true nature of these problems is unknowable, thus requiring the assistance of a therapist to recognize them. According to Freud, there is a pact between therapist and patient calling for "complete candour on one side and strict discretion on the other" (p. 31).[6]

The core dynamics of psychoanalytic treatment are *remembering* (i.e., recalling childhood experiences) and *reliving* through the transference relationship with the analyst. Strengthening a weak ego requires self-knowledge. Insight and understanding based on remembering and reliving act to strengthen the ego through providing this self-knowledge. They are thus viewed as the crux of basic personality change in therapy.

The nature of treatment outcomes is not considered to be amenable to measurement by current research techniques. Similarly, symptom alleviation is not considered to be the most important outcome of treatment. The ability to derive happiness from life, to deal with normal life stresses, to relate in satisfying ways with others, and, most importantly, the release of the individual's potential which was previously blocked by neurotic conflicts are typical descriptions of preferred treatment outcomes.[5]

Given the personally and intellectually demanding nature of psychoanalysis, it is considered useful only with relatively high functioning patients. It is generally believed to be most valuable with those who are highly motivated to overcome more infantile manifestations of behavior, are able to think logically, have adequate ego strength to endure short-term frustration and anxiety in the interest of long-term benefits, are flexible, have functional assets such as good school or work performance, and maintain an "honest skepticism" about the success of therapy rather than being overly exuberant (p. 266).[5] Additionally, the following patient characteristics are predictive of successful therapy: discipline, ability to verbally express thoughts and feelings, basic honesty, and ability to test reality. Psychoanalysis is considered best suited to those with the disorders of hysteria, anxiety hysteria, obsessive-compulsive neurosis, and other disorders characterized by anxiety. Freud himself saw psychoanalysis as valuable for those with neurotic disorders and as having little benefit for those with psychotic disorders.

CRITICISMS AND LIMITATIONS

Freud acknowledged limitations of his own approach: "It may be that there are other still undreamt-of possibilities of therapy. But for the moment, we have nothing better at our disposal than the technique of psycho-analysis, and for that reason, in spite of its limitations, it should not be despised" (p. 39).[6]

As Freud anticipated, there have been criticisms and reformulations of both his theory and therapeutic technique. Typical examples of criticisms of the psychoanalytic approach are found in Glasser's[7] writings on reality therapy and are implied in the work of behaviorists. Glasser claims that six of the most basic tenets of psychoanalytic theory are invalid: the belief in mental illness and its classification; the probing of the personal, historical roots of the problem; the encouragement and use of transference in treatment; the belief in understanding and insight to effect personality change; the avoidance of the issues related to moral responsibility for behavior; and the disdain of the teaching role of the therapist. He challenges all six points on the basis that psychoanalytic treatment promotes a view of mental illness and therapy that is illness-focused, promotes irresponsible patient behavior, and is mystical and backward-looking rather than focused on the future and the development of adaptive behavior.[7]

Behaviorally oriented therapists criticize the lack of research evidence for effectiveness of psychoanalytic, insight-oriented approaches. These writers note both that there is a lack of research to support the effectiveness of classical psychoanalysis, and that it is expensive and time consuming.[8]

White[12] and other writers have challenged the psychoanalytic view that all motivation springs from tension reduction, libidinal energy, and conflicts. These critics stress that humans have tension-seeking drives that are focused on productivity, control, creativity, and other behaviors having little or nothing to do with sex. Many other criticisms of Freud's exclusive focus on sexual drives have been levied.

Systems theorists criticize psychoanalysis for its overly mechanistic and homeostatic view of humans and for its failure to acknowledge the processes by which humans grow, change, acquire skills and values, and so forth.[11] Finally, psychoanalysis has been criticized as not being relevant to the majority of persons who experience mental disorders and who are not capable of the insight process and verbal demands or who cannot afford its costly treatment.

The work of psychoanalysis has made an important contribution to the understanding of human behavior and motives and cannot be discounted out of hand despite its very clear limitations, errors, and incompleteness. Chapter 3 (The Neo-Freudians) chronicles many of the new ideas that were generated by the insights and discoveries as well as the limitations and weaknesses of classical psychoanalysis.

COMMENTARY

The psychoanalytic approach has been incorporated into some occupational therapy treatment. This occurred in part because of pressure by psychiatry to make psychoanalysis the sole perspective of all mental health workers. Occupational therapists were told explicitly that their use of occupations to influence health could only be explained by psychoanalysis.[9]

In response, therapists developed methods by which crafts could be used to reveal emotions and symbolic themes and as methods to work out feelings and conflicts, as well as to receive gratification at regressed levels of psychosexual development. However, this approach to occupational therapy has been criticized as both abandoning the field's original mission to use occupations to organize behavior and as selling short the real value of occupation. Thus it has been challenged by therapists for being in opposition to both the development of a unique identity for the profession of occupational therapy and to the original tenets of the field. The use of activities as a means of expressing unconscious material and pent-up emotions directly contradicts the use of activities to challenge and promote adaptive behavior. While this issue is taken up later in the chapter on occupational therapy, it appears that classic psychoanalysis has little in common with occupational therapy.

Reilly[10] suggests that occupational therapists can coexist with those using an analytic approach. She points out that the occupational therapist is concerned with the nonsexual areas of motivation and productivity and as such offers its own unique orientation to the problems of psychosocial dysfunction.

Those who have criticized the wholesale transformation of occupational therapy activities into psychoanalytic tools have suggested that as occupational therapy builds an alternate conceptualization of its use of occupations, some useful ideas from psychoanalysis may be revised and retained.[9] The Fidlers,[4] who originally contributed to the development of psychoanalytic applications of occupational therapy, have proposed one such reconceptualization. They incorporate some ideas from psychoanalysis into a newer framework which acknowledges a much broader and nonsexually focused view of occupations— one which conceptualizes occupation as facilitating the growth, development, and integrity of skills, roles, and a positive sense of self. Their work is exemplary for those who wish to examine this issue further.

SUMMARY

History and Purpose	Psychoanalysis was initiated and developed by Sigmund Freud in the late 19th and early 20th centuries. It was influenced by cause-and-effect sequential thinking and the belief that human psychological functioning could be explained in terms of scientific laws.
	Concepts of infantile sexuality, mental conflict, the topographic theory (consciousness as layered), and the structural theory (id, ego and superego) characterize this approach.
View of Order	The view of order paradoxically developed largely in response to and from observation of pathological processes. Although psychoanalysis emphasizes disordered states, some indications of order can be discerned by looking at the theory of how mental processes develop and interrelate.
	Order is a function of drives that emanate from biological inheritances, which are mediated and interrelated at different levels of consciousness. Order involves the process of reducing conflict.
	For order to exist the ego must protect the mind from an upsurge of conflictual material by use of defense mechanisms. Mental health is related to how well the ego manages this task.

View of Disorder	Disorder occurs when psychic forces are in conflict and out of balance, when the person cannot appropriately release tension through defenses, when serious conflicts prevent the normal progression through psychosexual stages of development, and when libidinal drives are misplaced. The disorder most commonly dealt with in classical psychoanalysis is neurosis. Childhood conflicts are believed to be largely responsible for later emergence of neurotic behavior by making the person vulnerable in adulthood to excessive ego demands.
Action Implications	The therapy process involves bringing repressed mental content back to conscious awareness for the purposes of increasing insight into past conflicts and current behavior and to enable the patient to work through conflicts. Thus psychoanalytic treatment is a process whereby the patient is led to talk about feelings, recollections, dreams, and thoughts and to develop a relationship with the therapist who analyzes both the patient's verbal renderings and behavior in the relationship. Therapeutic techniques include free association, analysis of transference, analysis of resistance, and interpretation. Psychoanalysis is believed to be most useful for those with neurotic disorders rather than with psychotic problems.

Criticisms and Limitations	Psychoanalysis has been criticized for promoting a view of therapy that is illness-focused, promotes irresponsible client behavior, and is mystical and backward-looking.
	It is also criticized for lack of research supporting effectiveness and for being inaccessible to many in need due to time and expense requirements.
	Other authors see the view of motivation as emanating purely from tension as an incomplete view. Critics have argued against Freud's strong emphasis on sexual drives.
	Systems theorists criticize psychoanalysis for its overly mechanistic and homeostatic view of humans.
	It has been criticized as being of little use for individuals incapable of the demands for insight and verbal expression.
Commentary	For a while, psychoanalytic concepts were incorporated into occupational therapy practices. This has been criticized as abandoning the field's original commitment to the use of occupations. Classic psychoanalytic knowledge and occupational therapy have little in common although they can coexist.

TERMS AND CONCEPTS

aggressive instinct	a primary motivating force which tends toward destruction. In interaction with libidinal energies, aggression creates conflict.
analysis of transference	the therapist's continued deepening of the patient's understanding of the transference. During this, the patient comes to distinguish current reality from past events and begins to align more mature, appropriate responses with the present.
analytic process	the actual therapy process, which includes the steps of initiation and establishment of the analytic situation, transference and its analysis, and termination.

analytic situation	the patient/therapist relationship in which the expectation is set for the patient to openly express all mental content and for the therapist to listen without influencing the flow of the patient's thoughts.
anxiety	the general negative feeling of uneasiness, fear, and/or apprehension recognized as a common symptom of neurosis. It acts as a warning signal to the ego of mental imbalance, indicating the need to activate defensive strategies for self-protection.
cathartic abreaction	an early treatment technique for hysteria used by Freud in which the patient was helped to recall unpleasant memories from the unconscious and express the related emotion to effect emotional relief and release of undischarged energy.
conscious	mental content of which one is lucidly aware.
drives	tension states that motivate the organism to act in order to reduce tension. The sources of these drives are the love instinct and the aggressive instinct.
dynamic viewpoint	a principle of psychoanalytic theory that refers to the forces that interact, stimulating the mind to function and change. These forces are libidinal and aggressive drives that emanate from the human biological endowment.
ego	a collection of functions characterized by concern with self-preservation through avoiding pain while seeking pleasure. It serves as mediator between the id and superego demands and reality factors.
erotogenic zones	body areas that are sensitive and provide a sense of pleasure.
free association	the process of making the unconscious conscious by having the patient report all thoughts, uncensored and regardless of their seeming insignificance.
genetic viewpoint	a principle of psychoanalytic theory that places the sources of conflict, character traits, symptoms, and the entire psychological configuration in key childhood events.

id	a disorganized collection of instinctual drives and related energy that is genetically inherited.
interpretation	the therapist's understanding of all observed patient behavior and verbalization. These insights are carefully timed, being shared by the therapist at the time when the patient is perceived as being on the brink of understanding them.
libidinal energies	sexual drives. These are a primary source of motivation in Freudian theory and derive from the love instinct (Eros), which tends to bind together. In interaction with the aggressive instinct, libidinal energies create conflict.
neurosis	disorder that results from an imbalance between psychic structures and is characterized by anxiety and the use of immature responses to current situations.
preconscious	mental content that is easily remembered, but which is not foremost in awareness.
psychic determinism	the belief that mental events, such as feelings and thoughts, have specific causes that are often unconscious and related to earlier life events.
repression	the process of keeping mental material from conscious awareness to avoid unpleasant events.
resistance	the process in which the ego of the patient in analysis persistently opposes the perceived threat of the analysis process and the necessary moving of unconscious content to levels of greater awareness.
structural theory	a theory of the mind's organization in which components of mental function (the id, ego, and superego) are identified by the roles they play in conflict.
superego	the mental structure that functions as the moral agent. It is influenced by parental training and contains ideals for action.

topographic theory	a description of mental events as being organized into layers of consciousness—the conscious, preconscious, and unconscious.
transference	the emotional bond between the therapist and patient in which the patient begins to relate to the therapist as though the therapist were another significant person from the patient's life.
unconscious	mental content that is inaccessible to keen awareness and must be inferred or otherwise recognized as being in the unconscious.

REFERENCES

1. Arlow, J. A. Psychoanalysis. In R. Corsini (Ed.), *Current psychotherapies* (2nd ed.). Itasca, Ill.: F. E. Peacock, 1979.
2. Bischof, L. J. *Interpreting personality theory* (2nd ed.). New York: Harper & Row, 1970.
3. Brenner, C. *An elementary textbook of psychoanalysis.* New York: Anchor Books, 1974.
4. Fidler, G., & Fidler, J. Doing and becoming: Purposeful action and self-actualization. *American Journal of Occupational Therapy*, 1978, *32*, 305–310.
5. Freedman, A. M., Kaplan, H. I., & Sadock, B. J. Theories of personality and psychopathology: Freudian schools/Sigmund Freud and classical psychoanalysis. *Modern synopsis of comprehensive textbook of psychiatry* (2nd ed.). Baltimore: Williams & Wilkins, 1976. Pp. 227–270.
6. Freud, S. [*An outline of psychoanalysis*] (J. Strachey, trans., rev. ed.). New York: W. W. Norton & Co., 1969.
7. Glasser, W. *Reality therapy: A new approach to psychiatry.* New York: Harper & Row, Perennial Library, 1975.
8. Kanfer, F. H., & Goldstein, A. P. (Eds.). *Helping people change.* New York: Pergamon Press, 1975.
9. Kielhofner, G., & Burke, J. The evolution of knowledge and practice in occupational therapy: Past, present and future. In G. Kielhofner (Ed.), *Health through occupation: Theory and practice in occupational therapy.* Philadelphia: F. A. Davis, 1983.
10. Reilly, M. Occupational therapy can be one of the great ideas of 20th century medicine. *American Journal of Occupational Therapy*, 1962, *16*, 1–9.
11. von Bertalanffay, L. General system theory and psychiatry. In S. Arieti

(Ed.), *American handbook of psychiatry* (Vol. 3). New York: Basic Books, 1969.

12. White, R. Motivation reconsidered: The concept of competence. In H. Proshansky, W. Ittelson, & L. Rivlin (Eds.), *Environmental psychology*. New York: Holt, Rinehart & Winston, 1970.

3
The Neo-Freudians: Adler, Horney, Fromm, and Sullivan

Some of Freud's successors, although still linked with the analytic tradition, did not accept certain key facets of classic psychoanalysis and thus proposed their own revisions and extensions of psychoanalysis.[4] Despite a lack of unanimity among these neo-Freudians, there are global themes that unite their theories. While neo-Freudian thought today is represented by various therapists, four prominent neo-Freudians—Adler, Horney, Fromm, and Sullivan—have been chosen to illustrate the themes and orientation of neo-Freudian thought.

Probably the most basic of neo-Freudian themes is the emphasis placed on understanding behavior within a cultural and interpersonal context, as opposed to understanding it primarily in terms of the libido and the transformation of infantile oral sexuality into a mature heterogenous sexuality.[6,7] Adler, the first to break with Freud, called his school Individual Psychology. He constructed a unified theory of personality development and dynamics that focuses on the person's attitudes toward self and other persons.[6] Similarly, Horney and Sullivan repudiated the primacy of the libidinal and destructive drives so heavily stressed by Freud,[6] and accentuated interpersonal relations, cultural values, and a drive toward self-actualization as key determinants of human behavior.[4,6] Fromm, also considered to be a member of the dynamic-

---

Some readers may question why Jung was not included in this chapter. Although a neo-Freudian in the sense that Jung broke with Freud to found his own school, analytic psychotherapy, he is generally not linked with any of the other neo-Freudians. His theories are permeated with religion and philosophy, and in this country, he appears to have had more of an influence on literary and philosophical thinking than on psychotherapeutic practices. With the recent growth of mysticism and religious movements, Jung's ideas have become more popular; however, it seems less likely that occupational therapists will encounter Jungian therapists in their settings than therapists who have been following in the traditions of the theorists included in this chapter.

cultural school along with Horney and Sullivan, did not wholly reject Freud's drive theory. However, he criticized it for not recognizing that drives can also be socially determined and that people, unlike animals, are not obliged to solely follow their instincts.[8] Thus, these neo-Freudians disagreed with Freud over his accentuation of the biologically driven nature of the person and his corresponding deemphasis of the role of society and culture in influencing behavior.

In addition, the neo-Freudians objected to the overly reductionist and mechanistic view of personality suggested by Freud's structural theory of the mind. Whereas Freud proposed the tripartite structure of id, ego, and superego, the neo-Freudians proposed concepts that reflected a more holistic view of personality development.

Neo-Freudians also criticized classical psychoanalysis for its pessimistic view of human potential and the required use of nondirective therapeutic techniques, such as free association. In addition, Horney rejected the devaluation of female sexuality associated with the analytic tradition.[7]

The neo-Freudians were primarily concerned with the neurotic individual. Horney's writings explicitly refer to the "neurotic personality," although she loosely applied the concept of neurosis to all maladaptive behavior, including behaviors that psychiatrists would be more apt to label psychotic.[2] Sullivan had extensive clinical experience with both hospitalized schizophrenics and predominantly neurotic private clients; in his lectures he emphasized the necessity of differentiating which treatment techniques were applicable to specific disorders. Adler's influence has been felt in many arenas, partly because he lectured widely and encouraged implementation of his ideas in varied and nontraditional settings such as mental clinics, schools, and juvenile courts.[2] Fromm's writing is less directed to clinical pathologies than to the problems of living encountered by the contemporary person in an industrial society.

HISTORY AND PURPOSE

Adler, a Viennese physician, joined Freud's psychoanalytic circle in 1902. After several years of close association, theoretical differences began to emerge between the two. Adler, convinced that their ideas were fundamentally different, broke with Freud to found a school of Individual Psychology. His theoretical system was probably one of the earliest phenomenological psychologies, in that it focused attention on the importance of subjective interpretation of events.[2] Adler believed that behavior must be studied from the perspective of the individual; that is, that a person's perceptions and interpretations of events direct future behavior; and that values, attitudes, and interests represent the kinds of thoughts one has about reality.[2] By breaking with Freud, Adler set the stage for dissension by other adherents to psycho-analysis. His influence has pervaded the thinking of most neo-Freudians, as well as existentialists, humanists, and cognitive therapists.[5]

Horney also trained as a psychiatrist and classic psychoanalyst. An excellent clinician, her practice led her to doubt certain clinical and theoretical aspects of the classical psychoanalytic system. She gradually developed her own line of thought, rejecting the notion that behavior is determined by a drive toward sexual fulfillment (i.e., the libidinal drive) and contending instead that culture and interpersonal relationships were the clue to understanding neurosis.

Sullivan, a native American, was influenced by Adolph Meyer's theories of psychosocial behavior (elaborated in the occupational therapy chapter) and the thinking of early American humanists.[4] Sullivan's early clinical work was in hospital settings with schizophrenics. After he moved into private practice, he began to develop his own theoretical system, believed by many to rival Freud's in comprehensiveness.[2,4] Among Sullivan's major contributions are his emphasis on the situational determinants (particularly interpersonal) of behavior, his attempt to understand the phenomena of attention and aware-ness, and his description of the therapist as a "participant-observer" in the therapeutic session.[2]

Fromm's writings anticipate the ideas of existentialism (see Chapter 4), while still drawing freely on the ideas of Freud and other schools of psycho-analysis.[4] Trained as a psychologist, sociologist, and psychoanalyst, he used eclectic ideas to influence students of varied traditions. Fromm did not develop a complete theoretical system, nor did he write specifically about psycho-therapeutic processes. Nevertheless, he is generally associated with the dy-namic-cultural theories of Horney and Sullivan because of his belief that the major issue facing the individual is to achieve a loving and productive rela-tionship with one's fellow beings, and that success or failure in this goal will be largely shaped by one's response to the prevailing culture.[4]

VIEW OF ORDER

These neo-Freudians propose a considerably more optimistic view of the person than found in classical psychoanalytic doctrine. They agree that human behavior is culturally embedded and that both positive and negative personal qualities may be environmentally nurtured.[7] Another commonality is a shared emphasis on the unity of behavior. However, each of the neo-Freudians proposed a different set of terminology and events to explain the development of both ordered and disordered behavior.

Three concepts are central to the Adlerian view of order. First is the belief that all people are born with a capacity for "social interest," or a propensity and desire for cooperation with other persons.[1] Second, Adler emphasized that behavior is goal-directed. Personal goals are neither determined by the environment nor by innate drives, but are chosen by the individual on the basis of a "private logic"—the personal truths, convictions, and fictions (or subjective representations of reality) that the individual lives by.[1] Thus, in contrast to Freud's emphasis on innate, biological drives as motivators of behavior, Adler stresses thinking and planning. The third important concept is that, although individuals have certain genetic endowments and encounter various environmental conditions, their use of or response to these givens is a more important determinant of present and future behavior than either the genetic or the environmental conditions. Thus, he espouses a view of human order that relies on personal responsibility and choice rather than uncontrollable inner and external forces.

In Adler's view, the developing child is subject to influences ranging from constitutional to familial. These influences are met with assumptions and interpretations accumulated by the child through experience. From these interpretations, the child creates his or her own version of reality, one which includes priorities for action and/or inaction. These priorities become recognizable as the individual's "life-style."[1]

The life-style includes a hierarchy of goals and plans which underlie one's actions and enable one to meet new situations. The core of the life-style is a "fictional goal," or a subjective image of what the person would like to be.[5] Adler uses the concept of the life-style to explain what he saw as an underlying tendency toward coherence of an individual's behavior. In other words, the life-style comprises a predominantly non-conscious cognitive plan or organization for coping with life events, without being a rigid or predetermined pattern of behavior.[5] Ultimately, Adler's view of order was one in which the psychologically healthy individual developed an altruistic and flexible interest in others and was capable of replacing false values promoted by society with values representing an honest commitment to life and to humanity.[5]

Horney believed that behavior is largely learned in a sociocultural context and that individuals develop response patterns, building on smaller units until larger organizational sets are formed.[2] She saw the basic determinant of behavior as being a need for security, rising from an anxiety common to all infants: "the feeling a child has of being isolated and helpless in a potentially hostile world" (p. 344).[6] This need for security could lead to either adaptive or maladaptive responses. Horney postulated that people have a central "real" self, which, if given appropriate conditions, would become actualized by the individual.[2] This concept presages the belief of humanistic psychologists in an innate drive toward self-actualization (see Chapter 4).

Horney did not write extensively about normal behavior or psychosocial order. However, her concept of conflict and its personal resolution does imply a view of order. Conflict may exist because of discrepancies between one's "ideal" image of what one should be and one's "actual" self. In this sense, it is an intrapersonal concept. But Horney also believed that intrapersonal conflict reflected cultural ambiguities and inconsistencies about values.[2] For instance, in the United States achievement and getting ahead are highly valued at the same time that brotherhood, democracy, and cooperation are praised by religion, schools, and the government. All people incorporate these cultural inconsistencies and experience conflict as a result. It is not the presence or absence of conflict, then, that characterizes order, but the way in which it is handled. Order, therefore, derives from the ability to reconcile discrepancies between the ideal and actual selves, and between oneself and society, in such a way that the "real" self can become actualized.

Sullivan's view of order is the most comprehensive and introduces many new terms. Like Horney and Adler, Sullivan believed that behavior must be understood within the context of interpersonal relations, and like most analysts, he believed that childhood experiences could induce feelings of either anxiety or security.

According to Sullivan, behavior emerges to satisfy two sets of needs. Biological needs lead to the pursuit of satisfactions, while the need to maintain a state of emotional well-being leads to the pursuit of security and a concomitant feeling of euphoria. Because children experience feelings of security and euphoria for behaving in socially valued ways, they become socialized to the mores of their culture. A child's experiences of security, and the behavior associated with them, become privately labeled as the "good me." Experiences that have led to anxiety become known as the "bad me." If the child is surrounded by people who love and respect him or her, then the "good me" predominates and order exists in the child.[6]

Sullivan believed that interpersonal relationships encompassed the attitudes, fantasies, and daydreams that one has about real people, as well as the visible manifestations of these relationships. He therefore was interested in the development of thought patterns and identified three cognitive models through which people progress. The first mode, called "prototaxic," is one in which children experience random, seemingly unconnected sensations and do not perceive themselves as separate from the environment. In the "parataxic" mode children develop an illogical kind of cause-and-effect reasoning, relating events because of the sequence of their occurrence rather than because of logic or reason. The highest mode, "syntaxic," is characterized by the logical and rational use of publicly accepted symbols.[7]

As children mature, different needs emerge, determining what will and will not receive their attention. Children who are not overly anxious learn to fill these needs successfully, become capable of self-respect and respect for others, and develop the inner freedom and resources that will allow them to question or adapt to the current social structure and values.[8]

Fromm's picture of the development of order emphasizes coming to terms with humanity's existential and historical dichotomies. The existential dichotomies facing people are the knowledge of death while we live and the awareness that we will not be able to realize our potentials in our life span. Historical dichotomies refer to contradictions that have been created by society, but to which solutions could be found.[3] An example of a historical dichotomy is the equal potential for good and harm to result from the development of superior technical knowledge and skills, such as nuclear science. Historical contradictions can be rationalized or explained away, denied or ignored, or annulled and canceled through one's actions; existential dichotomies can be buried or faced.[3] Accepting responsibility for one's part in annulling historical dichotomies and facing the truth about existence leads to the realization that meaning in life can only be found through one's own choices and actions.[3] For Fromm, order in life is thus conferred through productive living. Productivity, embodied by an attitude of relatedness to all forms of human activity and by the individual's sense of being in control of his or her abilities, is the only way in which meaning can be created in life.[3] Interestingly, Fromm rejected fewer of Freud's concepts than Adler, Horney, or Sullivan; however, he believed that the essence of human conflict derived not from the biologically driven nature of the person, but from the necessity for each person to find his or her own solution to the historical and existential contradictions of life.[6] The historical and existential dynamic is Fromm's major contribution to understanding human order.

A synthesis of these neo-Freudians' views of order leads to the following conclusions: (1) order must be seen as part of the cultural context; (2) order involves a progression toward fulfilling goals and actualizing one's potentials; and (3) order derives from individual choices and directions. This view of order is one which focuses on a high level of wellness; it goes beyond an ability to meet the basic requirements of life.

VIEW OF DISORDER

The view of disorder that is described by the neo-Freudians is dominated by a focus on neurotic behavior. Neuroses, in general, are seen as resulting from a constricting or rigid approach to life in which the individual inflexibly approaches new situations with old behavioral and cognitive patterns. Further, disordered behavior is seen to differ from order more in degree than in kind. These neo-Freudians place varying amounts of emphasis on the role of interpersonal conflict, or anxiety, in precipitating neurotic behavior, but they agree that the primary manifestation of neurotic behavior is difficulty in interpersonal relationships.

In Adler's conceptualization, disorder arises from a faulty or constricting life-style (i.e., the individual's cognitive plan for coping with life) or from the choices for action made within the context of the life-style. The same life-style can lead to useful or useless behavior; however, disorder occurs when the individual makes poor behavioral choices within the frame of the life-style. On the other hand, the life-style itself may be the source of disorder.[5] A constricting life-style is one which is rigid and limiting in terms of the individual's goals and behavioral repertoire. However, even a constricting life-style (for example, one in which the individual refuses to take risks or experiment with new ways of behaving) will not necessarily cause problems of living, unless it is challenged by reality.[5]

A faulty life-style is organized around certain distorted perceptions. There are six categories of distortions, or "basic mistakes," that people may hold: distorted attitudes about one's self and capabilities; distorted attitudes about the world and people; distorted goals, such as "I must be perfect"; distorted methods of achieving goals; distorted ideas about life; and distorted conclusions about other people or about what will happen in particular situations.[1] These distorted beliefs reflect faulty learning or the avoidance of common sense.

Adler introduced the notion of an inferiority complex. When individuals feel inferior—socially or biologically—they subsequently compensate by over-emphasizing some other trait or tendency. Adler was less concerned with the role of anxiety than other neo-Freudians. He acknowledged that anxiety would contribute to the development of neurotic behavior, primarily through the possibility of leading to the overemphasis of certain behavioral responses (those which were not anxiety-provoking to the individual) at the expense of others.

One of Horney's major contributions to understanding disorder was to locate neurotic behavior within a cultural context. She asserted that neurotic behavior was culturally relevant, and that what might be considered neurotic in one society would not necessarily be so in another. For her, neurotic disorders were characterized by rigidity and compulsiveness, that is, the indiscriminate application of one response to many events. The inflexibility of these responses prevents realization of the person's potential.

Horney placed the development of disorder in infancy, with the experience of basic anxiety. The need to overcome this anxiety leads to three categories of interpersonal responses: moving toward people or seeking safety in relationships; moving away from people—becoming self-reliant; and moving against people—rejecting the advances or advice of others.[6] Whereas the normal person achieves a balance among these responses, the neurotic prefers and uses one pattern exclusively. Succeeding in the use of one pattern, however, means repressing the needs that relate to the unchosen patterns while idealizing the needs of the predominating pattern. For instance, the person who always moves toward people might believe that there is virtue in passively acquiescing to others' wishes and not making waves. This imbalance of interpersonal responses inevitably leads to conflict between the person's idealized self and "actual" self. This conflict cannot be resolved until the person recognizes the *ideal* self as neurotic.

Thus, Horney's view of disorder involves an overly rigid set of behavioral responses that concentrate on one mode of interpersonal relationships to the exclusion of others. This condition, precipitated by childhood anxiety, prevents development of potential in adult life and eventually leads to conflict within the person.

Sullivan also believed that disorder represented attempts to overcome or dispel anxiety.[2] This anxiety might be elicited by proximity to anxious or malevolent persons, rejection, ridicule, punishment in a malevolent context, and inconsistencies of significant adults. In these situations, the child first responds with avoidance and later ceases to use behaviors relevant to such situations. For instance, a child who is ridiculed for something said in school may eventually stop speaking up in class. When the child cannot avoid these settings, or needs to use behaviors that are associated with settings in order to reduce need tensions, conflict develops. The conflict may be handled by substituting ineffective behaviors, by selective inattention to situations that cannot be physically ignored, or by mental preoccupations that preclude the possibility of making the distressing responses. The child ridiculed in school might thus begin to act the role of clown, not pay attention to the teacher, or daydream during class. The consequences of these attempts at conflict resolution are a constricted life-style, interference with interpersonal relationships that are necessary to satisfying needs, ineffectiveness in interpersonal relationships, and dissociation or deletion of certain responses from one's behavioral repertoire.

Sullivan, along with Adler and Horney, therefore traced disorder to a life-style dominated by one set of behavioral responses at the expense of others. Sullivan considered that the anxiety that resulted from inconsistencies or rejection in interpersonal situations was a crucial factor in leading to a rigid life-style and future inability to satisfy interpersonal needs.

Fromm considered neurosis to be more a philosophical than a clinical dilemma, although he did delineate various neurotic character types. He viewed neurosis as the outcome of the individual's fear of freedom and corresponding choice of a nonproductive orientation to life. An example of a nonproductive orientation is the "receptive" orientation, dominated by the need to conform and the belief that experts exist to tell one how to do things. Fromm believed that certain character orientations were more likely to be found in particular societies and at particular times than others. For instance, the receptive orientation is more often found in societies with social inequities, where one group or class habitually exploits the rights of another.[3] The marketing orientation, in which the person experiences and evaluates himself and others as a salable commodity, is a product of modern times. Thus, in his view, disorder is closely tied to the meanings available in a given culture. Society provides both the conflict and the modes for its expression in the neurotic personality.

In their views of disorder, the neo-Freudians, with the exception of Adler, did not wholly reject the notion of biological drives and tension reduction as motivating behavior. However, they sought new ways to encapsulate this concept—for instance, as a need for safety or a need for security and well-being. In addition, they included with this need an inherent urge toward actualization of one's potentials or inner self. Disorder was then seen as impinging upon this actualization and creating conflict between the realities and possibilities of one's life. The neo-Freudians considered social and environmental circumstances to be crucial factors in determining whether or not a constricting or actualizing life-style would develop. Finally, the concept of conflict, a classical Freudian concept, continues to dominate this view of disorder. The neo-Freudians ultimately remain true to their heritage by linking their conception of disorder to thwarted drives, distorted response patterns, and intrapersonal conflict.

ACTION IMPLICATIONS

The neo-Freudians as a whole realized that classical psychoanalytic treatment was too inflexible to be used for all patients. In particular, they objected to emphasis on daily or almost daily treatment, the establishment of a transference neurosis as a vital part of treatment, and the operating criterion of free association.[7] Because of their common belief that behavior was learned in interpersonal relationships, they saw the therapeutic setting as a special class of interpersonal relationships in which the therapist's behavior contributed actively to the patient's learning.

Adler conceptualized the therapeutic process as an educational experience potentially involving more than one therapist and more than one patient. The goal of this cooperative process was to develop the patient's interest and investment in social relationships.[5]

He delineated four aims of therapy that have since been expanded upon by his followers. The first aim of therapy was to strive for a friendly relationship between equals. To achieve this, it was necessary for the therapist and patient to align their goals. This meant that the therapist could not arbitrarily determine treatment goals for the patient and that the patient might have to modify or clarify his or her own initial plans for therapy. Therefore, the model for the therapeutic relationship could not be based on the medical model (see Chapter 1), which posited a relationship in which the therapist directed the course of treatment because of his or her superior knowledge and understanding of pathology while the patient willingly complied with the suggested treatment.

Second, since the ultimate goal of therapy concerned the development of social interest, therapy investigated the patient's life-style and how it affected current functioning. Because the life-style is dynamic, the client's current behavior in the context of the therapeutic setting was as relevant as his or her history. In fact, the importance of childhood recollections lay in their ability to enhance understanding of the life-style. Because people tend to sift through their past, selectively remembering only those incidents that are consistent with their present life-style, memories served as clues to understanding the life-style of the patient.[5] Free association was discouraged by Adler, but he believed that dreams offered relevant material. However, unlike Freud's notion of dreams as replays of old problems, in Adlerian therapy dreams are viewed as problem solving or rehearsing for the future.[5]

The third aim of Adlerian therapy was to achieve insight, or "understanding translated into constructive action" (p. 70).[5] The therapist might use interpretation or explanation of the patient's behavior, humor, parables, and paradox to facilitate insight. Paradox, also used by communication/interaction theorists and logotherapists (see Chapters 4 and 8), involves a seemingly contradictory statement or situation, which, through its inherent contradictions, leads to understanding or to the desired behavior. Telling someone afraid of fainting in public places to deliberately faint the next time he or she enters a store is an example of paradoxical treatment.

The last step in Adlerian therapy was reorientation, or taking the risk to change. Reorientation involves "motivation-modification" (p. 100),[2] that is, establishing new or more realistic goals for behavior and identifying new or more functional alternatives to one's present actions.

Contemporary Adlerians use a variety of techniques, including role playing, role modeling by the therapist, setting either achievable or paradoxical tasks for the client, group therapy, therapeutic social clubs, and marriage and family counseling.[1,5]

Horney's descriptions of the therapeutic process seem quite conservative and not substantially different from classical analysis. She emphasized the development of insight and understanding by clients in recognizing their response patterns, their ineffectiveness, and their relationship to symptoms.

Free association was an important part of the patient's role, and "observation, understanding, interpretation, help in resistance, and general human help" were the mainstay of the therapist's role (p. 511).[2]

In her later writings, Horney specified a set of four therapeutic goals: (1) assumption of responsibility for one's actions and decisions; (2) inner dependence, or recognition of and belief in one's own hierarchy of values; (3) spontaneity of feeling; and (4) wholeheartedness, or a total commitment to one's feelings, work, and beliefs.[2]

Sullivan, along with Adler and Horney, believed that although childhood socialization needed to be examined to discern the roots of anxiety, subsequent maladaptive thinking and behavior patterns needed to be directly attacked in therapy. In particular, Sullivan considered the "psychiatric interview," or treatment session, to represent an interpersonal relationship between the client and therapist. As a member of this relationship, the therapist both contributed to and responded to the client's behaviors. Sullivan called the therapist a "participant-observer" to denote this role as a cause of, respondent to, and observer of the client's behavior.[2]

Sullivan conceptualized the psychiatric interview as a single session or a series of sessions, consisting of four stages. In the first stage, or inception, observation was the primary function of the therapist. Even at this early point, however, Sullivan thought that clients should feel they are learning something. The second stage, or reconnaissance, referred to the gathering of extensive and intensive biographical material. Following the reconnaissance, the therapist would proceed with detailed inquiry, or the testing of hypotheses about how the person might think, act, or feel in various situations. Finally, the interview should be terminated with suggestions for future problem solving on the client's part.[4]

Fromm's picture of therapy was, in a sense, that of a religion, with its ultimate goal being to remove the individual's "blocks to loving and being loved" and to resolve his or her "strictures on productivity and creativity" (p. 211).[7] To this end, the therapist's role was to help the client understand irrational needs for authority by examining the relationship with the therapist. In this process, the client would discover healthy parts of the self that had been condemned or ignored by the patient.[7]

Again, we see that the neo-Freudians both diverged from and converged with classical psychoanalysis. Therapy, for the most part, involves a verbal session in which the client presents information about the present and past and the therapist interprets this information in order to help the client develop new ways of satisfying interpersonal needs. Unlike classical psychoanalysts, the neo-Freudians believed that the client's current functioning within the context of the treatment session was as important a source of material as past history for analysis. Neo-Freudians were both directive in their approach—by their willingness to give suggestions, to guide the course of the session, and to acknowledge their impact on the client's behavior—and cooperative, in their emphasis on sharing responsibility for setting goals.

CRITICISMS AND LIMITATIONS

Neo-Freudians have been subject to criticisms from both classical psychoanalysts and writers outside the psychoanalytic tradition. Orthodox analysts criticize the neo-Freudians for substituting Freud's libido theory with equally ambiguous concepts, such as Horney's "real," "ideal," and "actual" selves. According to one writer, "there is a tendency to recast Freudian formulations in novel, excruciatingly complicated neologisms; to concentrate on nuances, torturing these into broad theorems" (p. 220).[7] The neo-Freudians have been further criticized for tendencies to overgeneralize.[2] Adler, for instance, attributes all behavior to one ultimate fictional goal, while Horney regards large organizational sets of behavior responses as obvious and clearly cohesive response patterns.[2]

The neo-Freudians are ambivalent about the role of biological drives, and while they postulate a motive or force toward self-actualization, their treatment of it as an unconscious drive seems more similar to libido theory than to concepts of effectance motivation or intrinsic motivation. The latter concepts propose that the individual engages in activity in order to feel effective and competent in his or her environment. In this sense, although an innate drive, effectance motivation involves conscious decisions on the individual's part. The neo-Freudians' drive toward self-actualization seems closer in spirit to an unconscious force that determines behavior by virtue of its being unimpeded by external events.

Although refusing to attribute behavior to either solely intrinsic or solely extrinsic determinants, the neo-Freudians nevertheless remain elusive about the ways in which a person might respond to or act on the environment. This major limitation seems to come from their position as a bridge between orthodox Freudian theory and environmental/sociological perspectives on behavior. Not willing to totally give up the constructs of psychoanalysis, they were unable to resolve some of the paradoxes that Freudian theory had raised for them. Thus, although they rejected the mechanistic view of the mind proposed by Freud, they did not reject the most fundamental mechanistic ideas underlying Freudian thought. Retaining the notion of an unconscious force that drives persons to act perpetuated the view of persons as tension-releasing organisms. In some ways their work resembles a situation in which theorists attempt to resolve problems within a dominant paradigm of theory by revision of that theory, when what is really required is a major reorientation and shift in fundamental views and precepts. The work of the neo-Freudians is therefore more like surface or cosmetic repair than reconstruction and reconceptualization.

COMMENTARY

The impact of neo-Freudian thinking on occupational therapy has been more subtle than that of classical psychoanalytic thinking. Because psychiatrists have continued to dominate mental health settings, as they have incorporated the ideas of the neo-Freudians, other mental health workers have been under pressure to do so as well. To the extent that this has meant an increasing awareness of sociocultural influences on psychosocial order and disorder, this has been beneficial to occupational therapy.

Likewise, the contributions of neo-Freudians to understanding the goal-oriented nature of the person and the importance of work in giving meaning to life supports the concept that the purpose of occupational therapy is broader than activity prescribed for symptom relief (i.e., reduction of anxiety). That is, they pave the way for asserting that occupations can be used to reach goals, generate meaning, and so on. Interestingly, the development of these kinds of themes in occupational therapy have not relied on neo-Freudian thought, but rather on the work of humanistic/existential writers and ego psychologists. This may be because the most fundamental Freudian tenets remain intact in neo-Freudian thought, producing a deep incompatibility with occupational therapy. Thus, if one does not closely examine the bases of these theories, they may appear more overtly similar to current occupational therapy than they really are. It should be noted, for example, that the occupational therapy view of order and disorder that we describe in this text is substantially different from that of the neo-Freudians. Issues that form the crux of occupational therapy thinking, such as locus of control, effectance motivation, and maintenance of habits of work, leisure, and self-care in everyday life, are virtually ignored by the neo-Freudians. Similarly, the techniques used by neo-Freudians have mostly continued in the mainstream of other psychoanalytic techniques. Verbal, insight-oriented therapy is radically different from the action-oriented techniques used by occupational therapists.

SUMMARY

History and Purpose	Adler broke with Freud to found a school of Interpersonal Psychology, setting the stage for dissension by other pscyhoanalysts.
	Horney and Sullivan each developed theoretical systems emphasizing cultural and interpersonal determinants of mental health.
	Fromm incorporated existential, sociological, and psychoanalytic ideas into a perspective on psychosocial order.
	Neo-Freudians as a whole protested Freudian drive theory and its mechanistic view of personality.
View of Order	Human behavior is culturally embedded and environmentally nurtured. Behavior is unified and integrated.
	Adler's view of order stresses an altruistic and goal-oriented life-style.
	Horney stresses the ability to reconcile one's ideal and actual selves in order to allow "real" self to become actualized.
	Sullivan emphasizes the role of interpersonal relationships in letting the child (or adult) develop psychological order.
	Fromm emphasizes coming to terms with historical and existential crises in order to live productively.
Disorder	Generally, neo-Freudians believe that disorder is precipitated by childhood anxiety; their focus is on neurotic behavior.
	Social and cultural conditions contribute to the development of neurotic behavior.
	Neuroses are manifested in poor interpersonal relationships, the use of one pattern or mode of behavior responses for all experiences, and the inability to satisfy personal needs.

Action Implications	Behavior is learned in the context of interpersonal relationships; the therapeutic setting is a type of interpersonal relationship.
	The therapist responds to, causes, and observes the client's behavior; the relationship between client and therapist is as important a source of information as is past history.
	The therapeutic process is an educational experience with the goals of understanding and changing one's life-style, setting more realistic goals for action, and becoming committed to one's feelings, work, and to other people.
Criticisms and Limitations	Neo-Freudians introduced complicated new terminology whose meanings may not differ very much from Freudian concepts.
	The neo-Freudians postulate a force toward self-actualization, but they treat it as an unconscious drive similar to Freud's concept of libidinal drive.
	Their contributions tend to be surface or cosmetic repair to Freudian ideas.
Commentary	Emphasis on goal-oriented nature of persons and importance of work in giving meaning to life is compatible with a view of occupational therapy as being more than tension reduction.
	Neo-Freudian theories for the most part ignore themes that are crucial to occupational therapy theory.
	Fundamental Freudian tenets, left intact in neo-Freudian thinking, are incompatible with occupational therapy.

TERMS AND CONCEPTS

actual self	the way in which a person is experienced and perceived by others.
bad me	behaviors or experiences that the child associates with anxiety.

faulty life-style   one in which the individual's choices for action are limited, due to distorted perceptions or beliefs about oneself, other people, and life.

free association   the process of making the unconscious conscious by having the person report all thoughts, uncensored and regardless of their seeming insignificance.

good me   behaviors or experiences that the child associates with feelings of security.

ideal self   the way a person thinks he or she should "ideally" be.

life-style   a primarily nonconscious plan for coping with life events that includes an ideal image of oneself, and a hierarchy of goals or priorities for action.

parataxic mode   pattern of thinking in which cause and effect of events is based solely on their sequential occurrence.

phenomenological psychology the study of behavior from the perspective of the individual's experience; a person's behaviors cannot be understood without understanding this person's interpretations and personal framework for these behaviors.

private logic   a complex of personally held beliefs that direct an individual's life goals.

prototaxic mode   pattern of thought in which the child (individual) does not perceive self as separate from the environment.

psychiatric interview   Sullivan's conceptualization of the treatment session, as well as a series of sessions. In both cases, the psychiatric interview moves through four stages, from observation to data gathering, to detailed inquiry, to suggestions for future problem solving.

real self   one's central being, which, given appropriate conditions, becomes actualized by the individual.

social interest   a desire and tendency to cooperate with other people for the good of society.

syntaxic mode   pattern of thought characterized by logic, reasoning, and the use of publicly accepted symbols.

transference   the emotional bond that forms between the therapist and client; the client begins to relate to the therapist as though the therapist were another significant person in the client's life.

REFERENCES

1. Dinkmeyer, D. C., Pew, W. L., & Dinkmeyer, D. C., Jr. *Adlerian counseling and psychotherapy*. Monterey, Calif.: Brooks/Cole, 1979.
2. Ford, D. H., & Urban, H. B. *Systems of psychotherapy: A comparative study*. New York: Wiley, 1963.
3. Fromm, E. *Man for himself*. New York: Holt, Rinehart & Winston, 1947.
4. Harper, R. A. *Psychoanalysis and psychotherapy: 36 systems*. New York: Jason Aaronson, 1974.
5. Mosak, H. H. Adlerian psychotherapy. In R. J. Corsini (Ed.), *Current psychotherapies* (2nd ed.). Itasca, Ill.: Peacock, 1979.
6. Munroe, R. A. *Schools of psychoanalytic thought*. New York: Holt, Rinehart & Winston, 1955.
7. Wolberg, L. R. *The technique of psychotherapy. Part one* (3rd ed.). New York: Grune & Stratton, 1977.
8. Wyss, D. *Psychoanalytic schools from the beginning to the present*. New York: Jason Aaronson, 1973.

ADDITIONAL READINGS

Adler, A. *The practice and theory of individual psychology*. New York: Harcourt, Brace, 1924.
Adler, A. *Social interest*. New York: Putnam, 1939.
Clinebell, H. *Contemporary growth therapies*. Nashville: Abingdon, 1981.
Fromm, E. *The sane society*. New York: Rinehart, 1955.
Horney, K. *Neurosis and human growth*. New York: Norton, 1950.
Progoff, I. *The death and rebirth of psychology*. New York: Julian Press, 1956.
Sullivan, H. S. *The interpersonal theory of psychiatry*. New York: Norton, 1953.
Sullivan, H. S. *The psychiatric interview*. New York: Norton, 1954.

4
Existential-Humanist Bodies of Thought

The existential-humanist tradition is united by a fundamental vision of the nature of human existence. Logotherapy, client-centered therapy, humanistic and existential psychotherapy, gestalt therapy, and the human potential movement all have been influenced by existential and phenomenological philosophy, and all share a concern for helping the individual to find meaning in life. The differences among these approaches result primarily from the emphases of the key individual associated with each body of knowledge: Carl Rogers with client-centered therapy, Victor Frankl with logotherapy, Abraham Maslow with humanistic psychology. Inevitably, these pairings have led to the association of special techniques with particular streams of thought. Therefore, while the overall goals for each of these psychosocial therapies may be similar, their action implications often differ.

Because of the concern for helping the individual to transcend the "givens" of life,[2] the target of these therapies is rarely the psychotic patient, the chronically mentally ill, or the deinstitutionalized schizophrenic. These therapies do not focus on symptom relief, nor are they concerned with the development of adaptive daily living skills per se. Instead, they attempt to fill a spiritual gap believed to be ignored by psychotherapy. What Frankl says of logotherapy is essentially true for all the existential-humanistic approaches:

> Logotherapy must *supplement* psychotherapy. . . . By the use of logotherapy we are equipped to deal with philosophical questions within their own frame of reference, and can embark on objective discussion of the spiritual distress of human beings suffering from psychic disturbances. (p. 17)[6]

Because its target is the spiritual or existential dissatisfaction and alienation of individuals in modern society, existential-humanistic psychology has been applied to the parts of society that may contribute to or potentially alleviate this distress—industry and education—as well as to psychotherapy.[10]

This chapter covers the general themes of the existential-humanist tradition and highlights Frankl's logotherapy and Rogers' client-centered therapy. These two therapies are emphasized because of the unique action implications of logotherapy and the particular relevance of Frankl's discussion of meaning to occupational therapy, and because of Rogers' pervasive influence on helping professionals' relationship and interviewing techniques.

A semantic problem arises in this chapter in that the terms *existential* and *humanistic* have been used by different writers to refer to both disparate bodies of knowledge and to one tradition. This chapter, when referring to general themes, will use both terms in a hyphenated form; when referring to specific contributions from either school of thought the appropriate term will be used alone.

HISTORY AND PURPOSE

Drawing on phenomenology, existential philosophy, and humanistic themes in philosophy, literature, and religion, existential-humanistic psychology arose in response to mechanistic and reductionist currents in twentieth century psychology. These trends ignored the inner experience of humans and sought generalizations about human behavior from the study of rats and pigeons.[10,14] Existential-humanistic psychology attempted to counterbalance these trends by stressing the importance of understanding human experience from each individual's perspective, that is, by understanding the personal meaning that an individual attaches to behavior.

William James and G. Stanley Hall, two nineteenth century American psychologists, are usually identified as early humanists because of their belief that psychology should stress the wholeness, unique passions, and individuality of persons.[14] This orientation was later reiterated in the 1930s by Goldstein, Allport, and Maslow. Significantly, the period prior and subsequent to World War II was a time when many European scholars emigrated to the United States. These scholars brought with them a school of thought—phenomenology—that stressed the importance of subjectivity and intuition as the keys to understanding a person's experience and knowledge of the world.[10] In other words, knowledge, according to phenomenologists, not only differs for each person, but is also continually shaped by each individual's experiences and subsequent interpretations of these experiences. The influence of this philosophy was felt in terms of the methods used to study behavior—phenomenology emphasized the unbiased recording of human experience from the subject's perspective, rather than the objective description of external, observable behavior.

During this period, existentialism was also attracting many adherents. Resting on a phenomenological foundation, existentialism focused on the individual's subjective awareness of existence and the way in which one came to terms with the knowledge of one's inevitable nonexistence (death).[10] In Europe, Binswanger was one of the first psychoanalysts to examine patients' experiences in terms of existential issues. He did not, however, develop a comprehensive system of therapy, so although he may be considered a "founder" of existential analysis, his influence is less directly felt today.[11]

Frankl, another European therapist, is associated with a specific form of existential therapy—logotherapy. Logotherapy clearly reflects Frankl's personal history. Before World War II, Frankl was the medical director of a large mental hospital. During the war, imprisoned in a Nazi concentration camp, he struggled to find meaning in suffering and to retain the freedom to choose his attitude toward his fate. The idea that freedom remains in the most dire of circumstances was to become a central concept of logotherapy.

In the 1950s, several Americans were responsible for the systematic application of existential principles to psychology. Rollo May, James Bugental, and Carl Rogers particularly helped to consolidate the existential-humanistic movement. Rogers was profoundly influenced by Otto Rank's conceptualization of the treatment process. For Rank, the therapist's qualities as a human being and the relationship with the patient far outweighed the therapist's technical skills in guiding the patient toward health.[9] Building on this, Rogers proposed a nondirective, person-centered form of therapy, which for many individuals came to epitomize existential-humanist psychology.

In the 1950s and 1960s certain sociocultural trends further contributed to the emergence of the existential-humanist movement as a viable school of psychology.[14] The increasing alienation of people from their feelings and from their communities, the loss of tradition and continuity in modern life, and the compartmentalization of life, fostered by the domination of technology all fueled both the 1960s counterculture movement and existential-humanist psychology. Both groups espoused many of the same values—freedom, authenticity, and openness to experience and to others. Existential-humanist psychology perceived itself as offering individuals a chance to reconnect with themselves and with each other. To this end, sensitivity groups and encounter groups, which brought people together to examine their interpersonal behavior in intensive group experiences, became the cultural panacea of the 1960s.[14]

Many of the more unorthodox forms of therapy such as the marathon encounter groups which proliferated in the 1960s under the auspices of humanism and the human potential movement are no longer in vogue. Existential-humanist psychology, nevertheless, continues to be a strong force today.

VIEW OF ORDER

Three themes are central to the view of order in the existential-humanist body of knowledge: the urge toward wholeness, intentionality, and authenticity in one's relationships. The urge toward wholeness describes the belief that behavior is motivated by something more than unconscious drives or needs. Although not denying the presence of these needs, this body of knowledge sees the ultimate motivation as being an urge for unity and wholeness, manifested in the individual's search for self-actualization.[14]

The phenomenological focus of this tradition and its emphasis on an innate drive toward self-actualization converge in the concept of "intentionality." Intentionality refers to the idea that our experiences, and our perceptions of these experiences, derive from our goals or intentions.[14] In other words, not only do we have our own private interpretations of our experiences, but our personal intentions or goals lead us to choose these experiences in the first place.

Authenticity in one's relationship comes from the willingness to remain open to experience and to others and to not see oneself or others as fixed, immutable entities.[11,14] This authenticity is difficult to achieve, however, because of our awareness of conditions of "nonbeing." Conditions of nonbeing that fill us with existential anxiety are death, the realization that ultimately we are all alone, and a sense of meaninglessness in what we do. Existential anxiety is common to everyone; what determines order (or disorder) is the individual's response to it. The "ordered" individual is one who, despite this existential anxiety, persists in the active pursuit of goals that will lead to self-actualization. In this way, the individual achieves authenticity as well.[11,14]

Logotherapy and client-centered therapy incorporate and extend these central tenets, each in its own way. Although logotherapy draws on fundamental existential concepts, Frankl stated that it goes further because it is concerned not just with *being*, but also with *meaning*. For logotherapy, the person's life is dominated by the goal of finding meaning.[4]

Logotherapy bases its philosophy on three assumptions: freedom of will, an innate will to meaning, and the phenomenological meaning of life.[7,16] The first, freedom of will, is a freedom within the constraints or conditions of one's existence. People can assert themselves and take responsibility for their actions, or if they cannot choose their actions, then they can take responsibility for their attitudes. This freedom implies a moral responsibility of the individual, either to society, to religious beliefs, or to one's own conscience.[7]

The "will to meaning" is not a drive or need, but an innate search that shapes one's life. Meaning is found through the discovery of values that are relevant to one's life and through the commitment to a cause of greater significance than one's immediate, daily, and personal concerns.[7] Frankl's attitude toward self-actualization differs from other existential-humanists in that he does not consider it to be a motivating force, but an effect: Self-actualization and pleasure may result from the search for meaning, but they cannot be obtained as long as they are directly pursued as ends in and of themselves. According to Frankl, then, psychosocial order does not come from the pursuit of self-actualization but from the attainment of meaning.

The third assumption of logotherapy is that meaning is experienced subjectively and, therefore, differently for each person. There are three ways in which life may become meaningful for the individual:

> First, through *what we give* to life (in terms of our creative works); second, by *what we take* from the world (in terms of our experiencing values); and third, through the *stand we take* toward a fate we no longer can change (an incurable disease, an inoperable cancer, or the like). (p. 15)[7]

For Frankl, existential anxiety comes from the doubt that life has meaning and the tension that is created by the gap between existence and the *essence* or meaning of one's existence. This tension is a vital part of being human and is resolved by directing one's life toward a commitment or significant goal.[7]

Client-centered therapy is essentially a theory describing the optimal conditions for growth in human development and in the therapeutic relationship. Rogers' view of human order shares with Frankl's an emphasis on values and the individual's subjective experiences, but it has little to say about meaning or existential anxiety. Rogers' first interest was in the creation of an empathetic, therapeutic environment, and his theory of personality, derived from his observations of the therapeutic relationship, reflects the same emphasis.[12,14]

Maslow's hierarchy of needs is central to Rogers' view of development.[9] Maslow postulated the existence of five levels of needs. The first three levels comprise "deficiency" needs, needs that are essential for immediate maintenance of the organism. These include physiological and safety needs, and the need to belong to a social group and to be loved. The higher two levels, termed "metaneeds," are long-term and forever active. These are the needs for esteem and for self-actualization. The salience and potency of each level changes with the person's time of life, environmental circumstances, and so on, but generally, the individual will not concentrate on higher level needs until lower levels are met. Rogers believed, as did Maslow, that psychosocial order represented the realization of these higher level needs.

According to Rogers, the organism has a basic, innate goal to grow and enhance and actualize its capacities. Through this process, the individual develops an increasingly differentiated self-concept. As the individual interacts with the environment and with other people, new experiences are either perceived and organized in some relationship to oneself, or ignored and distorted. Rejection or distortion of these perceptions occurs because they are inconsistent with the view of self that one has begun to hold, whereas the acceptance of perceptions occurs when these are consistent with one's self-image. For instance, an adolescent girl who thinks of herself as unattractive may ignore feedback from family or friends that contradicts her self-image. On the other hand, if she sees herself as possibly being in an awkward stage, yet going through a process of growth and change, then she may be able to accept feedback from others on both her strengths and weaknesses. Consequently, for psychosocial order to exist, the person must have a flexible and realistic self-image that allows for the assimilation of new experiences. For the child, this will occur naturally when the parent's love has been unconditional, or not selectively given and withdrawn according to what behaviors the child exhibits.[12]

In Rogers' view of human order, individuals will naturally value such ideas as freedom, communality, and respect for others, unless they are contaminated by the false values of other people. Well-adjusted persons, however, being open to new experiences and constantly reexamining their perceptions of these experiences, will not hold fixed, rigid values, but will realize that valuing is an ongoing process.

The overall view of order in the existential-humanist tradition is one in which the individual makes responsible choices for action in the face of a universal sense of aloneness and meaninglessness in life. These decisions to act reflect an innate motivation for self-actualization and the individual's subjective interpretation of experience. Finally, self-actualization and meaning in life come from and imply a willingness to remain flexible and open in one's attitudes toward and perceptions of others, experiences, and oneself.

Rogers and Frankl are both clearly in the existential-humanist tradition; yet their theories diverge from one another in significant ways. The most important difference between the two theories is the emphasis Frankl gives to meaning. Rogers' belief in the self-actualizing tendency of the person fits more closely with the tradition as a whole. For Frankl, the need for self-actualization is not enough to shape one's life; it is the will to meaning that makes life more than just mere existence.

VIEW OF DISORDER

Existential anxiety is an inevitable component of life; the way one faces this anxiety, however, can create psychopathology. Lying, or not admitting to oneself that death and finitude are ultimately part of life, results in neurotic as opposed to existential anxiety. Existential anxiety is an inescapable response to our awareness of death; neurotic anxiety, however, is an unrealistic response that arises from an attempt to deny our eventual aloneness and the certainty of death.[11] Herein lies a paradox, however, because to some extent, denial of the conditions of nonbeing is precisely what enables people to live a "normal" life:

> The individual has to protect himself against the world, and he can do this only as any other animal would: by narrowing down the world, shutting off experience, developing an obliviousness both to the terrors of the world and to his own anxieties. . . . We can say that the essence of normality is the *refusal of reality*. (p. 178)[1]

Persons who are called neurotic, though, have carried this denial too far: they have chosen a life-style that has so many restrictions and limitations that they can no longer make active choices or grow in their understanding of themselves and their lives.[1]

In Frankl's perspective, disorder comes from the loss of meaning in life.[6] As with existential anxiety, the loss of meaning is precipitated both by our awareness of the conditions of nonbeing and our unwillingness to accept responsibility for the way in which we respond to these conditions. Frankl hypothesizes that this loss of meaning, or the existential vacuum, is a concomitant of industrialization, which contributes to the meaninglessness of work[6] and to unemployment. He notes: "Having no work, [a person] thinks life has no meaning. . . . Unemployment becomes a culture medium for the proliferation of neuroses" (p. 121).[6]

Despite this abstract view of disorder, Frankl describes two very concrete forms of neurotic behavior: anticipatory anxiety and excessive self-observation, or excessive intention. When someone fears that he or she will stammer or sweat during a speech, the anticipation of this is enough to bring about precisely what the person has dreaded will happen; this is anticipatory anxiety.[7] Excessive self-observation or excessive intention have the opposite effect— the more one wants to achieve a certain state, the more it eludes the person. (It is for this reason that Frankl states that one cannot pursue pleasure or self-actualization as ends in themselves.)

Rogers' discussion of disorder is quite discrepant from the existentialists' and does not relate pathology to a conscious decision to lie to oneself about life experiences or to a loss of meaning. Instead, he attributes it to a tragic development in infancy.[11] When the parent's love is conditionally given for certain behaviors and attitudes, the child soon becomes estranged from the characteristics or behaviors that are not rewarded by the parents. These behaviors are pushed out of the self-concept or the child's idealized self-image, because to admit them would mean admitting that certain parts of the child were not valued or loved by the parents. Further, the child develops certain defensive reactions or mechanisms that make it possible to ignore experiences that are incongruent with this self-image. As long as people are able to ignore incongruous information, they will not feel internal conflict or seek therapy. Once someone begins to admit that there is substantial contradictory evidence to the self-image, internal tension will begin to grow.[12]

Rogers is more concerned with *why* someone will feel discomfort than with what the manifestations of this discomfort may be. Similarly, the connections between neurotic anxiety, the existential vacuum, and the development of specific pathological behavior are somewhat unclear. While the concepts of existential and neurotic anxiety are intuitively meaningful, why they should result in particular symptoms is less so. In both cases, the avoidance of a clear-cut discussion of pathology no doubt reflects the focus of this body of knowledge on the phenomenological meaning of existence. In addition, the strong philosophical background of the existential-humanist tradition is probably responsible for the rather nonclinical approach it presents to disorder.

ACTION IMPLICATIONS

Existential-humanist therapy is characterized by four distinguishing features. These are:

1. a concern for the autonomous, "being" aspects of the client;
2. emphasis on the here-and-now experiences of both the client and the therapist;
3. the belief that the existential quest (whether for self-actualization or finding meaning in life) is as important as any instinctual needs or drives; and
4. a focus on the "real" aspects of the therapeutic relationship, not just its transference aspects.[14]

Taken together, these features imply the overall goal of helping the client to achieve an authentic existence, one in which the individual can dynamically and openly "be" in the physical and social worlds and in his or her own personal world.

Traditionally, specific techniques have been deemphasized by the existential-humanists. They believe that to do otherwise leads to treating the client as an object in a treatment category, with the therapist deciding on the best means for changing the client.[11] In actuality, many existentialists draw on psychoanalytic techniques, but they differ from classical analysis primarily in their belief that the client has the right to freely choose to be influenced by or to resist the therapist. In addition, the therapist and client recognize that meaning is not absolute and that it may differ for each of them.[14]

Although Rogers' client-centered therapy embodies these beliefs, he strongly felt that components of the ideal therapeutic relationship could and should be identified and that the model for this relationship was not classical analysis. Rogers' dominant interest has been in the creation of an environment in which the client would feel safe to explore unwanted perceptions and to reorganize his or her life structure in a less defensive fashion. To this end, client-centered therapy involves a process in which the client, unsettled by the contradictions between his or her experiences and self-concept, finds that both the certain and uncertain parts of self are accepted by the therapist. This acceptance offers clients the freedom to reexamine self-perceptions and shape a new self-concept.[12] Clients change because within the context of a genuine, empathic relationship with the therapist, they are able to achieve a new self-awareness and see that both their right and wrong decisions, their certainties and uncertainties, can be accepted by another person.

Positive regard, one of the key elements in this relationship, is a form of liking and respect for another person that acknowledges one's individuality and does not trivialize a person's feelings. Another important aspect of the relationship is the feedback provided by the therapist. Although Rogers initially conceptualized the therapist's role as being nondirective, more recently he has come to believe that the therapist's feedback is useful in helping the client process information or attend to things that might otherwise have been screened out.[11] Congruence, another key therapeutic element, refers to the therapist's attempts to share subjective reactions to the client with the client. In other words, the therapist does not maintain a facade, but allows his or her true responses to be perceived by the client. Only in this way can the therapist and client relate to one another as unique individuals, rather than as objects. Finally, the therapist also helps the client begin to process his or her experiences in a more vital, evocative, and potent language. As the client's mode of expression becomes more enhancing and actualizing, experiences become so as well.[11]

Logotherapy means "therapy through meaning" (p. 11).[4] In some respects, logotherapy is more unusual than other existential therapies. First, Frankl is careful to note that logotherapy is not intended for all problems and that it can be a supplement to other types of treatment. Second, logotherapy is girded by the belief that engaging in meaningful activity may be the most effective form of therapy for people confronting an existential vacuum.[13] Third, it has developed two unique tools that stand somewhat apart from the rest of the existential tradition. *Paradoxical intention**⋆* and *dereflection*, specifically applied

---

*The use of paradox in therapy is not unique to logotherapy; this technique is also discussed in Chapters 3 and 8.

to the problems of anticipatory anxiety and excessive intention, are considered to be effective treatment tools because of people's ability to step back and be detached from their behaviors. Through the use of paradoxical intention, the person is able "to develop a sense of detachment toward his neurosis by laughing at it" (p. 147).[6] Paradoxical intention encourages the client to do precisely what is feared, while dereflection encourages the person to be less self-observant and to ignore the trouble. Instead of withdrawing from situations that produce anxiety, the individual laughs at the symptoms, and instead of fighting against obsessive ideas and compulsive behaviors, or conversely, trying too hard to achieve something that remains unattainable, he or she focuses attention away from the self and toward potential meanings and values in life.[6]

Logotherapy is not practiced solely by psychotherapists. Because of its emphasis on helping the client to clarify and actualize values, Frankl believes that it provides a structure of ideas that can be used by many people who want to find direction and assume responsibility in their lives.[4]

CRITICISMS AND LIMITATIONS

A major criticism of the existential-humanistic movement is that it is not really a unified tradition but is more of a fad or slogan serving to unite—poorly—many divergent strands.[10] As a fad, it has contributed to the proliferation of many eccentric forms of encounter groups, some of whose benefits are dubious at best. Further, because of the emphasis on self-growth, this movement has been called a "cult of the self" (p. 126).[10]

It has also been criticized for lacking scientific character. Proponents of client-centered therapy have carried out quite a few research experiments in their attempts to identify the features of the therapeutic relationship that enable the client to change. Nevertheless, much of the research is seriously flawed.[11] For example, controls are often not matched to subjects in terms of their need for therapy; in some of the experiments the controls are untreated; and measures of change are often ambiguous self-report instruments. However, because the existential-humanist movement does not espouse any one technique and generally rejects scientific evaluation, it probably cannot be evaluated by prevailing scientific methods.[11]

Existential-humanism has been accused of contributing to a breakdown in the social order by its "emphasis on the freedom to choose our own rules for living" (p. 105),[11] and it has been accused of sanctioning despair and suicide.[3] But, as Dunning[3] points out, careful analysis shows that this is a life-affirming, and not a life-denying, philosophy, because the only way in which we can reconcile our eventual death is to live in a meaningful relationship with the world and ourselves.

Another criticism that has been made is that existential-humanistic psychology is often indistinguishable from classical analysis. Certainly, it shares much—philosophically and technically—with the neo-Freudian tradition, and in terms of practice, it continues in the tradition of verbal therapy that is best-suited to an articulate, highly functioning individual.

Perhaps the most relevant limitation of the existential-humanist tradition is that its view of order and disorder seems inadequate and unsatisfactory for describing the very concrete problems of daily living that are common to the chronic mentally ill persons often seen by occupational therapists.

COMMENTARY

The themes of existential-humanist psychology are relevant to occupational therapy in their provision of a perspective for understanding the value of occupation. Humanistic and existential ideas shaped the thinking of early occupational therapy leaders. Meyer and Slagle both emphasized the subjective or phenomenological aspects of performance, and the value of work and play in giving meaning to one's existence.[15]

The overriding concern of the existentialists for the individual's search for meaning in life is the backbone of the occupational therapy clinic. Yerxa, explicitly relating existentialist literature to occupational therapy, states that "authentic occupational therapy is based upon a *commitment* to the client's realization of his own particular meaning" (p. 8).[17] In this statement she captures both the phenomenological nature of disability and the actualizing potential of engaging in occupation. Clients can confront the reality of their disability in occupational therapy because they are not treated as objects with fixed limitations. Faced with the choice of doing or not doing, they are given the chance to choose their attitudes toward disability and ability, and through this choice, to find meaning in life.[17]

The idea that the client both creates and refines an understanding of self in occupational therapy is reiterated by Dunning and later by the Fidlers. In describing the occupational therapist as a humanist, Dunning notes that because "the patient must define himself, his preferences, and his skills by personal choice" (p. 476),[3] self-clarification through activity can be achieved. Likewise, the Fidlers explore the relationship of "doing" to "becoming."[5] Doing verifies one's place as a productive member of society and enables the individual to truly relate to oneself, to the physical world, and to others.

There is a growing emphasis in occupational therapy and the occupational behavior tradition on existential themes. Sharrott and Yerxa see existential thought as forming the philosophical basis of occupational therapy.[15] In the sense that the ultimate purposefulness of human occupation is the generation of meaning through personal creativity or doing, occupational therapy does serve an existential need in human beings.

The belief of occupational therapists, that patients find meaning in work, rest, and play, is inherent in the existential-humanist tradition, and makes sense only if occupational therapy is practiced within the philosophical framework of this tradition.[15] As Yerxa notes,

> Occupational therapy's use of "meaningful" and "purposeful" activity places value upon the *patient's* view of meaning. . . . In sum, the occupational therapy value system requires that our service depend upon the patient, child, or client acting in some new and personally meaningful way that moves him or her to a new state of healthfulness. (p. 27)[18]

In order to synthesize existential thought in occupational therapy with the concern for human occupation, there will have to be an interweaving of ideas concerning the biological basis of the human urge for exploration and personal mastery and ideas concerning the human experience of meaning. The volition subsystem of the Model of Human Occupation[8] is one step in this direction, as it identifies an underlying energizing component (the urge to explore and master and its biological basis in the nervous system) along with personal experience of self-ability, interests, and value.

SUMMARY

History and Purpose	European existential philosophy and phenomenological psychology are important roots of this tradition; it arose in response to mechanistic and reductionist explanations of human behavior.
View of Order	The underlying motivation for behavior is a search for self-actualization.
	Experiences and perceptions are "intentional," or shaped by one's goals.
	Authenticity, the mark of order in life, comes from an openness to experience, to oneself, and to others, and from the active pursuit of goals.
	Frankl, the founder of logotherapy, posits a "will to meaning" that leads to the discovery and choice of values, and commitment to a significant cause in life.
	For Rogers, psychosocial order is epitomized by a flexible and realistic self-image that allows for the perception and assimilation of new experiences.

View of Disorder	Neurotic anxiety is the response of the individual who cannot face the certainty of death—this anxiety manifests itself in symptomatic behavior.
	Rogers proposes that disorder occurs when the parents' love is given conditionally to the child, causing the child to reject the parts of the self-image that the parents do not seem to love.
Action Implications	Therapy emphasizes here-and-now experiences within the therapeutic relationship.
	Rogers described client-centered therapy as being the creation of an environment in which the client feels safe to re-examine self-perceptions and achieve a new self-awareness.
	Logotherapy proposes that engagement in meaningful activity helps the individual confront the existential vacuum.
	Paradoxical intention and dereflection are two techniques associated with logotherapy.
Criticisms and Limitations	The existential-humanistic movement has been considered a "cult of the self."
	It has been criticized for rejecting scientific evaluation and for using methods that are highly similar to classical analysis.
	Therapy is limited to neurotic individuals for the most part.
Commentary	Existential-humanistic themes provide a perspective for understanding the value of occupation.
	"Doing" in occupational therapy enables the individual to choose one's attitude toward one's abilities and disabilities, to relate to oneself and the world, and to find meaning in life.

TERMS AND CONCEPTS

congruence   the therapist's attempts to share honest reactions to the client with the client.

dereflection   a technique that encourages the client to direct attention to something other than the problem, to focus on other goals.

existential anxiety   feelings associated with our awareness of impending death and a sense of meaninglessness in life.

existential vacuum   the loss of meaning in life.

intentionality   the existential concept that one's goals influence both the choice and interpretation of one's experiences.

neurotic anxiety   feelings and behaviors that arise from denying to oneself that death is part of life.

paradoxical intention a technique that encourages the client to do precisely what is feared.

phenomenology   a philosophy and psychology that stresses the importance of understanding human experience from the perspective of each individual, i.e., reality is subjective, not objective.

positive regard   freely given and unconditional liking for another person as an individual, without placing demands or requirements on that person's behavior.

REFERENCES

1. Becker, E. *The denial of death*. New York: Free Press, 1973.
2. Bugental, J. F. T. *Psychotherapy and process: The fundamentals of an existentialist-humanist approach*. Reading, Mass: Addison-Wesley, 1978.
3. Dunning, R. E. The occupational therapist as counselor. *American Journal of Occupational Therapy*, 1973, *27*, 473–476.
4. Fabry, J. B. Logotherapy in action: An overview. In J. B. Fabry, R. P. Bueka, & W. S. Sahakian (Eds.), *Logotherapy in action*. New York: Jason Aronson, 1979.
5. Fidler, G. S., & Fidler, J. W. Doing and becoming: Purposeful action and self-actualization. *American Journal of Occupational Therapy*, 1978, *32*, 305–310.
6. Frankl, V. E. *The doctor and the soul*. New York: Alfred Knopf, 1972.

7. Frankl, V. E. *Psychotherapy and existential papers on logotherapy.* New York: Square Press, 1967.
8. Kielhofner, G., & Burke, J. P. A model of human occupation. *American Journal of Occupational Therapy*, 1980, *34*, 572–581.
9. Meador, B. D., & Rogers, C. R. Person-centered therapy. In R. J. Corsini (Ed.), *Current psychotherapies* (2nd ed.). Itasca, Ill.: Peacock, 1979.
10. Misiak, H., & Sexton, V. S. *Phenomenological, existential, and humanistic psychologies: A historical survey.* New York: Grune & Stratton, 1973.
11. Prochaska, J. O. *Systems of psychotherapy: A transtheoretical analysis.* Homewood, Ill.: Dorsey, 1979.
12. Rogers, C. R. *Client-centered therapy.* Boston: Houghton Mifflin, 1961.
13. Sahakian, W. S. Logotherapy—For whom? In J. B. Fabry, R. P. Bueka, & W. S. Sahakian (Eds.), *Logotherapy in action.* New York: Jason Aronson, 1979.
14. Shaffer, J. B. P. *Humanistic psychology.* Englewood Cliffs, N.J.: Prentice-Hall, 1978.
15. Sharrott, G. W., & Yerxa, E. J. *Existentialism as the philosophical base of occupational therapy, Parts I and II.* Unpublished paper, Department of Occupational Therapy, University of Southern California, 1982.
16. Ungersma, A. J. *The search for meaning.* Philadelphia: Westminster Press, 1961.
17. Yerxa, E. J. Authentic occupational therapy. *American Journal of Occupational Therapy*, 1967, *21*, 1–9.
18. Yerxa, E. J. The philosophical base of occupational therapy. In *Occupational Therapy—2001*. Rockville, Md.: American Occupational Therapy Assoc., 1979.

ADDITIONAL READINGS

Bugental, J. F. T. (Ed.). *Challenges of humanistic psychology.* New York: McGraw-Hill, 1967.
Ellul, J. [*The technological society.*] (J. Wilkinson, trans.). New York: Knopf, 1964.
Frankl, V. E. *The unheard cry for meaning.* New York: Simon & Schuster, 1978.
Koestembaum, P. *The new image of the person.* Westport, Conn.: Greenwood Press, 1978.
Rogers, C. R. *On becoming a person.* Boston: Houghton Mifflin, 1961.
Tillich, P. *The courage to be.* New Haven: Yale Press, 1952.

5
Behavioral Approaches

Behavioral approaches represent a substantial body of knowledge and techniques developed to treat a wide range of problems. While there are several focuses within the behavioral tradition, they all share a concern for the use of research-supported methods; a view of behavior as being strongly influenced by reinforcing conditions; and a belief that changes in behavior precede changes in thought, attitude, and emotion. Proponents of behavioral approaches argue that they provide the most effective and efficient way to change overt behavior and eventually to have an impact on cognition and affect.[2]

Behavioral techniques have developed from experimental research on principles of reinforcement (learning principles). Both theory and practice are rigorously grounded in quantitative animal and human research. Careful attention is given to operationally (behaviorally) defining target behaviors for treatment, quantifying behavior, and measuring treatment outcomes. This foundation in research supports behaviorists' confidence in the effectiveness and efficiency of their techniques.

The behavioral approach, regardless of the "brand" practiced, typically focuses on outward behavior, rather than inner psychological processes, and views adaptive and maladaptive behaviors as learned through reinforcement. However, more recently, some behavioral theorists and practitioners have become concerned with the relationship between cognitive processes and behavioral changes.[5]

At its inception, this approach, being unique among therapies for psychosocial dysfunction, created excitement and greatly increased clinical research. On the other hand, it stirred controversy and distrust among adherents of more traditional approaches that emphasized the emotional disorder underlying observable behavior and the therapeutic relationship.

The use of behavioral techniques has been investigated with many different problematic behaviors. Its clinical applications are myriad, ranging from people with mild phobias to psychotic children and adults needing to learn skills. Behaviorists do not consider psychiatric diagnoses to be useful guides for treatment. Any maladaptive behavior believed to be amenable to relearning is accepted by behaviorists as a legitimate target for treatment.

HISTORY AND PURPOSE

Since the beginning of time, people have "commonsensically" used certain behavioral principles learned from everyday experiences. However, behaviorism as an identifiable body of knowledge with scientific hypothesis testing and statement of lawful relationships is commonly traced back to Pavlov, a turn of the century Russian physiologist.

The methods of the behavioral tradition are modeled on the physical sciences (e.g., chemistry) in the interest of achieving similarly precise scientific techniques. Behaviorists reduce human behaviors to their smallest observable units in an effort to understand their characteristics and functions. Just as chemists analyze atoms and molecules to understand complex chemical reactions, behaviorists study the units of response and stimulus that eventually add up to complex individual and social behaviors.[10] Wolpe[16] defines a response simply as "a behavioral event" and a stimulus as "the antecedent of a response" (p. 14). Complex behavior is accordingly seen as the simultaneous interaction of many responses, each of which becomes the stimulus for future events.[16] As one behaviorist notes, learning has occurred

> . . . if a response has been evoked in temporal contiguity with a given sensory stimulus and it is subsequently found that the stimulus can evoke the response although it could not have done so before. If the stimulus could have evoked the response before but subsequently evokes it more strongly, then, too, learning may be said to have occurred. (p. 260)[15]

Thus, behaviorists seek to analyze and understand complex human actions through the study of component parts and their causal relations. Two major traditions have evolved to make up the behavioral approach: classical and operant conditioning.

Classical Conditioning

Pavlov was interested in the process by which a new stimulus would come to elicit the response previously associated with another stimulus. The new stimulus is referred to as a conditioned stimulus. Unconditioned stimuli are typically connected to smooth muscle functioning such as glandular operations. Pavlov found that dogs salivated (an unconditioned response) at the sight of food. By pairing the unconditioned stimulus of food with another stimulus such as the sound of a bell, the latter eventually elicited salivation—now a conditioned response—without the presence of food. The sound of the bell, then, became a conditioned stimulus.[10] Pavlov therefore concluded that if two stimuli were repeatedly and simultaneously presented, the weaker, secondary stimulus came to elicit the same response that only the stronger (unconditioned) stimulus previously elicited alone. This model is called Pavlovian or classical conditioning.

A significant development out of the classical conditioning model is counterconditioning. In this process, a subject learns a fear-inhibiting response such as calmness. The connection between fear (or anxiety) and the stimulus that produces fear is weakened as the subject experiences the incompatible response (calmness) in the presence of the stimulus.[16] In 1958, Wolpe presented the principle that describes how counterconditioning occurs.[17] Pavlov, Wolpe, and others developed one tradition within behaviorism based on the original classical conditioning model and extended this in the counterconditioning model to form the tradition of "behavior therapy."

Operant Conditioning

The works of Thorndike and Skinner characterize the other major tradition within behaviorism. Their similar observations that behavior was controlled by consequences[7] led to the development of a technology based on operant methods. The model derived from their works is called instrumental, operant, or Skinnerian conditioning.

Skinner's work in the 1930s was built on the simple principle that all responses had consequences.[10] He demonstrated that by manipulating consequences, one could control the occurrence of particular behaviors. For example, if one provided food pellets to hungry rats when they pressed a lever, their lever-pressing behavior increased. The behavior that increased was said to have been positively reinforced. Negative reinforcement works on the principle that unpleasant consequences (e.g., shock) could increase frequency of avoidance or escape behaviors. The name operant conditioning was applied because the organism's response (for example, lever pressing) *operated* on the environment to achieve the desired effect.[10] Such early observations led to experiments seeking ways to establish, eliminate, increase, or decrease the frequency of behaviors. A science of positive and negative reinforcement with delineation of schedules of reinforcement was thus developed.

Further Developments

In the 1950s, Wolpe began to apply behavioral methods to the treatment of neurotic patients. He developed an approach called reciprocal inhibition through systematic desensitization.[17] He believed neurotic behavior was learned in the presence of fear-producing stimuli, and he conceptualized treatment as the reversal of this learning.[6] In other words, the patient needed to learn to produce relaxed, nonneurotic behavior in the presence of the original stimuli. To do this, Wolpe used progressive relaxation techniques, assertion training, and the operant conditioning methods of positive and negative reinforcement and extinction.[16]

Bandura represents another significant direction of behavior theory, research, and practice: social learning theory. He studied the impact of modeling and other vicarious learning processes, rather than the direct effects of reinforcement.[1]

Throughout this discussion, the behavioral tradition will be presented as a whole. However, a distinction is sometimes made between two broad focuses of the behavioral tradition: behavior modification and behavior therapy. Whenever someone exerts a degree of control over others, as in such varied interpersonal situations as the classroom, advertising, and political campaigns, behavior influence has occurred. Behavior modification is a special type of behavior influence based on the Skinnerian principle that persons' behaviors are influenced by consequences.[13] Behavior modification is mainly an operant approach that has developed in inpatient institutional settings, especially from work with mentally retarded and severely mentally ill patients. Principles of positive and negative reinforcement, punishment and extinction; techniques of shaping, chaining, fading, and prompting; and programs such as the token economy are characteristic of a behavior modification approach.[6]

Some writers speak of behavior therapy as a type of behavior modification used in a one-to-one clinical relationship.[13] Others see behavior therapy as the behavioral treatment of neurotic behavior developed in outpatient settings and not as a subset of behavior modification. In it, the classical conditioning model is more prevalent. This is evidenced by the concern for counterconditioning anxiety or the relearning of more adaptive emotional responses and fear reduction techniques.[6] While behavior modification and behavior therapy are separate branches of behavioral treatment, their uses of models and techniques overlap.

VIEW OF ORDER

The view of order in behaviorism incorporates several interrelated themes. It is heavily influenced by the fact that behaviorists have incorporated the world view of the physical sciences into their understanding of human order. Consequently, the themes relating to order are: (1) humans, like machines, are causally and environmentally determined entities; (2) humans are hedonistic, drive-centered beings; and (3) humans are homeostatic and moved by cause-and-effect forces. From this foundation, other themes emerge.

The fundamental operating principle in human behavior is thought to be a process of seeking a state of nontension (homeostasis). From a purist behavioral viewpoint, tension arises from disruptions in tissue states (e.g., hunger). Behavior is oriented to reducing these tensions (e.g., by obtaining and consuming food). In this sense, all behavior is goal-oriented (i.e., oriented to achieving a reduction in tension), and stimuli are viewed in terms of their relevance to goals programmed into the organism. Consequences of behavior that reduce tension reinforce and shape behavior. For example, a rat comes to press a lever because this action leads to getting food (a goal-oriented behavior) which when consumed reduces the tension of hunger. These underlying tensions are also referred to as drives.

The concept of drives arising from disturbances of homeostasis is central to early behaviorist thought. It is from the underlying drives that the stimuli and consequent behavior derive their relevance to the organism's behavior. Stimuli exist and have meaning to the organism only as they complement drive states. While more recent thought and practice in behaviorism is not as strictly bound to the concept of drives, the idea of the human being as a goal-oriented, tension-reducing organism still tends to permeate behaviorist thinking. Related to drive theory is the assumption that the motivation for human behavior is basically hedonistic or pleasure-seeking in nature; that is, humans act to satisfy their drives, avoid discomforts, and attain the pleasure associated with tension-reduction. In addition, behaviorist thought stresses the degree to which humans are shaped by their environments, because environmental conditions will either allow or prevent the organism's tension-reduction.

In behaviorism, ordered behavior is a function of the causal laws that determine how environmental stimuli and consequences influence behavior. These laws or principles seek to explain how the environment shapes and determines behavior, and they are equally applicable to the explanation of disorder and order. The distinction between order and disorder, therefore, does not lie in how behavior is acquired, but in the eventual success of this behavior in meeting the organism's needs and in its social acceptability.

While a large number of these causal laws exist describing how behavior is influenced by the environment, only two will be described here to illustrate the general nature of these laws. The first is the law of intermittent reinforcement. It has been found that the timing of reinforcement presentation is one of the most important factors in the effectiveness of a reinforcer's influence on behavior. Continuous reinforcement exists when every behavioral response is reinforced; this method is generally used when the researcher seeks to establish a new behavior. Intermittent reinforcement occurs when not every behavior is reinforced; reinforcement may be random or on some schedule, such as every second or third response. The law of intermittent reinforcement states that behavior that is reinforced periodically (intermittently) rather than constantly is less likely to subside or be extinguished once reinforcement is withdrawn.[7]

Reciprocal inhibition is another causal law; this refers to a situation in which two incompatible responses are elicited by the same stimulus, leading to the extinction of one of the responses. For instance, "if a response inhibiting anxiety can be made to occur in the presence of anxiety-evoking stimuli, it will weaken the bond between these stimuli and the anxiety" (p. 17).[16] This principle is the most frequently used to inhibit anxiety or fear responses in the treatment of neurotic behavior with methods of counterconditioning.

Such laws as intermittent reinforcement and reciprocal inhibition describe the many ways in which stimuli and consequences (reinforcers) influence behavior. Together these principles constitute a network of lawful relations that describe how human behavior is ordered.

Most of these principles have been generated from experimental situations and, therefore, are more exact than the way such principles operate in everyday life. For example, the principle of intermittent reinforcement refers to how the timing of reinforcement affects behavior in the laboratory, yet its application is generalized to all human situations. Intermittent reinforcement, like all behavioral principles, is assumed to be one of the causal laws operating in human life. Importantly, the view of order in behaviorism comes from laboratory experiments rather than from naturalistic observation of human beings in their everyday settings.

As previously noted, the theme of environmental determination is implicit in this view of human behavior as influenced by cause-and-effect laws. Humans are viewed as passive respondents to events, having learned, or having been shaped, conditioned, or molded by environmental events. As Skinner, a radical behaviorist, argues, human freedom is simply an illusion, a form of wishful thinking.[12] No mention is made of humans creating their experiences, originating events, or acting out of a natural desire simply to act. Goldstein states this view straightforwardly:

> Determinism, the concept that every behavior is completely determined by antecedent factors, is the most basic concept relative to the development or change of personality. Behavior therapists absolutely deny the concept of free will in that sense that one ever behaves in a way which is not contingent upon antecedent events. (p. 219)[6]

Classically, little attention has been given to inner processes, although some behaviorists have more recently acknowledged the role of cognition and blended their practice with cognitive restructuring methods. This is an important shift to the recognition of the influence of cognitive processes, attitudes, and thoughts on behavior.[6]

Finally, in the behavioral tradition order is recognizable by its adaptive consequences which:

> take the form of progress toward the satisfaction of a need . . . or the avoidance of possible damage or deprivation. . . . All this may be summarized by saying that behavior is adaptive to the extent that it is "worth while." (p. 32)[17]

A person in a state of order, then, is one who satisfies basic drives in a socially acceptable fashion while reacting to environmental influences.

VIEW OF DISORDER

The behaviorist views disorder not in terms of inner conflicts and diagnoses, but rather as maladaptive behaviors resulting from faulty learning. That is to say, the disordered individual was reinforced or conditioned to act in ways that did not meet the individual's needs or which were not socially acceptable. Faulty learning may refer either to failure to acquire a particular skill or to acquisition of a socially disruptive behavior. Socially disruptive behavior may be self-satisfying but shows little regard for others' needs and hampers others' adaptive performance. In this case, the behavior will eventually interfere with the subject's adaptation. In other cases, the appropriate behavioral cues (stimuli) may not have been learned, so that an individual expresses a certain skilled behavior at inappropriate times or in inappropriate settings.

Examples of the range of behaviors addressed by the behaviorist help to clarify the scope of disorders dealt with and the behavioral approach to classifying disorders as either the presence of undesirable behaviors or the absence of desired behaviors. For instance, behavior modification techniques are used with retarded persons to counteract unwanted behaviors such as self-abuse, head banging, masturbation, undressing, kicking, screaming, and biting; to teach new behaviors such as the self-help skills of dressing, showering, and speech; to treat "odd behaviors" such as tics and mutism; and to treat substance abuse behavior.[10] Behavior therapy is used to reduce anxiety responses and phobias; to treat learned maladaptive habits such as nail biting and tantrums; and to correct the maladaptive habits of schizophrenic and psychopathic people. As the examples illustrate, behaviorally oriented practitioners rely on commonsense definitions of what is inappropriate. They explain all these "disorders" as products of faulty learning, meaning that in the past, behaviors were not appropriately paired with stimuli and reinforced.

ACTION IMPLICATIONS

Defining disorder in terms of outward behavioral responses yields a treatment focus on changing behaviors and modifying the observable, measurable manifestations of emotional responses associated with objects and events. The emphasis on the overriding role of environmental impact on the person is reflected in the goals of therapy and in the role of the behavioral therapist.

The general goal of behavioral treatment is to provide environments that promote learning or relearning for a person in whom the learning of effective behavior previously never took place or was lost. Through the treatment process, the patient is not made to feel ill or symptomatic, but simply is viewed as the recipient of faulty learning. This puts the responsibility on the therapist to treat the patient effectively as measured by target behavior changes or to revise the treatment program. When therapy does not work, the therapist admits personal inability to devise effective behavior change strategies, rather than blaming issues such as patient resistance.

Behavioral treatment is generally characterized by two types of evaluation. First, the therapist does an analysis of the problematic behavior and its antecedent and contingent surrounding events (stimuli and reinforcing behavior).[2] Second, the effectiveness of treatment techniques and programs is evaluated.

In the patient evaluation phase of treatment, the therapist seeks to determine what typically happens before and after those behaviors targeted for treatment. This may involve a history-taking interview, recording of baseline data of observed behaviors, and/or administration of a standard test. The goal is to identify maladaptive behaviors ("target behaviors") and the set of circumstances in which they occur. This careful analysis is performed for the purpose of understanding the stimulus-response relationships that support the behaviors.

The next phase of treatment involves continued information gathering, formation of hypotheses about the target behaviors (i.e., how they came about and how they can be changed), and further development of the cooperative working relationship with the identified patient or patient representative (as in the case of a child or severely cognitively impaired patient). This phase has been referred to as a relationship-building phase of therapy and involves development of a cooperative working relationship between the therapist and patient, leading to the design of a treatment program.[6]

Treatment methods for establishing new behaviors, both simple and complex, include shaping by successive approximation, chaining, prompting, fading, modeling, role playing, and behavioral rehearsal. *Shaping by successive approximation* is an operant method that uses reinforcement of incremental steps, building from the absence of the desired behavior to its free expression. In this process, behavior is shaped by reinforcing closer and more exact expressions of the final preferred performance.[10] *Chaining* is another operant technique in which a series of related simple behaviors are reinforced to establish a larger more complex behavioral unit (chain). These chains are typically taught in reverse order. For example, with dressing, all but the last event—putting shoes on—will be performed for the person. The subject will be taught the last step first, since it is most reinforcing for the subject to have completed a complex behavior. The subject then continues learning in this "backward" sequence until the entire chain of behaviors called dressing is mastered.[7] *Prompting* involves simply directing the subject's attention to the task. This may be done by physically guiding the learner to perform a given behavior or through more subtle use of verbal cues or signals. *Fading* refers to the gradual cessation of these prompts so that natural, more subtle elements in the environment will come to evoke appropriate behavior without the learner's reliance on artificial prompts.[7] *Modeling* involves demonstrating the desired behavior for the learner and can communicate the subtle or expressive qualities of complex behavior.[8] In *role playing*, the person practices a role he or she normally does not perform without the risks of being in a "real life" situation.[4] *Behavioral rehearsal* combines modeling techniques with role playing.[8,9] In these techniques, positive and negative reinforcement and stimulus control (which involves manipulation of antecedents of behavior to effect the likelihood of the behavioral event's occurring) are used to increase the frequency of desirable behavior.[7]

To decrease undesirable behaviors, the techniques of punishment, response cost, time out, extinction, and satiation are used. *Punishment* involves either presenting an aversive stimulus, removing a positive reinforcer, or presenting a neutral stimulus to decrease or stop the frequency of a particular behavior.[7] It is properly used to decrease immediately dangerous behavior or to control behaviors that cannot be modified by manipulating cues or consequences. *Response cost* is a type of punishment in which known reinforcers are taken away when undesirable behavior is expressed. In *time out*, the subject is removed from the setting in which he or she might receive reinforcers. Thus, it is time out from reinforcement. Time out is used when the attention that is given to disruptive behaviors may be unintentionally serving as a positive reinforcement. *Extinction* involves withdrawing the reinforcement to eliminate a behavior. *Satiation* involves continuous reinforcement over a brief time period so that the subject becomes tired of responding and the reinforcer becomes less powerful as it becomes readily accessible.[7]

Behavioral techniques are used with individuals, in group settings such as in assertion training groups, and as an integral part of the structure of ward culture, as in token economies.

CRITICISMS AND LIMITATIONS

Three main criticisms of behaviorism found in the literature are: (1) the inadequacy of the behavioral approach on the issue of motivation; (2) the limitations of the reductionist nature of the approach; and (3) the concerns over ethical issues in the control of behavior.

Florey[3] and White[14] have pointed out the inadequacy of behaviorism for explaining much spontaneous human behavior. The behaviorist approach refers solely to extrinsic sources of motivation in which behavior occurs because it serves a goal outside itself (e.g., eating to reduce hunger). However, not all behavior occurs because of such extrinsic rewards or reinforcements. There is a class of spontaneously occurring, creative, initiative actions which are performed for the simple pleasure of action itself, for having an impact on one's surroundings, and for the feelings of competence accrued from having effects on the environment. Such behavior is said to be intrinsically motivated (i.e., the motive lies within the behavior itself). In addition, these writers reject the idea that all behavior is tension-reducing.[3,14] White postulates a tension-seeking drive for competence. This urge for competence leads the organism to act for action itself or for the pleasure of being a cause or having competence. Skinner[11] rebuts the notion of intrinsic motivation, claiming that the scientific approach to the study of behavior cannot admit to the "self as a true originator or initiator of action" (p. 225).

A criticism of radical behaviorism is the inadequacy of its scientific methods for the study of complex human behavior. Based on the methods of physical science, behaviorists practice reductionism, analyzing the causal relationships of behavioral components, then providing treatment with the expectation that these remediated components when reassembled will yield functional, adaptive performance and a healthy, ordered individual. Critics of this approach point out that human behavior is a gestalt that must be studied in a more holistic fashion.[14]

Thus, both of these criticisms argue that the behaviorist approach oversimplifies the explanation of human behavior. However, the problem may not be one of simplicity versus complexity but rather of adequacy. In its view of motivation and its reductionistic approach, behavioral theory is incomplete and, therefore, inadequate for fully understanding behavior.

A third issue is the ethical considerations that arise over treatment and research aimed at behavior control, especially with involuntarily confined patients. These concerns are typically countered by behaviorists who state that *all* therapy involves some control of behavior and that people control each other daily. Behaviorists argue that they are simply more straightforward and systematic in addressing the issue of manipulation. Other rebuttals suggest that the behavioral treatment is really offering a person more control of his or her life by introducing greater access to tools of self-control.[10,13]

Another criticism frequently voiced by practitioners from other theoretical orientations is that behavioral techniques effect only a superficial change and that underlying cognitive and affective symptoms will reappear in new contexts. Still others accept the evidence of behavioral changes but believe that cognitive mediating processes, and not simply the behavioral techniques, are the reason changes occur in "behavioral treatment." This criticism has led to extensions of behavioral theory and methods to include concerns with cognition. While cognitive approaches grew out of some behavorists' works, they differ significantly and, thus, are treated in the following chapter.

Criticisms of behaviorism abound, and their validity is at times difficult to discern. The charge of inadequacy of the behavioral view of motivation seems to be a reasonable concern. Daily experience provides numerous examples of activities that are difficult if not impossible to explain in terms of behavioral theory (e.g., those who enjoy the sport of rock climbing, a highly risky venture to physical integrity). The charge of reductionism appears to be a debate of magnitude. Skinner argues that what is lost when one focuses on components is minor,[11] while critics see the loss of perspective as significant. Ethical debates must always be kept in the fore, reminding all who work in the helping professions to be cognizant not only of the direct impact of treatment intervention, but also of the possibility of the incidental impact of therapy on patients and the implications of whether one covertly or overtly attempts to change people. Finally, the practical concerns of whether the most important, in depth, lasting, and meaningful changes are being effected in patients, as well as teasing out the exact reasons for behavior change, are the most difficult to judge and remain to be demonstrated.

COMMENTARY

Decisions about the value and compatibility of behaviorism with occupational therapy must be considered from the perspective of whether behaviorism matches the goals and processes of the field. Occupational therapy has as a fundamental theoretical concept a belief in the naturally motivating quality of activity. Initially, this appears incompatible with the behavorist premise that behavior is extrinsically motivated. However, a more adequate perspective for the occupational therapist is to recognize that both extrinsic and intrinsic motives for behavior exist. In that sense, occupational therapy approaches that stress activity for its own sake and behavioral approaches that change behavior through reinforcement can be seen as complementary. Similarly, the use of some behavioral technology adjunctively with occupational therapy can supplement treatment.

Based on the occupational therapy tradition, theory, and practice, it is not the role of the therapist to participate in the development of a purely behavioristic overall treatment program or to design an occupational therapy program based on behavioral principles. However, a dilemma sometimes arises for occupational therapists who find themselves working within a total treatment milieu (e.g., a ward or total program) that is based on behavioral principles. Here the therapist must ask how the occupational therapy approach can fit into such a program. In such a situation, the therapist should recognize the utility of building a program that uses extrinsic rewards to alter behavior, while developing an occupational therapy approach that provides activities that are motivating because of their intrinsic interest and meaning. Even within a predominantly behavioral approach, it is important to recognize that persons are motivated by and do some activities simply because they provide stimulation and a feeling of competence. Thus, the occupational therapy program can add balance to the overall program.

This is not to suggest that techniques developed by behaviorists or which reflect behaviorist principles never enter into the occupational therapy process. There are really two points to consider. First, a number of techniques have been developed by behaviorists that neither solely reflect nor strictly originate from behavioral principles. Such processes as modeling, relaxation techniques, role playing, and giving praise are techniques that behaviorists write about, use, and have refined in practice. However, these methods are not exclusively behavioral techniques. Other theoretical writers and practitioners, including occupational therapists using nonbehaviorist orientations have described and used similar techniques. For instance, relaxation techniques help to manage anxiety and may thus be used to provide clients with a self-help tool to calm themselves and maximize the benefits of involvement in occupational therapy. In similar ways occupational therapists use role playing to enhance occupational therapy activities. Thus, the therapist will undoubtedly find himself or herself using techniques that have been used by behaviorists. However, this does not mean the therapist is using a behavioral approach.

Second, there are instances when occupational therapists will find it compatible to use techniques based on behavioral principles in concert with their own approach. For instance, an adolescent boy with behavioral problems may be in the woodshop to explore, to pursue interests, and to develop competence. These are all processes that are defined by a different (nonbehavioral) theoretical tradition of promoting competence and health. That same adolescent may be told that if he acts out while in the woodshop, he will experience certain negative consequences. Here, the healthy behavior (i.e., woodworking) is motivated through the intrinsic motives of interest and challenge, while the unhealthy behavior is controlled by extrinsic motives (the threat of punishment). An inappropriate use of behavioral techniques in this case would be to reward the adolescent for working in the woodshop.

It is worth noting additionally that the behavioral approach to treatment is more than its learning-based techniques. Thus, other dimensions of behaviorism may have relevance for occupational therapists. Careful determination of target behaviors, clear specification of treatment procedures through clear goal setting and progress measures, and reliance on objective, verifiable data to evaluate treatment outcomes are valuable for any approach to treatment and, indeed, are advocated by other traditions as well.

Behaviorists and occupational therapists focus on different aspects of human behavior (i.e., intrinsically versus extrinsically motivated behavior). Complex psychosocial problems typically require the efforts and techniques available through collaboration of disciplines. An important contribution of the occupational therapist to overall program design is to point out the necessity of a balanced approach in which both intrinsic and extrinsic motives for behavior are recognized and nourished.

SUMMARY

History and Purpose

Behaviorism is a research- and learning theory-based science of behavior with a systematic approach to analyzing and treating observable behaviors, rather than inner psychological processes. Any maladaptive behavior amenable to relearning is considered treatable by behaviorists.

It is based on models of the physical sciences, and its origin is commonly traced back to the work of Pavlov and his model of classical conditioning. The operant conditioning model associated with Skinner, counterconditioning associated with Wolpe, and social learning theories of Bandura are further significant developments.

Two broad areas within behaviorism are behavior therapy, based on classical conditioning, and behavior modification, based on an operant model.

View of Order	Behaviorists tend to view people reductionistically, as machine-like, moved by cause-and-effect forces, and as being homeostatic in nature. Thus, people are seen as goal oriented, seeking tension reduction, and acting hedonistically.
	Human actions are believed to be environmentally determined, that is, shaped by the environment to the degree that all behavior is understood as the result of laws of conditioning and reinforcement and as dependent on environmental cues for its enactment.
	Numerous principles describe how order comes about. These include reinforcement schedules and reciprocal inhibition, among others.
	A person in a state of order is one who satisfies basic drives while reacting to environmental influences.
View of Disorder	Disorder is viewed as the result of faulty learning. Disordered overt behavior, not inner processes, is the object of behavioral treatment interventions.
Action Implications	Behavior theory and research have been translated into numerous systematic principles and techniques for changing outward behavior. The goal of behavioral treatment is, then, to provide environments that promote learning or relearning. The evaluation phase is well-developed, characterized by (1) careful gathering of data on behavior and the events that support it and (2) evaluation of treatment techniques and program effectiveness.
	There are specific techniques to establish new behaviors, increase the frequency of desired behaviors, and decrease the frequency of undesired behaviors.

Criticisms and Limitations	Behaviorism has been criticized for its exclusively extrinsic view of motivation, for its narrow reductionistic approach, and for ethical concerns with behavior control. Additionally, nonbehavioral clinicians charge that the changes in behavior are superficial. Those who may be considered cognitive-behavioral in orientation suggest that the behavior changes occur, but some cognitive process is really influencing the change.
Commentary	Occupational therapy uses techniques which are similar to those discussed in behavioral literature. Some of these include modeling, role playing, relaxation techniques, and giving praise. However, these do not belong exclusively to behaviorism. The fundamental importance of intrinsic motivation to the occupational therapy process is the key principle to keep in mind. Occupational therapy per se does not rely on deliberate, planned use of extrinsic rewards.

TERMS AND CONCEPTS

behavior modification	a major branch of behaviorism based on the Skinnerian principle that behaviors are influenced by consequences. It is mainly an operant approach.
behavior therapy	a major branch of behaviorism associated with the behavioral treatment of neurotic behavior. In it, the classical conditioning model is more prevalent.
behavioral rehearsal	a combination of modeling techniques with role playing used to teach new, complex behaviors.
chaining	an operant technique in which a series of related simple behaviors are reinforced to establish a larger more complex unit (chain). These chains are typically taught in reverse order.
classical conditioning	the early behavioral model based on Pavlov's studies. The basic law of this model states that a previously neutral event will come to elicit the same response as an event that naturally elicits that response when the two events are repeatedly paired.

counterconditioning   a further development after classical conditioning based on the principle of reciprocal inhibition explained by Wolpe. This is a process in which the subject learns a fear-inhibiting response so that the connection between fear and the stimulus object producing fear is weakened as the subject experiences the incompatible response in the presence of the stimulus.

environmental determinism   a basic behaviorist belief that humans passively respond to and are shaped by the environment.

extinction   a technique that involves withdrawing the reinforcement to eliminate a behavior.

fading   the gradual cessation of prompts so that natural, more subtle elements in the environment will come to evoke appropriate behavior without the learner's reliance on artificial prompts.

faulty learning   occurs when the individual is reinforced or conditioned to act in ways that do not meet the individual's needs or are not socially acceptable.

modeling   demonstrating desired behavior for the learner in order to communicate the subtle or expressive qualities of complex behavior.

operant conditioning   a behaviorist model characterized in the writings of Skinner which state that all responses have consequences and behavior is controlled by these. Thus, by manipulating the consequences, one could control the occurrence of particular behavior. Also called Skinnerian and instrumental conditioning.

prompting   involves simply directing the subject's attention to a task. This may be done by physically guiding the learner to perform a given behavior or through more subtle use of verbal cues or signals.

punishment   involves either presenting an aversive stimulus, removing a positive reinforcer, or presenting a neutral stimulus to decrease or stop the frequency of a particular behavior.

reciprocal inhibition   eliciting two incompatible responses leading to the extinction of one of the responses. This principle is the most frequently used to inhibit anxiety or fear responses in the treatment of neurotic behavior using methods of counterconditioning.

reinforcer   a stimulus which, when contingent on an operant response, will maintain or enhance the likelihood of that operant response occurring.

response   one of two basic units of behavioral study. A response is the behavioral event that follows a stimulus. The stimulus and response together constitute the next larger unit of behavioral study.

response cost   a type of punishment in which known reinforcers are taken away when undesirable behavior is expressed.

role playing   a technique to establish new behaviors that requires that the client practice a role in the treatment setting which he or she normally does not perform, without the risks of being in a "real life" situation.

satiation   a technique to decrease undesirable behaviors that involves continuous reinforcement over a brief time period so that the subject becomes tired of responding and the reinforcer becomes less powerful as it becomes readily accessible.

schedules of reinforcement   the timing of reinforcement presentation. This has an important influence on the effectiveness of the reinforcement.

social learning theory   an area of behavioral study associated with Bandura in which the impact of modeling and other vicarious learning processes are studied rather than the direct effects of reinforcement.

shaping by successive approximation   an operant method that uses reinforcement of incremental steps along a continuum, building from the absence of the desired behavior to its expression. Behavior is viewed as being shaped by the process of reinforcing closer and more exact expressions of the final preferred performance.

stimulus	one of two basic units of behavioral study. A stimulus is the event that precedes a response. The stimulus and response together constitute the next larger unit of behavioral study.
tension reduction	an underlying belief of behaviorists that the human organism acts to decrease tension arising from disruption of tissue states (e.g., hunger). Behavior is believed to occur for the purpose of relieving such tension.
time out	a technique for decreasing undesirable behaviors in which the subject is removed from the setting in which he or she might receive reinforcers.

REFERENCES

1. Bandura, A. *Principles of behavior modification*. New York: Holt, Rinehart & Winston, 1969.
2. Freedman, A. M., Kaplan, H. I., & Sadock, B. J. *Modern synopsis of comprehensive textbook of psychiatry* (2nd ed.). Baltimore: Williams & Wilkins, 1976.
3. Florey, L. L. Intrinsic motivation: The dynamics of occupational therapy. *American Journal of Occupational Therapy*, 1969, *23*, 319–322.
4. Flowers, J. V. Simulation and role playing methods. In F. H. Kanfer & A. P. Goldstein (Eds.), *Helping people change*. New York: Pergamon, 1975.
5. Goldfried, M. R., & Goldfried, A. P. Cognitive change methods. In F. H. Kanfer & A. P. Goldstein (Eds.), *Helping people change*. New York: Pergamon, 1975.
6. Goldstein, A. Behavior therapy. In R. Corsini (Ed.), *Current psychotherapies*. Itasca, Ill.: F. E. Peacock Publishers, 1973.
7. Karoly, P. Operant methods. In F. H. Kanfer & A. P. Goldstein (Eds.), *Helping people change*. New York: Pergamon, 1975.
8. Liberman, R. P., King, L. W., DeRisi, W. J., & McCann, M. *Personal effectiveness: Guiding people to assert themselves and improve their social skills*. Champaign, Ill.: Research Press, 1975.
9. Marlatt, G. A., & Perry, M. H. Modeling methods. In F. H. Kanfer & A. P. Goldstein (Eds.), *Helping people change*. New York: Pergamon, 1975.
10. Schaefer, H. H., & Martin, P. L. *Behavior therapy* (2nd ed.). New York: McGraw-Hill, 1975.

11. Skinner, B. F. *About behaviorism*. New York: Alfred A. Knopf, 1974.
12. Skinner, B. F. *Beyond freedom and dignity*. New York: Alfred A. Knopf, 1971.
13. Stolz, S. B., Wienckowski, L. A., & Brown, B. S. Behavior modification: A perspective on critical issues. *American Psychologist*, 1975, *30*, 1027–1947.
14. White, R. W. The urge towards competence. *American Journal of Occupational Therapy*, 1971, *25*, 271–274.
15. Wolpe, J. Experimental neuroses as learned behaviour. *British Journal of Psychology*, 1952, *43*, 243–268.
16. Wolpe, J. *The practice of behavior therapy* (2nd ed.). Oxford: Pergamon, 1973.
17. Wolpe, J. *Psychotherapy by reciprocal inhibition*. Stanford, Calif.: Stanford University Press, 1958.

ADDITIONAL READINGS

Buckholdt, D. R., & Gubrium, J. F. *Caretakers: Treating emotionally disturbed children*. Beverly Hills, Calif.: Sage, 1979.

Corsini, R., & Contributors. *Current psychotherapies* (2nd ed.). Itasca, Ill.: F. E. Peacock Publishers, 1979.

Kanfer, F. H., & Goldstein, A. P. (Eds.). *Helping people change*. New York: Pergamon, 1975.

Lange, A. J., & Jakubowski, P. *Responsible assertive behavior: Cognitive/behavioral procedures for trainees*. Champaign, Ill.: Research Press, 1976.

Mosey, A. C. *Three frames of reference for mental health*. Thorofare, N. J.: Charles B. Slack, 1971.

6
Cognitive Approaches to Therapy

The cognitive approaches to therapy, sometimes called semantic therapies, are relatively new and represent a collection of varied techniques from divergent traditions. Yet, they all share concern for the impact that cognitive functions such as beliefs, attributions, assumptions, and expectations have on affect and behavior. In addition, this concern is combined with the use of research-based techniques of behaviorism.[6] In theory, these approaches may be viewed as existing on a continuum from purely cognitive to a combination of cognitive-behavioral treatment; however the exact boundaries of this body of knowledge are not agreed upon. While there are some common concerns shared by cognitive therapists, the field is still in the process of definition and seeking to prove its effectiveness and gain respectability.

While some theorists see cognitive therapy as a recent model in the behavioral tradition,[14] there are others who consider cognitive therapy to be totally distinct.[7] A crucial difference between cognitive and behavioral therapies is the importance given to cognitive processes. Whereas behaviorists typically ignored beliefs, expectations, and other cognitive functions, the cognitive therapists believe that thoughts fundamentally influence emotions and behavior.

The cognitive therapies include cognitive restructuring techniques, coping skills therapies, and problem solving therapies.[8] Certain areas of shared beliefs unite these approaches. These beliefs suggest that adaptive and maladaptive behavioral patterns are mediated by cognition. In addition, they suggest that there are identifiable learning experiences that can activate or alter cognitive processes. Hence,

[the] resultant task of the therapist is that of a diagnostician-educator who assesses maladaptive cognitive processes and subsequently arranges learning experiences

that will alter cognitions and the behavior and affect patterns with which they correlate. (p. 692)[8]

The *cognitive restructuring approaches*, also called systematic rational restructuring, are those approaches in which the therapist helps the client identify maladaptive thoughts, acknowledge their negative effects, and replace them with more adaptive patterns.[1,4,8,10] Rational-emotive therapy (RET)[3] is an example of these approaches. *Coping skills therapies* are a collection of diverse methods characterized by their focus on using techniques to help the individual deal (cope) with stressful situations.[5,8] They represent a new way of using existing techniques. A third category consists of *problem solving therapies*, which likewise contain varied principles and techniques. These focus on presenting a general way of approaching and dealing with a range of life problems.[2]

Cognitive approaches have been used effectively in the treatment of anxiety, anger, chronic pain, self-control, obesity, sexual dysfunction, and depression with a cognitive component.[6,9] They are believed to be helpful in treating obsessional thoughts, phobias, and, in general, (learned) neurotic disorders.[9] Cognitive approaches are not recommended for use with clients with limited ability to remember and express feelings and thoughts, those with difficulty recognizing the existence of personal problems, and those with limited ability to imagine solutions. The use of cognitive approaches is generally ruled out with individuals who are out of touch with reality and who cannot communicate. This may include most psychotic individuals, severely retarded people, drug abusers who are not reality oriented, very young children, and people who are severely brain damaged.[13] Specialized knowledge is required for use of cognitive therapy with children and adolescents.[6,10]

This chapter will highlight RET, one of the earliest cognitive therapies developed. It has been widely promoted through publications, workshops, and a training institute, and many clinicians are familiar with and use its methods. Therefore, RET stands as a popular example of the cognitive therapy approach.

HISTORY AND PURPOSE

Cognitive interventions arose from an attempt to find a synthesis between insight-oriented therapies and the behavioral movement. Whereas psychoanalytic and traditional psychotherapies focused on the development of insight and merely assumed that behavioral change would follow, behavioral therapies emphasized observable changes in behavior, while ignoring unobservable mental processes. The cognitive approaches, as a meeting ground between these two polarities, take for granted the involvement of cognitive phenomena in behavior, and at the same time seek to incorporate experimentally derived behavioral interventions and scientifically based assessment of effectiveness.[6]

The earliest reference to a cognitive influence on behavior is credited to the Greek Stoic philosopher Epictetus, who observed in the first century A.D. that "men are disturbed not by things, but by the view which they take of them" (quoted in Ellis,[3] p. 167). This is the understanding that Adler achieved in 1911 as he branched out from close association with Freud and came to view human conflicts as grounded in distorted thinking. Adler's ideas eventually influenced European and American thinking and theorizing. Although others sporadically referred to the role of thinking in the development of mental illness, no systematic scheme of the relationship between cognition and behavior was proposed until 1955. Then, Ellis formally presented his ideas on rational psychotherapy.[11] In the 1970s literature on cognitive therapy proliferated, presenting a challenge to the strict behavioral views that explained behavior in stimulus-response terms and to behavioral ideas of environmental determinism. The thesis of these writings was that stimulus-response explanations of human behavior were unable to account for complex human actions, and that cognitions, or thoughts, were the primary determinants of emotion and behavior.[13] In part, the challenge to environmental determinism was the result of developing methods of self-control. This new focus on self-control opened the way for consideration of internal or cognitive mediating processes and a view of humans in a more complex, reciprocal relationship with the environment—called reciprocal determinism.[8] Further, behavioral scientists themselves were becoming more interested in "private events," or thoughts. Interestingly, although thought processes were beginning to be the target of behavioral therapies, they were considered and explained in traditional stimulus-response terminology.[8]

Interest in cognitive therapies spread to other mental health workers, as well as to the lay person. Ellis[3] and Beck,[1] among others, were particularly influential in promoting the development of cognitive models. In a short time span, the blending of cognitive and behavioral theories had taken place, and new models emphasizing the mediative role of cognitions in the influence on emotions and behavior were developed.[8]

VIEW OF ORDER

From the perspective of RET, humans are seen as being neither good nor bad. Humans are objectively viewed as limited, and acceptance of human limitations is believed to be important to a rational life-style. At the same time, people are seen as capable of creating and guiding their own lives. Thus, humans are important simply because they exist and are in most instances able to direct their lives, guided by experience and personal values. While individuals are limited, they nevertheless have creative potential. In particular, this potential is important in the creation of emotional states, or in how one responds to positive and negative life events. Humans have, if they choose, control over their emotions and the option to decide to deal with life rationally.[11] Thus, RET philosophy views humans as responsible for their emotions and behavior, as having the potential to create personal meaning, and as behaving in ways influenced by thought processes rather than determined by unconscious forces.[3,11]

This view of humans offers no description of an ideal state of order, because people are viewed as limited and fallible while still capable of being basically well-functioning. The well-functioning (ordered) person is simply one who chooses to act in ways compatible with life satisfaction and positive social interaction and who has a few intimate relationships and involvement in personally satisfying activity.[12]

VIEW OF DISORDER

Typical of the RET view of disorder is the belief that clients have faults in their thinking patterns. Ellis called these faulty thinking patterns irrational. By this, he meant that individuals tended to think of simple desires or wishes for approval, success, and so on as needs, or essential conditions, rather than as the "simple preferences" that they are. Such irrational thinking leads to the conclusion that one *must* have certain things, and that life is awful if these hoped for events do not occur. Ellis coined the term "awfulizing" to describe this irrational process.[3,11]

Ellis developed the ABC theory of personality (later expanded to the ABCDE model) to explain the relationship among thoughts, feelings, and behavior. The components of this model are:

A—activating event (e.g., "I'll have to tell my wife I've lost the house keys");

B—belief system (beliefs may be rational or irrational; e.g., "A husband should be more responsible; I'm a failure and she will think I am an oaf");

C—emotional consequences (largely created by B; e.g., "Now I'm really feeling like a dummy and I'm anxious");

D—disputation or rational challenges to B, which may eliminate disturbing Cs (e.g., "Anyone can misplace keys. That certainly does not mean I'm a dummy"); and

E—new effects, "a more rational philosophy, a level of affect compatible with effective problem solving"(p. 21)[12] (e.g., "I'll tell her my keys are misplaced, we'll look around for them, and if necessary make a new set").

Ellis theorizes that A does not directly cause C. The beliefs, thoughts, or meanings we attribute to events determine the relationship between the activating event and the emotional response. This emphasis on the intervening influence of the belief system on emotions and behavior is central to the RET approach.[3,12]

Ellis suggests that there are a limited number of basic irrational beliefs that are responsible for an individual's emotional discomfort. These irrational beliefs are characterized as: untrue, commanding, leading to disturbed emotions, and not helpful in meeting goals. Some of these result from a category of thinking that Ellis calls the "Major Musts":

I must: (do well, get approval, etc.)
You must: (treat me well, love me, etc.)
The world must: (give me what I want quickly and easily, treat me fairly, etc.). (p. 74)[12]

A core irrational belief reflects the notion that people can be evaluated or rated in terms of their worth, goodness, and so on, and that people have certain obligations or needs. For example, the beliefs that if one is not loved then life is awful, or that one must always be treated fairly by others, are typical core irrational beliefs.[12] These core beliefs are then embellished and individualized to reflect the particular circumstances of a person's life. Disorder thus becomes the use of invalidated, irrational thinking to deal with the events of daily life. The emotional outcome of this pattern of thinking is emotional distress.

The theory of RET acknowledges genetic, environmental, and sociocultural impacts on the development of irrational thinking but puts these in perspective by saying that genetic and environmental influences do not maintain irrational thinking—people do this to themselves by "self-indoctrination."[3,12] It is the "here and now" faulty thinking that needs to and can be abandoned. No excuses based on personal history or environmental influences are acceptable. The focus is the present and the future.

ACTION IMPLICATIONS

Cognitive treatment in RET consists of logical, straightforward challenging of irrational beliefs. It is directed toward changing "faulty thinking" and is guided by the ABC model. Activating events, the belief system (especially core irrational beliefs), and emotional consequences are identified, and the therapeutic change centers on the client's recognizing illogical thinking and learning to dispute irrational beliefs. Thus, the ultimate goal of the RET process is to help the client learn to become his or her own therapist.[3,12]

Ellis speaks of the use of the ABC model and how the focus of RET differs from other traditional psychotherapies:

Most major psychotherapies also concentrate either on A, the Activating Events in the individual's life or on C, the emotional Consequences experienced subsequent to the occurrence of these events. But this is precisely what the individual wrongheadedly does himself: over-focuses on A and/or C and rarely deeply considers B, his Belief System, which is the vital factor in the creation of his symptoms. (p. 178)[3]

The treatment process begins with some type of evaluation. This is probably the least developed area of RET, because there are few evaluations available that identify basic irrational ideas.[3,12] Information is gathered through the use of psychological tests, history-taking, and general discussion of the model components.[13] The therapist assumes that clients can identify their problems; this is in contrast to psychoanalytic approaches in which people are believed to be incapable of truly knowing what their problems are.

The therapist's role is typically active-directive, persuasive, straightforward, and challenging. This role combines a perception of the client as an individual with "a ruthless, hardheaded campaign against [the client's] self-defeating *ideas, traits,* and *performances*" (p. 169).[3]

The components of the treatment process include: (1) direct education and persuasion to the RET belief in irrational thoughts as the cause of distress; (2) use of the client to self-monitor thoughts; (3) therapist modeling of rational thinking; (4) use of straightforward feedback, challenge, confrontation, and redirection of client thoughts and beliefs; and (5) use of homework assignments and practice sessions in which new rational self-statements and behaviors are performed.[8] A variety of methods such as discussion, behavioral techniques, reading assignments, and audiovisuals are employed to achieve profound cognitive changes. All treatment techniques are aimed at enabling the client to replace a self-defeating outlook with a more tolerant life philosophy.[3] Typical of the cognitive restructuring techniques, RET helps people learn to identify and attack their irrational, perfectionistic thoughts, abandon absolutist thinking, and be more realistic about human limitations.[3]

CRITICISMS AND LIMITATIONS

A major criticism of the cognitive body of knowledge is that research is inadequate to determine the relative effectiveness of cognitive and behavioral techniques for achieving change. Currently research support for behavioral techniques appears to outweigh that for cognitive techniques.[7]

Another criticism concerns the combining of cognitive and behavioral practice models. Debate continues over the degree to which these approaches can or should be combined to accurately reflect the complexity of human functioning.[8,14]

Finally, the population which can benefit from these techniques is clearly limited to a reality-oriented, insightful, and verbally expressive population.

COMMENTARY

Occupational therapists seek to understand persons' occupational performances in the context of their values, interests, and sense of effectiveness in daily life. These motivational components may reflect and interact with belief systems, whether faulty or rational. As such, occupational therapy and cognitive techniques can be complementary, supporting therapies. Occupational therapists already use some of the techniques developed by cognitive therapists. This is particularly true in the area of developing interpersonal skills. Thus, both occupational and cognitive therapists can work together to reinforce therapeutic goals related to enhancing the patient's sense of control in life, to learning more adaptive ways to interact socially, and to recognizing and acknowledging one's abilities, strengths, successes, and potentials. In the area of identifying personally valued ideas, as opposed to family or culturally promoted ideas, both cognitive and occupational therapists intervene to help the client to clarify and to enact personal values.

As the cognitive therapist helps the client to identify the thought processes that are impeding satisfying participation in life, the occupational therapist can challenge the client to explore and learn more about his or her abilities and everyday behavior. Both therapies share a common focus on the present and future and an emphasis on positive ways to be involved in and interpret the meaning of life events.

SUMMARY

History and Purpose	Cognitive approaches to therapy all share concern for the influence that cognitive functions have on affect and behavior. While their relationship to behaviorism is debatable, many acknowledge that cognitive therapies developed from discontent with behaviorists' general disregard of the effect that cognitive processes have on emotion and behavior. This examination of the role of thoughts on emotions and behavior emerged in the 1960s.

View of Order	In RET, individuals are viewed as limited by their humanity, yet possessing creative potential, enabling much individual control over emotional states and life choices. An ordered or well-functioning person chooses to act in ways compatible with: life satisfaction; positive social interaction; having a few intimate relationships; and involvement in personally satisfying activities.
View of Disorder	According to RET, the use of invalidated, irrational thinking to deal with the events of daily life constitutes disorder. The emotional outcome is distress.
Action Implications	The RET treatment process is directed toward changing faulty thought patterns and is guided by the ABC model of personality. The therapist directly challenges the client's maladaptive beliefs. Treatment aims at helping the client learn to be his own therapist.
Criticisms and Limitations	One criticism of cognitive approaches concerns the lack of evidence of clinical effectiveness to support a major role for cognitions in influencing behavior. Another major criticism concerns the relationship to behaviorism and the degree to which models of human functioning should reflect cognitive and behavioral events to accurately describe complex human functioning. Finally, cognitive therapies are limited, serving a reality-oriented, insightful, and verbally expressive population.
Commentary	Occupational therapists should have general knowledge of cognitive approaches as a complementary, supporting therapy. Occupational therapists already use some cognitive techniques. The two approaches can be used compatibly with clients to enhance their sense of control; to learn socially adaptive routines; and to confront values, abilities, strengths, successes, and potentials. Primarily, the cognitive therapist may help identify faulty thought processes while the occupational therapist can challenge clients to explore and learn about their abilities and their everyday behavior.

TERMS AND CONCEPTS

ABC theory

the personality theory on which RET is based in which the relationship among thoughts, feelings, and behavior is explained. It has been expanded to the ABCDE model. The components of the model are: A-Activating events; B—Belief system; C—emotional Consequences; D—Disputation or rational challenges to B; and E—new Effects.

"awfulizing"

a coined term used to describe irrational thought processes.

cognitions

conscious thought processes such as beliefs, attributions, expectations, and assumptions.

cognitive restructuring

a category of cognitive therapy in which the therapist helps the client identify maladaptive thoughts, acknowledge their negative effects, and replace them with more adaptive patterns. Also called systematic rational restructuring. Rational-emotive therapy is one example of this type of therapy.

cognitive therapies

a collection of varied therapy techniques from divergent traditions all sharing concern for the impact that cognitive functions have on affect and behavior. In a pure sense, cognitive therapists believe that changes in cognitions will lead to changes in affect and behavior. These are also called semantic therapies and include: cognitive restructuring therapies, coping skills therapies, and problem solving therapies.

coping skills therapies

a category of cognitive therapy containing a collection of diverse methods characterized by their focus on using techniques to help the individual deal (cope) with stressful life situations.

irrational thoughts

a term used in RET for thought patterns that reflect personal beliefs that are unrealistic, illogical, or exaggerated in importance. Such thinking leads to emotional discomfort.

problem solving
therapies

a category of cognitive therapy containing varied principles and techniques that focus on presenting a way to approach and deal with a range of life problems.

rational emotive
therapy (RET)

a cognitive restructuring therapy developed by Albert Ellis in the 1950s in which people are considered responsible for their emotions and behavior, able to lead creative lives and behave in ways influenced by thought processes, not by unconscious forces. This approach is characterized by emphasis on the intervening influence of personal belief systems on emotions and behavior. Treatment consists of direct challenging of the interfering beliefs.

REFERENCES

1. Beck, A. T. *Cognitive therapy and the emotional disorders*. New York: International Universities Press, 1976.
2. D'Zurilla, T. J., & Goldfried, M. R. Problem solving and behavior modification. *Journal of Abnormal Psychology*, 1971, 78, 107–126.
3. Ellis, A. Rational-emotive therapy. In R. Corsini (Ed.), *Current psychotherapies*. Itasca, Ill.: F. E. Peacock, Publishers, 1973.
4. Goldfried, M. R., & Goldfried, A. P. Cognitive change methods. In F. H. Kanfer & A. P. Goldstein (Eds.), *Helping people change*. New York: Pergamon, 1975.
5. Kanfer, F. H. Self-management methods. In F. H. Kanfer & A. P. Goldstein (Eds.), *Helping people change*. New York: Pergamon Press, 1975.
6. Kendall, P. C., & Hollon, S. D. (Eds.). *Cognitive-behavioral interventions: Theory, research, and procedures*. New York: Academic Press, 1979.
7. Ledwidge, B. Cognitive behavior modification: A step in the wrong direction? *Psychological Bulletin*, 1978, 85, 353–375.
8. Mahoney, M. J., & Arnkoff, D. B. Cognitive and self-control therapies. In S. I. Garfield & A. E. Bergin (Eds.), *Handbook of psychotherapy and behavior change: An empirical analysis* (2nd ed.). New York: John Wiley and Sons, 1978.
9. McMullin, R. E., & Giles, T. R. *Cognitive-behavior therapy: A restructuring approach*. New York: Grune & Stratton, 1981.
10. Meichenbaum, P. Self-instructional methods. In F. H. Kanfer & A. P. Goldstein (Eds.), *Helping people change*. New York: Pergamon Press, 1975.

11. Morris, K. T., & Kanitz, H. M. *Rational-emotive therapy*. Boston: Houghton Mifflin, 1975.
12. Walen, S. R., DiGiuseppe, R., & Wessler, R. L. *A practitioner's guide to rational-emotive therapy*. New York: Oxford University Press, 1980.
13. Werner, H. D. *Cognitive therapy: A humanistic approach*. New York: The Free Press, 1982.
14. Wilson, T. G. Cognitive behavior therapy: Paradigm shift or passing phase? In J. B. Foreyt & D. P. Rathjen (Eds.), *Cognitive behavior therapy: Research and application*. New York: Plenum Press, 1978.

ADDITIONAL READINGS

Ellis, A. The basic clinical theory of RET. In A. Ellis & R. Grieger (Eds.), *Handbook of RET*. New York: Springer, 1977.

Lazarus, A., & Fay, A. *I can if I want to*. New York: Warner Books, 1977.

Mahoney, M. J. *Cognition and behavior modification*. Cambridge, Mass.: Ballinger Publishing Co., 1974.

Schwartz, A. *The behavior therapies: Theories and applications*. New York: The Free Press, 1982.

7
Reality Therapy

Reality therapy is an approach to behavior change developed by William Glasser in the 1950s. It stresses the responsibility that individuals should take for their own behavior. It also focuses on current behavior and on specific planning for more responsible future actions.[4,8] The therapeutic process depends on developing a relationship of caring involvement between the therapist and client, coupled with the therapist's consistent, firm requirement that clients clarify values and standards for behavior and judge their own behaviors as responsible or irresponsible.[8] Reality therapy deliberately deemphasizes psychiatric diagnostic labels. Psychosocial health and illness are understood primarily as manifestations of responsible or irresponsible behavior.[5] Reality therapy "depends upon what might be called a psychiatric version of the three R's, namely, *reality*, *responsibility*, and *right-and-wrong*" (p. xii).[9] Reality therapy is considered to be a commonsense therapy, easily learned and applicable to a wide range of people in a variety of situations.[8] Its principles have been used widely with delinquent and emotionally disturbed adolescents. They have been broadly applied to grade school classes as preventive intervention to promote successful identities in young children and to prevent failure and irresponsible behavior.[6] They have been successfully used in individual and group therapy for bereavement, marital discord, anxiety, and psychosis. Because it depends on a flow of effective communication, reality therapy is of little benefit to autistic or severely retarded clients.[8] The format for its use varies from group and individual psychotherapy to classroom discussion groups. Likewise, reality therapy principles are used in a wide range of settings, from mental hospitals to correctional facilities, halfway houses, and schools.[2]

HISTORY AND PURPOSE

Glasser considers reality therapy to be his unique creation which happens to be compatible with the thinking of several predecessors. For instance, the

Swiss physician Paul DuBois emphasized the role of the physician as an interested "friendly counselor," in which he helped the patient to focus on healthy thoughts as a replacement for ruminations on illness. Many similar early 20th century themes that emphasize healthy behavior and the sincere, friendly therapist presage modern reality therapy principles.[8] For instance, Adolf Meyer, an American psychiatrist, promoted such a commonsense approach, which stressed reality and responsibility. However, Glasser argues that the intervening "pansexual views" of Sigmund Freud came to overshadow these rational approaches.[8]

Reality therapy represents a reaction to many Freudian-oriented teachings. While in a psychiatric residency, Glasser and his supervisor, Harrington, who both shared doubts about traditional psychotherapy, jointly developed and applied the concepts of reality therapy with chronically psychotic veterans and seriously delinquent adolescent girls. Both programs were viewed as successful and led to applications in school settings and to the founding of the Institute for Reality Therapy. The reality therapy principles that grew out of this process are described in *Reality Therapy*[5] and *Schools Without Failure*.[6] The latest concern of reality therapy is with societal changes in the Western world around the 1950s. As the focus of contemporary life has moved from an emphasis on individual achievement (a job, diploma, etc.) to a concern with meaningful life roles, there have been corresponding repercussions in family life, the experience and meaning of success and failure, and those major institutions that deal with people experiencing chronic failures—the welfare system, hospitals, and the justice system. These changes have concomitantly affected the thinking and focuses of reality therapists.[7]

In comparing reality therapy with traditional analytically oriented psychotherapy, Glasser aims to invalidate the latter's claims of effectiveness. He states six points of reality therapy that are in fundamental disagreement with traditional psychotherapy:

1. Because we do not accept the concept of mental illness, the patient cannot become involved with us as a mentally ill person who has no responsiblity for his behavior.
2. Working in the present and toward the future, we do not get involved with the patient's history because we can neither change what happened to him nor accept the fact that he is limited by his past.
3. We relate to patients as ourselves, not as transference figures.
4. We do not look for unconscious conflicts or the reasons for them. A patient cannot become involved with us by excusing his behavior on the basis of unconscious motivations
5. We emphasize the morality of behavior. We face the issue of right and wrong which we believe solidifies the involvement, in contrast to conventional psy-

chiatrists who do not make the distinction between right and wrong, feeling it would be detrimental to attaining the transference relationship they seek.

6. We teach patients better ways to fulfill their needs. The proper involvement will not be maintained unless the patient is helped to find more satisfactory patterns of behavior. Conventional therapists do not feel that teaching better behavior is a part of therapy. (p. 54)[5]

It is evident from these statements that reality therapy is radically different from conventional therapy.

Reality therapy is, in a sense, a very conservative approach, taking a stand on what is right and wrong and doggedly returning responsibility to the client. This is in contrast to many new therapies which stress the relativity of morality.

Although the principles have been developed by psychiatrists, current practitioners of reality therapy include such professionals as psychologists, clergymen, social workers, teachers, probation officers, nurses, policemen, lawyers, and judges.[8]

VIEW OF ORDER

Early in his career and before he formulated the principles of reality therapy, Glasser stated this basic assumption: "We are often given the illusion that we can change our surroundings when in fact either they change in their own inconsistent pattern and/or we change our position relative to the world" (p. 8).[4] Glasser's view of order stresses individual responsibility, the ability to take control of one's life and to change one's own behavior, and the inability to change other people to make them fulfill one's personal needs. The only alternatives to facing reality and acting responsibly are to change our surroundings by moving to another location (e.g., changing jobs) or to try to make others change to meet our needs. However, because personal needs still exist regardless of where we live or work and because we have little real power to change other people, Glasser concludes that people must face reality and accept control of their own lives, learn to meet their own needs appropriately, and act responsibly on their knowledge of reality.

The concept of identity is the first and most basic idea of reality therapy. It reflects the universal need of all people to feel unique. People have either a success identity or a failure identity, based on feedback from social interactions and personal experiences with people and objects. This self-image may or may not be the same view that others have of us; it is highly personal. Glasser and Zunin[8] assert that this identity forms at the age of 4 to 5 years. They note that people with success identities associate with others with success identities, and, similarly, those with failure identities seek the company of like peers. Thus, success breeds success, and failure breeds failure.

Individuals with success identities are believed to possess two traits. First, they know that at least one other person in the world loves them, and they love that person in return. Second, they know that they are worthwhile individuals and that at least one other person believes this to be true also. Those with failure identities share the common experience of loneliness and deal with this discomfort by either denying reality or ignoring it.[8] Therefore, the concept of order in reality therapy is directly related to an individual's self-image, or success identity, which is revealed in the way a person behaves— responsibly or irresponsibly.

The second major concept is responsibility, a pervasive theme in reality therapy. It is defined as "the ability to fulfill one's needs, and to do so in a way that does not deprive others of the ability to fulfill their needs" (p. 15).[5] Behaving responsibly enhances feelings of self-worth and one's sense of value to others. Responsibility is learned through a caring, involved relationship, and as one demonstrates the ability to handle limited responsibility, one is challenged to accept more responsibility and achieve new successes.[5]

Involvement is a third important concept. It is the process by which people naturally fulfill needs and develop self-images as successes. Involvement also refers to the genuine, caring therapist/client relationship (not as a transference relationship) and is also importantly recognized as the process through which therapeutic gains will be maintained after termination of treatment. Glasser and Zunin see the need for involvement as "the primary intrinsic driving force governing all behavior" (p. 296).[8]

These principles suggest a view of humans as self-determined; that is, given an individual's assets and limitations of biological and psychological inheritance and of the environment, people can make of themselves what they will. People are what they do, and they have a vast capacity to behave in many different ways. The way in which one behaves "depends upon decisions rather than conditions" (p. 306).[8] Glasser and Zunin further state that each person has a "health or growth force," meaning that people naturally want and strive toward successes, responsible behavior, and meaningful relationships with others (p. 297).[8]

VIEW OF DISORDER

Glasser disagrees with the concept of "mental illness" and prefers the medical analogy of "weakness" rather than "illness." Ideally, he would like to totally dispense with diagnosis and refer to all clients as simply irresponsible. In Glasser's view, all psychosocial disorders emanate from irresponsible behavior, leading to a lack of need fulfillment and unhappiness.[4,5] Irresponsible people either deny or ignore reality and consequently are unable to meet their own needs. The resulting behavior has been popularly called mental illness. People with a psychosis deny reality by viewing the world through their own private fantasy for the purpose of self-protection from feeling lonely and worthless. Those called delinquent, sociopathic, and personality disordered are all basically antisocial in their disregard of society's rules. They simply ignore the reality that they know exists.[8] Glasser and Zunin summarize the view of etiology in the assertion that "unhappiness is the result and not the cause of irresponsibility" (p. 292).[8]

This unconventional view of etiology suggests that people develop emotional discomfort "because their performance has been, and is, too low" (pp. xiii–xiv)[9] rather than because their standards have been excessively high; thus, the goal of therapy is to increase one's accomplishments. This *under*socialization is the basic problem in disorder, and it is manifested in irresponsibility and the failure to make commitments and the accompanying sacrifices required to achieve goals.[9]

ACTION IMPLICATIONS

Reality therapy attempts to challenge the client to be responsible, to make commitments, and, consequently, to achieve more. Its concepts are all designed to accomplish these goals, with the anticipated result that people who once viewed themselves as failures will accept increasing responsibility, accumulate accomplishments, and begin to feel successful. Persons with all diagnoses are treated using basically the same process to help the person to "fulfill his needs in the real world so that he will have no inclination in the future to deny its existence" (p. 7).[5] In short, the therapist teaches responsibility to those who did not learn it early in life.

Reality therapy is best described as a philosophy of treatment and a process of therapy rather than as a collection of techniques. A variety of accepted techniques such as role playing, contracting, and homework assignments may be used, but only as they fit within the basic philosophy of individual responsibility for behavior and the caring and involved relationship with the client.

Glasser and Zunin describe the reality therapy process as based on eight principles. First, the therapist is involved and cares; thus therapy is personal. Involvement takes place as the therapist relates to the client as a caring, genuine, and real person who acts to demonstrate responsibility and insists on the client's acting responsibly, while maintaining the caring relationship—a subtle and delicate balance.[5] The therapist is willing to share personal experiences and is open to having his or her values and standards challenged.

Second, the focus of therapy is on behavior and not feelings, because it has been observed that it is easier to intervene in a cycle of negative events through *doing* something different rather than by first *feeling* something different. Behavior is believed to be easier for an individual to control than feelings. Third, therapy deals mainly with the present. The past cannot be changed, and too much time is typically spent dwelling on past failures. In dealing with the present and future, discussion can turn to the more positive direction of what people are doing or can do to improve their situations. Fourth, reality therapists deal with value judgments. They expect clients to identify goals, values, and standards for behavior and to measure their own behavior against these. A fifth principle is that of planning. Once the client identifies general directions and ways to change behavior, the therapist has the client specify this change in terms of when, where, and with whom. The sixth principle is commitment. Early in therapy, the therapist encourages the client to follow through with plans "for the therapist" and later "for him- or herself." In both cases a commitment to action is required. The seventh principle simply states that no excuses are acceptable. The therapist realizes that plans fail at times, but concern is only for when the plan or an alternative will be tried again, not for the reasons of failure. The eighth and final principle is that of eliminating punishment. Punishment is not an effective way to help people with poor self-images to change.[5,8]

In addition to these eight principles, there are five identified stages of therapy that guide the client to clarify values, goals, and standards for behavior; to identify behaviors that interfere with their accomplishment; and to generate alternate behaviors.[1,8]

First, the problem solving process is initiated by asking "What are you doing?" and probing for details such as "What happened? Where? When? How?" but not "Why?" In the second stage, the therapist asks if the client's past actions accomplished any good. This question is commonly met with resistance. Thus, the therapist must be involved with the client if the client is to respond honestly to this crucial question. If the client maintains that he or she acted properly and would continue to behave in the same way, the therapist leaves the issue until the client expresses a desire to alter the behavior. Self-evaluation of behavior is essential since individual responsibility is the core of therapy. If the client admits that a behavior is negative, therapy continues, focusing on that behavior.

Assuming therapy progresses, the third stage begins the process of relearning as the therapist asks what the client's plan is for changing behavior. The plan of action is "pinned down." Alternatives are considered through a brainstorming process, role playing may be used, and future strategies, times, places, and backup plans are specified in detail. In the fourth and fifth stages, a contract stating details of the plan for behavior such as time, place, and so on is signed by the client and a follow-up session is scheduled for the client to report how the plan went or to revise the plan if necessary.[1]

Therapy may involve a lively verbal exchange, with the emphasis always on the client's positive points and potentials. The therapist's role is more like a teacher than a traditional therapist, and as such, the therapist is willing to be a real person, revealing personal information and being open to having values and opinions challenged.[1,5,8] Humor, confrontation, and debates may occur. Conversational content will likely range over a wide array of daily events as the therapist and client identify problems of social interaction and seek alternate ways for the client to become meaningfully involved with others.[8] As Glasser states, "When values, standards, and responsibility are in the background, all discussion is relevant to therapy. Continually stressing responsibility is artificial" (p. 38).[5]

The pivotal issue on which behavior change hinges is identifying the client's values:

> Where standards and values are not stressed, the most that therapy can accomplish is to help patients become more comfortable in their irresponsibility. Because our effort is always directed toward helping patients fulfill their needs, we insist on their striving to reach the highest possible standards. (p. 72)[5]

Thus, reality therapy involves a strong element of challenge to help the client live up to self-professed standards. The client maintains control of the pace of therapy by deciding whether or not to acknowledge irresponsible behavior. The therapist remains available to help at any time the client wishes to work further. Ideally, the trust nurtured through involvement, coupled with the client's natural urge to grow, will lead to change.

CRITICISMS AND LIMITATIONS

The point of view taken in reality therapy is typically in opposition to stands taken by two groups: (1) traditional psychoanalytically oriented individuals and (2) those who claim that there is an overemphasis on individual responsibility for personal misfortune when environmental factors may be more to blame. Those from a more classic psychoanalytic position are opposed to Glasser's stand that mental illness does not exist and criticize him for denying the emotional suffering of psychosocially dysfunctional persons. His unconventional theory and rebellion against traditional concepts of psychotherapy have resulted in a lack of support from some in the academic community who do not agree with his basic views of human behavior and its determinants.[10]

There has also been criticism of approaches to health care which emphasize the responsibility of the individual with a psychosocial problem who may be the "victim" of such factors as poverty, poor parenting, and the like. "Blaming the victim" is the phrase used to refer to these approaches. While the critics have not singled out Glasser's work per se, their criticisms appear to be relevant. In stressing the responsibility of the patient (especially with younger, poorer, and otherwise relatively powerless clients), the therapist may be overlooking familial and environmental factors that made the person's maladaptive behavior understandable and contributed to its maintenance. To the degree that the person is enjoined to shoulder all the responsibility, the responsibility that belongs to family, social agencies, and the like is ignored.[3,11]

A limitation of reality therapy is that it is not a complete system of treatment. Rather, it is a well-developed philosophy, with few clearly associated treatment techniques. Thus, practitioners are left to draw on a wide array of other techniques and apply them within their understanding of the theory. Glasser also notes the limitation of his theories to the Western culture and value system in which they were developed. In relationship to evaluations of treatment effectiveness, Glasser and Zunin note that research sophistication has not developed to a degree of refinement to meaningfully measure variables influenced by reality therapy.[8] While recidivism declined at the school for delinquent girls where reality therapy was applied, no controlled, long-term research study of outpatients has been conducted.[8] Overall, little research exists to support claims of treatment effectiveness.

Because reality therapy is primarily a verbal therapy, its application is limited to verbal, cognitively able clients. Another implication of the primarily verbal nature of reality therapy is that it involves talking about doing (i.e., planning for doing) but does not focus on learning skills for action.

COMMENTARY

Many of the themes of reality therapy are highly compatible with occupational therapy. The focus on establishing a relationship with the client where the therapist is a real multifaceted person (i.e., not a transference figure) is shared by both occupational therapy and reality therapy. Similarly, concern with providing a supportive, nonthreatening, but challenging environment for growth and the companion emphasis on the positive aspects of the client are common to both. Neither occupational therapy nor reality therapy encourages acting out negative behaviors. Instead, both encourage the development and expression of positive reality-based, socially acceptable, and need-satisfying actions. Both therapies approach clients with a challenging spirit to help them live up to their standards, fulfill their potential, and respond positively with accomplishment to the urge to grow and become competent. The reality therapy manner of introducing challenge to the patient and the dogged insistence that the patient plan and make a commitment to action are of special interest, since this theme of challenge is a shared philosophical area of agreement between the therapies. In occupational therapy practice, therapists might find the reality therapy orientation to be a useful guide for operationalizing the ideals of challenge and demands for performance in the clinic.

The focus on doing over feelings, behavior over attitudes, and the present and future over the past are common to both occupational therapy and reality therapy. Because of the compatibility of these themes, the shared common-sense orientation, and common interest in everyday situations as the content of therapy, the therapies may sound similar. However, there is one important difference. Reality therapy is a verbal therapy with homework assignments. Occupational therapy is activity-oriented and typically provides a setting for "hands-on" involvement in activities in which clients can test their abilities and become aware of the impact of these experiences on self-image. Therefore, there is potential for reality therapy and occupational therapy to be effectively used together.

SUMMARY

History and Purpose	Reality therapy is a commonsense approach to behavior change emphasizing reality and responsibility. It was developed by William Glasser in the 1950s in reaction to many Freudian-oriented teachings. It stresses the responsibility that individuals should take for their own behavior, current behavior, and specific planning for future actions.
View of Order	Humans naturally desire successful self-images and responsibility through a caring involvement with others. The formation of a successful self-image depends on being actively involved with others, meeting individual needs, and making responsible choices and actions.
View of Disorder	Individual diagnoses are not considered useful labels. All people with psychosocial disorders are viewed as irresponsible in their acknowledgement of reality. This irresponsibility leads to unhappiness as people either deny or ignore reality and are, thus, unable to meet their needs.

Action Implications	Reality therapy philosophy promotes individual responsibility for behavior and asserts the value of involvement with others to learn and maintain responsible behavior. A variety of techniques such as role playing, contracting, and homework assignments may be used, but only as they fit with the basic philosophy. Reality therapy attempts to challenge the client to be responsible, acknowledge personal values, make commitments, and achieve more. The key event on which behavior change is dependent is the acknowledgement of personal values.
Criticisms and Limitations	Reality therapy is criticized for denying the existence of painful emotional disturbance and overemphasizing individual responsibility when environmental factors may be more to blame. Its limitations include a lack of clearly associated treatment techniques, a lack of research, and the sole use of verbal therapy.
Commentary	Occupational therapy and reality therapy are compatible treatment approaches. Areas of agreement include establishing a genuine, caring client/therapist relationship; providing a supportive yet challenging environment for growth; focusing on health and positive issues; encouraging reality-based need-satisfying actions; and emphasizing doing in the present. The critical difference is in the treatment applications. Reality therapists work through verbal means. Occupational therapists use activities.

TERMS AND CONCEPTS

"blaming the victim" a phrase used by critics of treatment approaches that stress individual responsibility to refer to the unwarranted burdening of individuals (or clients) with responsibility for life events that have been beyond the individual's control.

failure identity an individual's self-image based on feelings of loneliness. Individuals with failure identities tend to deny or ignore reality as a way to cope with loneliness. Glasser believes that this self-image is formed by 4–5 years of age.

identity the basic cross-cultural need of all people to feel unique.

involvement the process by which people naturally fulfill needs and develop self-images as successes or failures. It refers to the genuine relationship with another person. The need for involvement is believed by reality therapists to be the intrinsic force behind all behavior.

irresponsible behavior the choices and actions that do not lead to need fulfillment or are disruptive to others' need fulfillment and lead to unhappiness, as people either deny or ignore reality and are unable to meet personal needs. Irresponsible behaviors are deemed the source of all psychosocial disorders.

responsibility the ability to meet individual needs while not interfering with others' ability to fulfill needs.

success identity an individual's self-image based on the knowledge that one is loved and that one loves others in return and that one feels worthwhile. Glasser believes that it is formed by 4–5 years of age.

REFERENCES

1. Bassin, A. The reality therapy paradigm. In A. Bassin, T. E. Bratter, & R. L. Rachin (Eds.), *The reality therapy reader: A survey of the work of William Glasser, M.D.* New York: Harper & Row, 1976.
2. Bassin, A., Bratter, T. E., & Rachin, R. L. (Eds.). *The reality therapy*

reader: A survey of the work of William Glasser, M.D. New York: Harper & Row, 1976.
3. Gaylin, W., Glasser, I., Marchus, S., & Rothman, D. *Doing good: The limits of benevolence.* New York: Pantheon Books, 1978.
4. Glasser, W. *Mental health or mental illness? Psychiatry for practical action.* New York: Harper & Row, 1960.
5. Glasser, W. *Reality therapy: A new approach to psychiatry.* New York: Perennial Library/Harper & Row, 1975.
6. Glasser, W. *Schools without failure.* New York: Harper & Row, 1969.
7. Glasser, W. *The identity society* (rev. ed.). New York: Harper & Row, 1972/75.
8. Glasser, W., & Zunin, L. M. Reality therapy. In R. Corsini (Ed.), *Current psychotherapies.* Itasca, Ill.: F. E. Peacock Publishers, 1973.
9. Mowrer, O. H. Foreword, in Glasser, W. *Reality therapy: A new approach to psychiatry.* New York: Perennial Library/Harper & Row, 1975.
10. Reilly, S. Dr. Glasser without failure. In A. Bassin, T. E. Bratter, & R. L. Rachin (Eds.), *The reality therapy reader: A survey of the work of William Glasser, M.D.* New York: Harper & Row, 1976.
11. Ryan, W. *Blaming the victim.* New York: Pantheon Books, 1971.

8
Communications/Interaction Theory

Communications/interaction theory is a relatively new body of knowledge that has arisen largely out of an attempt to understand the peculiar speech and thought patterns of people with schizophrenia. The stance of this theory is that behavior can be fully understood only if it is examined as part of the larger context, or framework, in which it is contained. This position is summarized by the following:

> A phenomenon remains unexplainable as long as the range of observation is not wide enough to include the context in which the phenomenon occurs. (p. 21)[13]

Because the context for most behavior generally involves relationships between and among people, this tradition of knowledge has been primarily concerned with seeking interpersonal or interactional explanations of disorder. Hence, its initial target client population was families with schizophrenic members, rather than schizophrenic persons themselves. However, many of the principles of treatment associated with this school have been more recently used with individual clients representing a variety of disorders.

HISTORY AND PURPOSE

Classical psychoanalysis (see Chapter 2) sought to explain behavior as individuals' attempts to satisfy inner needs or drives. Eventually, dissatisfaction with this exclusively inner-determined view of behavior led neo-Freudian theorists (see Chapter 3) to propose more socially or culturally oriented ex-

---

In some ways a confusing body of knowledge, the concepts in this tradition have frequently included new terminology, or used old, familiar terms in new and unusual ways. Whenever possible, this chapter will avoid this semantic problem by using more mundane ways of expressing the same ideas.

planations of behavior. Simultaneously, behaviorists were proceeding from the opposite direction, suggesting that behavior was a response to environmental stimuli (see Chapter 5). In all of these accounts, however, more emphasis was placed on explaining isolated acts of isolated individuals than on explaining patterns of behavior occurring during interactions between people. Further, these theories relied on relatively simple cause-and-effect explanations of behavior. For example, prolonged separation from one's mother during infancy was seen as the cause of becoming an insecure and untrusting adult. In addition, Freudian and neo-Freudian theories endowed people with inner structures, such as the superego or the id, that took on a life of their own.[13]

In the mid-twentieth century, the increased application of systems theory to the natural sciences and the development of information theory influenced an interdisciplinary group of social and behavioral scientists to begin describing both ordered and disordered human behavior purely in terms of patterns of interpersonal relationships. Because communication comprises the concrete or "observable manifestations of relationships" (p. 21),[13] a critical focus of this group was verbal and nonverbal communication. Along with the focus on observable events, communications/interaction theorists sought to understand the "what" and "how" of an event, instead of the "why," thereby precluding concern with mysterious inner structures as explanations of motivation and behavior.

VIEW OF ORDER

The view of order in this body of knowledge draws on four theoretical sources: information theory, cybernetics, systems theory, and Russel's Theory of Logical Types. Communications/interaction theorists have integrated ideas and concepts from these theories to develop an orientation to human behavior summarized by the belief that behavior can only be understood in the context of relationships.

Behavior as Information

Information theory enables human behavior to be seen as a process of "information exchange." What this means is that behavior is viewed as information passing between individuals as they act and react with reference to each other.[13] To amplify the notion of behavior as information, communications/interaction theories turned to the cybernetic concept of feedback.

Cybernetic theory focuses on processes of feedback and how they modify behavior. A common cybernetic process is the thermostat, which reads the temperature of the room (feedback) and, based on its reading, turns on or off a furnace or air conditioner (behavior) to achieve a preset goal. Such cybernetic processes of aiming for a goal, using feedback to monitor progress toward or maintenance of the goal, and altering ongoing behavior based on feedback are identified as an integral part of the information exchange that takes place when people interact. Thus, interaction and communication are circular processes in which one person transmits some "information" to another person, who then receives and reacts to this information. This reaction in turn sends new information to the first person. Each of the parties in the relationship continually judges the received information to determine whether or not it fits into his or her schema of acceptable responses.[13]

Because communication is a circular process, it is not always clear who is the initiator and who the respondent in a sequence of events. However, because people tend to look for beginnings and endings in their interactions, they figuratively add periods to the sequence of events in which they engage.[13] These figurative periods establish one event as beginning an interaction and another as a response to the first event. Thus, in some relationships, one person will consider his or her actions to always be a response to another's. For example, at the doctor's office, the patient frequently considers the doctor to be leading or directing the interaction. Similarly, one country may consider its escalation policies to be in response to another country's initiation of an arms build-up. In other situations, perhaps a problem-solving group, all parties may feel that they are equally leading and following.

Information exchange and feedback processes are used to explain how behavior and the external social order become stable, and thus accepted and expected by persons. The events of human behavior are recurrent; that is, they occur on a fairly routine basis in a fairly predictable fashion, giving out a constant stream of information about what behavior is acceptable in our social and cultural world. These repeated and recognizable patterns are construed by most people as indicative of normal or ordered behavior. For example, a pattern of ordered behavior in a relationship between an employer and employee may require the recognition that in this situation one person leads and another follows. Ordered behavior in other situations, however, may be characterized by equal leading and following on the part of both members of the relationship.[13]

Open Systems and Behavior

Systems theory adds a dynamic perspective to understanding behavior. Open systems theory seeks to go beyond the linear cause-and-effect thinking that characterizes closed systems concepts. An open system differs from a closed system in that it interacts with the environment and is capable of both maintaining and changing itself. As such, it is more complex than and incorporates cybernetic processes. Instead of maintaining a status quo, an open system evolves as it takes in information from the environment and puts out certain behaviors. Every event that affects an open system changes it in some way; thus, a system's response to present events reflects its past experiences.

In the communications/interaction body of knowledge, the family is described as an open system that incorporates cybernetic processes and information exchange. Looking at the family as a system implies that the family is more than just a collection of individuals. It is, in fact, an organization that is characterized by certain recurring patterns of behavior and that influences and responds as a whole to the external environment.[5]

Because the family is an open system, events proceed in a circular, rather than a linear, fashion. This means that the same behavior or result may arise from different causes. For instance, a teen-aged boy may be late to dinner because he was still doing homework, watching television, or angry with his parents. Similarly, behavior is also multidetermined; that is, there is not simply one antecedent to one response. Thus, a previous fight with his father may have caused the son to be unable to concentrate on his homework and not finish before dinnertime. Finally, positive events occurring outside the family system (such as a good teacher in school) may modulate or alleviate effects of family processes, while stress (say, failing a test) may exacerbate them, causing a "snowball" effect.[5]

Within the family system, just as within society, particular patterns of interaction occur on a regular basis. These characteristic patterns prescribe internally acceptable ways for family members to interact with one another.[5] For instance, an accepted pattern of behavior in one family may be for the mother to make all decisions about how late children should stay up. According to communications/interaction theorists, such patterns are unique to each family and are not to be judged in terms of external standards or norms, but rather in terms of their productiveness for the particular family.

Logical Types

The fourth major source of ideas for communications/interaction theory is the concept of logical types. This concept is concerned with the meaning of the information that is shared by persons and the way in which meaning is changed or influenced by context. The concept of logical types refers to the idea that not all communication is of the same kind. For instance, the comment, "This was an interesting conversation," is a statement *about* the talk and is clearly different from the communication given *during* the talk itself. Context refers to the overall setting or scene of behavior.[1] As the scene changes, the same words may take on totally different meanings. Thus the phrase "I love you" has a vastly different meaning when said between two persons celebrating their thirtieth wedding anniversary, between a parent and child, or between two people on their second date. Similarly, the game of baseball takes on two completely different meanings when played by major league teams or played at a picnic.

According to the theory of logical types, the context represents a different level of communication from the message occurring within it. It is a higher, or more abstract, class of communication. This is the same notion we use when we categorize animals, for instance. Mammals are a class that contains cats and dogs among others. Once we recognize that a cat is a mammal we immediately know certain facts about cats that are shared by all mammals. In the same way, by knowing the context of a behavior, certain information is communicated to us which helps to explain that behavior. This level of communication, being on a higher level than the immediate behavior itself, is called metacommunication; it is communication *about* communication.[1]

People recognize and manipulate contexts every day. For example, when two children agree to "play house," they are in effect saying that they will communicate and behave within the context of playing house. Should one child say something or behave in a fashion that does not suit playing house or the respective roles of mother, father, or child, his or her playmate will recognize and object to this behavior. This use of contexts is carried into adult life when persons behave and communicate in such varied contexts as a classroom, party, theater, walking down a street, dining out, praying in temple, and so on.

Context is not the only form of metacommunication that exists. Nonverbal communication, such as gestures, facial expressions, and distances between people, is a form of metacommunication that helps to define the relationship between communicating individuals.[4,8,9,13] For instance, we accept that doctors can freely touch patients, but it is quite unlikely that a patient will initiate contact with a doctor (unless it is to prevent some dreaded event such as a shot). At work, subordinates are much less likely to touch their bosses than vice versa.[4]

Nonverbal communication may be consistent with or contradictory to the verbal message. At times, the relationship between the two may be deliberately contradictory; this is often the case in play, fantasy, ritual, and humor.[1] For example, if one child says to another, "Let's shake hands," and then laughingly pulls his or her hand away at the last minute, a joking context of contradictory messages has been created. Further, the nonverbal communication within one context may be deliberately contradictory to that within another. To use our example of children playing house, if one child says to another, "Let's play house—I'll be the mommy and you be the baby," although the message *within* the game is that the children are *not* equal, the reality of the play situation is that the children *are indeed partners*.

Order

Ordered behavior, as conceptualized by this school, involves several components. First, it is behavior that meets certain acceptable standards for a given situation. To do this, individuals must recognize what is appropriate and required in different contexts. Second, order involves the ability to shift contexts, both as demanded by changes in the environment, and to fulfill one's own interpersonal goals. Order also derives from the ability to recognize and shift between relationships that involve leading and following, or sharing these functions on an equal basis. Finally, order involves the recognition of both stated and unstated meanings of communication and the ability to deliberately use nonverbal communication to lend meaning to contexts.

Communications/interaction theory thus explains order in human behavior as a form of information exchange in which people send and receive messages from each other, mutually adjusting their behavior as they go along. This process is aided by the ability to recognize different levels of communication, or metacommunication. In particular, the context in which the communication occurs influences participants' behavior, at the same time that their behavior helps to maintain the context. Further, this context gives meaning to behaviors that might otherwise appear to be senseless or puzzling. Order therefore involves a number of complex factors that simultaneously and dynamically affect any human interaction. To illustrate how these processes are manifested in a simple interaction, consider the following episode:

> A man approaches a cashier in a store to purchase an item. He hands her the item while smiling and looking directly into her eyes. She takes the item, ringing up the price and announcing the total. He takes a check out of his wallet while asking whether he has met her before. She responds negatively, displaying her ringless finger. She asks for his address and phone number to put on the back of the check he wrote, and he asks if he might not also have hers.

In this sequence of events two episodes occur simultaneously: the purchase and the meeting of a potential date. Both give messages that imply and derive their meaning from the two contexts that surround the events. The first context, the store, is immediately apparent and requires the behaviors of buying an item and waiting at the cash register. The second context is made obvious by virtue of actions that are clearly outside and even unnecessary to the first context—the eye contact, showing a ringless hand, the question of whether they have met before (which is not taken as a literal question, but as an indication of his interest in her), and the final request for her phone number. While neither the cashier nor the customer may believe they have initiated the interaction, both may interpret the other's actions as feedback to continue. Finally, behavior which might be puzzling in the wrong context is expected and consistent once both individuals have acknowledged the existence of a second context (flirting).

VIEW OF DISORDER

Communications/interaction theorists were initially concerned with understanding schizophrenia as a symptom of disordered family communication. Although they have since generalized from this work to explain other forms of psychopathology, schizophrenia, as a communication problem, is the focal point of their discussion of disorder.

In a basic form, disordered communication involves disagreement or confusion between the verbal intent of a message and the metacommunication accompanying the same message.[13] When such contradictions exist, the other party to the communication does not know what response to make. Because the nonverbal part of the message essentially serves to define the relationship between the two parties, it can say to the other person, "I accept you and our relationship as you see it"; "I do not accept you or our relationship"; or "I neither accept nor unaccept you—this relationship does not exist." The first two messages, while not equally desirable, are clearly understood, but the third is confusing and mystifying.[13] It is this third category that characterizes disordered communication. For instance, if a student requests an appointment with a professor, and the professor says either "I will meet with you next Tuesday" or "I will not meet with you next Tuesday," the message to the student is unambiguous. However, if the professor says, "Just drop in during office hours," but has no defined office hours and is never there, the student has received two contradictory messages—one of the professor's availability and one of his or her inaccessibility.

Although most people encounter this type of situation on an occasional basis, in some families it persists as the norm. When such contradictory or *double-bind* messages typify family communication, a potential setting for the development of schizophrenia exists. Communications/interaction theorists believe that the double-bind situation epitomizes pathological family communication.

The double-bind has five necessary ingredients. First, it involves two or more persons, one of whom is thought of as the "victim." Second, the double-bind generally begins with a primary negative injunction or command. For example, the child is told, "If you do not do what I say, you will be punished." Next, another negative message is given which conflicts with the first. Thus, the second message is of the sort that says, "Even though I am punishing you, I really love you." This conflicting message may be conveyed by nonverbal means, or it may be created by disagreement between two controlling parties (for instance, when parents disagree about what behavior is expected of the child). The fourth ingredient pertains to the inability of the victim, or child, to leave the setting. The last ingredient of the double-bind is that the combination of events represents a recurrent pattern of interaction. As the double-bind structure becomes the norm and is habitually expected by the child, any part of the sequence will suffice to precipitate the feelings and reactions associated with the entire sequence.[1,3,5,11]

The typical example given of a double-bind is a situation in which a mother feels threatened and anxious when her child responds to her as a loving parent. Because such feelings of anxiety are unacceptable to her, she counteracts her discomfort or hostility by simulating loving behavior. The first negative message given the child is, "If you are too affectionate, I will withdraw" (punish you). The second message, directly contradicting the first is, "Mothers are supposed to be loving and affectionate, so I will pretend to be that way with you and you must pretend to believe me." Both these messages are more likely to be communicated through actions or nonverbal behavior than through words. Finally, the child has no choice in the situation, other than to accept the double-bind. Either she or he perceives the initial truth, which will certainly not be pleasant, or the child deceives him- or herself in order to avoid the unpleasant truth. But deceiving oneself means denying one's own internal perceptions. In other words, if the child accurately perceives that the mother does not want the child to be affectionate, she or he will be hurt. But denying this first message will cause him or her to be hurt anyway, when the mother does withdraw.[1]

Because people caught in a double-bind learn to deny their perceptions, they eventually do *not* learn to interpret or manipulate the metacommunicative levels of interaction in the same way that others do. Instead, these people develop various maneuvers or strategies for dealing with the double-bind. These strategies make sense in their own universe, but not in anyone else's. For instance, they may respond literally to a metaphoric message, such as tasting a nonfood substance upon being told that it looks good enough to eat. They may insist that they are not there or that they are somebody else. They may continually search for hidden meanings in what others say, or they may treat all messages as unimportant and laughable. Sometimes, schizophrenics may use language as an attempt to *not* communicate. Because both agreeing and disagreeing with the messages being sent is dangerous, they may try to do neither, by using vague, incoherent, or tangential speech. Ultimately, they may simply avoid responding to all messages. These strategies parallel the bizarre behaviors of the different schizophrenias—paranoia, hebephrenia, catatonia, and speech peculiarities.

Disorder in the person therefore emanates from disorder in the family, in particular, from the "no win" and "no way out" communication of the double-bind. The victim of the double-bind escapes only by denying the reality of the communication in some fashion and is thereby forced out of the world of reality as others experience it.

ACTION IMPLICATIONS

The goal of communications/interaction therapy is to enable the family to identify the patterns maintaining the double-bind situation(s). Family members can then find more effective solutions to their problems and can replace the disordered communication patterns.

The communications/interaction theorists differentiate between two types of change—first-order change and second-order change.[14] First-order change refers to change made *within* a given context and tends to involve "more-of-the-same" or "less-of-the-same" behaviors. For example, two children playing house might get into a fight over the proper role of the "mother." To solve the fight, they eventually agree that the "mother" should do some, but not all, of the disputed behaviors. Another example would be a student's decision to study longer hours for an exam because of a previously low grade. Second-order change, however, involves a change of context, and thus a reconceptualization of the entire situation. The two children playing house might therefore decide that another game would be more enjoyable. Similarly, the student who made a low grade might decide that the problem was not one of poor study habits, but one of nervousness, and that practicing yoga before the next test would be more useful than extra cramming. To some extent, second-order change appears illogical because the connection between the solution and the problem is not immediately apparent.

Second-order change often involves the therapist's use of paradoxical instructions. Paradoxical instructions include such methods as telling someone to advertise something she or he has been concealing, to do something she or he has been afraid will happen; prescribing the symptom itself; or perhaps giving conflicting sets of instructions to the client.[12,14] An example of prescribing the symptom is telling an insomniac to try and stay up all night and not sleep for a month. This effectively changes the context from one of trying to sleep (which is not working) to one of trying to stay up. When this, as expected, fails, the objective of sleep is achieved. The result of techniques such as these is that the patient begins to formulate a new world view, to see that the inevitable is *not* inevitable, or that it is ludicrous and not frightening, or that it is something that can be controlled by the person. Bruner gives an example of treating a child's fear of making mistakes in school.[2] During tutoring sessions with the child, he changes the context from one of fear of being reprimanded, to a game in which the child deliberately tries to make mistakes:

The eleven-year old boy . . . said to the tutor that he was afraid to make an error in reading because his teacher yelled at him. The tutor asked whether his teacher yelled very loud, and upon being assured that she did, volunteered that he could yell louder than the teacher, and urged his patient to make a mistake and see. The boy did, and his tutor in mock voice yelled as loud as he could. The boy jumped. Tutor to patient: "Can she yell louder than that?" Patient: "Yes, lots." Tutor: "Make another error and I'll try to get louder still." (p. 482)[2]

The child was eventually able to treat mistakes playfully and to progress with and master his reading lessons.

In families, second-order change may involve relabeling a problem, and thereby shifting it from one individual to the family interaction system, or creating therapeutic double-binds.[3,14,15] The latter means that "the therapist must create situations that force the family into a bind. Either it continues its behavior, but does so under the command of the therapist, or it rebels, thus producing the desired change" (p. 482).[3] In either case, the family sees that its pathological interaction patterns or norms are subject to control and hence, can be changed. For instance, if the family norms consist of the father's setting limits or prescribing punishments while the mother plays the role of peace-maker or mediator, the therapist's interventions might be directed at helping the parents realize that the problem does not lie in the child's infraction of rules or the unfairness of punishments, but in the lack of an alliance between the parents.

Communications/interaction theorists, because of their belief that recurring patterns of behavior dominate family and social interaction, are especially interested in discovering family "rituals." A family ritual is a special pattern of behavior involving the entire family.[12] Eating together every night at 6 p.m. may be a family ritual. Some rituals, however, can be pathogenic or destructive—for instance, a weekly family bridge game in which the father consistently berates his partner. Replacing the pathogenic ritual with a therapeutic ritual is another type of second-order change.[12] Suggesting that the family try a noncompetitive activity instead of the bridge game might lead to the inculcation of a more positive ritual.

Both first-order and second-order changes are relevant to various problems, but to attempt either when the opposite is needed will create an impasse. The communications/interaction group therefore adheres to a problem-solving model of treatment for both individuals and families. This model begins with a concrete and clear specification of the problem. The next step is to determine what behaviors or patterns are maintaining the problem. From this, it is then possible to begin identifying whether first- or second-order change is needed.[14,15] If second-order change is necessary, attempts are made to relabel or re-context behavior, and to change behavior through paradoxical instructions, therapeutic double-binds, and therapeutic rituals.

CRITICISMS AND LIMITATIONS

One of the initial criticisms of the communications/interaction body of knowledge derives from its use of the "black box" analogy—that the mind can be compared to a black box, whose contents it is *not necessary to see* in order to understand behavior.[13] By not accounting for this unseen inner "structure," however, the role and importance of emotions and cognitions (concepts important to other schools of psychological thought) are minimized, while the importance of interaction as a focus increases.[3] Many critics also liken the theory to behaviorism and accuse its proponents of "a lack of understanding of the basic inner condition of the patient" (p. 134).[11] However, by limiting their domain to the behavioral effects of communication, communications/interaction theorists are not denying the existence of emotions, will, or motives; they are merely asserting that behavior can be changed without recourse to these phenomena. And, in fact, they very much believe in the individual's self-control. The ultimate goal of paradoxical treatment strategies is to lead people to seeing that they do have control over what they do.

Another source of criticism concerns the use of the Theory of Logical Types (i.e., different levels of communication) to explain the paradox created in a double-bind situation. One critic stated that "the double bind theory is 'an example of . . . mathematico-logical pseudo-psychologizing'" (p. 135),[11] and another indicated that what is described as levels of communication are more accurately a variety of dimensions, some pertaining to the actual communication while others are more descriptive of the individuals doing the communication.[10] Yet, the point of the communications/interaction theorists is that all communication does more than just convey a message; it also says something about the relationship between the people communicating. It is when this latter aspect of the communication is ignored, not correctly understood, or contradictory with the intent of the verbal message that pathology arises. Thus, this criticism either reflects an incomplete understanding of the premises of communications/interaction theory, or it must be taken as a rejection of communications/interaction theory as a whole.

The double-bind hypothesis is also criticized for lacking empirical research support. However, there is a plethora of published qualitative studies, transcripts, and case histories supporting the hypothesis. The deeper issue appears to be distrust of the qualitative/case *methods* used by the communications/interaction school to support the theory. Given the concerns of this school, extensive use of transcripts, cases, and qualitative data seems an appropriate methodological approach. The theory does not lend itself to experimental, correlational, or other quantitative methods.

This body of knowledge has limited itself to examination of observable phenomena and, in particular, communication. It has not sought to address issues such as motivation or drive-satisfaction, developmental stages, cognition, and a host of other phenomena. In addition, communications/interaction theorists do not accept role theory as being compatible with their views, because roles are seen as oriented toward individuals rather than interactions.[5] Further, these theorists do not comment on the external environment of the family system; although they acknowledge the potential impact of external events, their primary focus is on the family's interactional system.

In sum, criticism of this theory is aimed in part at the limitations of the theory, particularly its avoidance of psychodynamics. Nevertheless, communications/interaction theorists have addressed a prevalent phenomenon—communication—that had hitherto been given little attention, and they have done so in a unique manner.

COMMENTARY

Although this body of knowledge has targeted communication as its focus, some of its implications can enhance understanding of occupational performance and is therefore relevant to occupational therapy.

First, the focus on the family as an interactional system is relevant to understanding how exploration or play might be stifled in a child. In the family where the double-bind is a rule of life, a child might very quickly choose inaction as being safer than exploration. Eventually, the child may begin to avoid action in other settings as well, failing to learn the skills that other children acquire through play and exploration. However, occupational therapists also seek to understand the development of occupational behavior by examination of the adequacy of family members as role models, as well as by an examination of the resources and environment of the family.[7] Therefore, the communications/interaction perspective is only partially useful to an understanding of how pathological families might stifle childhood occupation.

The emphasis of communications/interaction theorists on the way in which ordered behavior reflects the *context* of that behavior is particularly relevant to occupational therapy treatment. A major role of the occupational therapist is the creation of contexts that give meaning to people's behaviors.[6] In other words, when the occupational therapist's goal is to enable someone to develop punctuality, discipline, and other work-appropriate behaviors, he or she tries to create a setting in which these behaviors are natural and expected. Thus, the therapist may involve this person in an assembly-line project, at the same hours every day, rather than in a once-a-week social games group. The latter context, however, might be right for someone needing to explore and experiment with new leisure interests.

Finally, on a practical level, occupational therapists are part of an interactional system with their clients and patients. Familiarity with the ambiguities and potentials of communication and metacommunication can only enhance therapeutic effectiveness and humanity. For instance, the nonverbal communication conveyed by a uniform and clipboard may be contrary to a stated message to a client that the therapist wants to *collaborate* with this person on goal setting. Similarly, the use of manipulative techniques may tell patients that therapists see themselves as authorities, even as they ask patients to share in guiding their own treatment.

In summary, then, the communications/interactional body of knowledge is one which can contribute to understanding the development of disordered occupational performance. At the same time, one must be aware of its limitations and different overall emphasis from that of occupational therapy. We have already incorporated some of its action implications into our own practice, in the form of creating therapeutic contexts; this body of knowledge provides an additional perspective for understanding the importance of doing so. Last, the recognition of how discrepancies between verbal and nonverbal communication may create double-binds for our clients is particularly relevant to understanding ourselves in therapeutic relationships.

SUMMARY

History and Purpose	Dissatisfaction with views of behavior as either exclusively inner-determined or environmentally determined led communications/interaction theorists to seek explanations of behavior in terms of communication patterns in interpersonal relationships.
	Theory is dominated by an interest in understanding peculiar speech patterns of people with schizophrenia.

View of Order	Theory base is derived from four sources: information theory, cybernetics, systems theory, and the theory of logical types.
	Ordered communication is a process of information exchange, in which frequently repeated events come to be recognized as socially expected.
	Behavior is understood in relationship to the context of that behavior; individuals recognize what behaviors are appropriate for different contexts (e.g., church, school, etc.) and are able to shift and manipulate contexts.
	Contexts and nonverbal communication are of a different logical type than the verbal content of communication; nonverbal communication lends meaning to the context.
	Families are open systems that can be characterized by unique communication patterns; these patterns prescribe acceptable, or ordered, behavior for the family.
View of Disorder	Schizophrenia, the primary concern of this school, is the outcome of disordered family communication.
	Disordered communication involves giving contradictory messages to a "victim" (usually the child), and creating a "no-win," "no-escape" situation known as the double-bind.
	The person caught in a double-bind learns to deny his or her perceptions instead of understanding and using metacommunication the same way others do.
	Bizarre schizophrenic behaviors are strategies for dealing with the double-bind.

Action Implications	Two types of change are distinguished: first-order change, which involves decreasing or increasing some behavior already present, and second-order change, which involves relabeling the problem, or placing it in a new context.
	In the family system, second-order change means shifting the problem from the individual to the family interaction system.
	The therapist seeks to uncover pathological interaction patterns and family rituals and to replace them with healthy patterns and rituals.
Criticisms and Limitations	The theory has been criticized for ignoring role of emotions, for use of complicated language and constructs, and for lack of empirical research support.
	Theory is limited to study of communication and does not address issues such as motivation or role theory.
Commentary	Double-bind phenomenon can add to our understanding of how family life might stifle the development of occupational behavior in children.
	Occupational therapy treatment involves the manipulation of contexts to give meaning to the activities of our clients; this theory increases our understanding of how ordered behavior relates to the context of that behavior.
	Therapists and their clients form a communication system; familiarity with ambiguities and potentials of communication and metacommunication can enhance the effectiveness of this communication system.

TERMS AND CONCEPTS

catatonia

in communications/interaction theory, a disorder in which a person attempts to *not* communicate with others.

context

total sum of the human and nonhuman components which comprise the scene in which a behavior occurs; sets the stage for behaviors.

cybernetics

the monitoring/regulation of behavior through the receipt of relevant feedback in order to maintain a predetermined goal or state, e.g., a thermostat.

double-bind

situation in which contradictory messages are conveyed to an individual by another person(s), providing an unclear message for expected behavior. Pathologically, these patterns of interaction occur repeatedly and the individual withdraws from the situation by developing bizarre behavior in response to it.

first-order change

behavioral change accomplished within a given context, generally by increasing or decreasing behaviors that already occur in that context.

hebephrenia

in communications/interaction theory, a disorder in which a person avoids communicating by laughing at all messages.

metacommunication

communication about communication; information conveyed through such phenomena as the context of behavior, body language, use of space, clothing, and so on, which gives added meaning to the verbal content of the communication.

open system

an organized complex of parts which dynamically interact in successive cycles of input, throughput, output, and feedback, in order to accomplish some purpose or goal in a coherent fashion.

paranoia

in communications/interaction theory, a disorder of communication in which a person continually searches for hidden meanings in what others say.

paradox situation in which individual is instructed to behave in what seems to be a contradictory or absurd manner in order to precipitate new ways of thinking about the situation. As a treatment technique, it is a form of bringing about second-order change.

second-order change behavioral change accomplished through reconceptualization of the context in which the behavior occurs. Therapeutically this may be achieved by using paradoxical instructions, therapeutic double-binds, and/or therapeutic rituals.

REFERENCES

1. Bateson, G., Jackson, D. D., Haley, J., & Weakland, J. H. Toward a theory of schizophrenia. In G. Bateson (Ed.), *Steps to an ecology of mind.* San Francisco: Chandler, 1972.
2. Bruner, J. S. On coping and defending. In J. Coleman (Ed.), *The psychology of effective behavior.* Glenview, Ill.: Scott, Foresman, 1969.
3. Foley, V. D. Family therapy. In R. J. Corsini (Ed.), *Current psychotherapies* (2nd ed.). Itasca, Ill.: Peacock, 1979.
4. Henley, N. M. *Body politics: Power, sex, and nonverbal communication.* Englewood Cliffs, N.J.: Prentice-Hall, 1977.
5. Jackson, D. D. The study of the family. In P. Watzlawick & J. H. Weakland (Eds.), *The interactional view.* New York: Norton, 1977.
6. Kielhofner, G. The art of occupational therapy. In G. Kielhofner (Ed.), *Health through occupation: Theory and practice in occupational therapy.* Philadelphia: F. A. Davis, 1983.
7. de Renne-Stephan, C. Imitation: A mechanism of play behavior. *American Journal of Occupational Therapy,* 1980, *34,* 95–102.
8. Ruesch, J., & Kees, W. *Nonverbal communication.* Berkeley: University of California, 1969.
9. Scheflen, A. E. *Body language and social order.* Englewood Cliffs, N.J.: Prentice-Hall, 1972.
10. Schuham, A. I. The double-bind hypothesis: A decade later. *Psychological Bulletin,* 1967, *68,* 409–416.
11. Watzlawick, P. A review of the double-bind theory. *Family Process,* 1963, *2,* 132–152.
12. Watzlawick, P. *The language of change.* New York: Basic Books, 1978.
13. Watzlawick, P., Beavin, J. H., & Jackson, D. D. *Pragmatics of human communication.* New York: Norton, 1967.

14. Watzlawick, P., Weakland, J. H., & Fisch, R. *Change: Principles of problem formation and problem resolution.* New York: Norton, 1974.
15. Weakland, J. H., Fisch, R., Watzlawick, P., & Bodin, A. M. Brief therapy: Focused problem resolution. In P. Watzlawick & J. H. Weakland (Eds.), *The interactional view.* New York: Norton, 1977.

ADDITIONAL READINGS

Ruesch, J., & Bateson, G. *Communication: The social matrix of psychiatry.* New York: Norton, 1951.
Weakland, J. H. The "double-bind" hypothesis of schizophrenia and three-party interaction. In D. D. Jackson (Ed.), *The etiology of schizophrenia.* New York: Basic Books, 1960.
Swenson, C. H. *Introduction to interpersonal relations.* Glenview, Ill.: Scott, Foresman, 1973.

9
Social Ecological Approaches

Approaches to psychosocial practice that emphasize the role of the environment, or milieu, in promoting health, can be grouped together under the rubric of social ecology. Included among these approaches are the therapeutic community, milieu therapy, and ecological psychology. Despite their common orientation to the environment as a critical dimension of health, these approaches are not a unified body of knowledge, and the reader would probably not find them grouped together in this way in other literature. Nevertheless, they share a fundamental difference from somatic or psychotherapeutic approaches to mental illness—their focus on the environment or context of treatment.[2] This chapter presents an amalgamation of these approaches in order to provide a perspective for understanding the contributions occupational therapists can make to the therapeutic use of the environment.

Some initial definitions will clarify the scope of this body of knowledge. Cummings[5] identifies the therapeutic community and milieu therapy as being two major approaches to the use of the environment in therapy. Traditionally, the therapeutic community designated an environment that focused on helping patients achieve insight and emotional control. As such, the social environment, or the roles of staff and patients, was the primary environmental concern, and various forms of therapy were incorporated into the therapeutic community as different means to the same end.[5] The therapeutic community was typically characterized by community meetings and an emphasis on achieving *insight* into one's problems or difficulties in interpersonal situations. Milieu therapy referred to a therapeutic environment that was organized around the goal of helping patients improve their competence in problem-solving and daily-living skills. Different therapies were incorporated into this context for their relevance to ordinary life and for their potential to present the patient with practical problems to solve.[5] Milieu therapy would thus be characterized by assigned tasks and chores for community maintenance, groups pertaining to the development of self-care skills, and an attempt to approximate the demands of the outside world.

The distinction represented by these terms is somewhat lost in present-day psychosocial settings. In some instances, writers use the terms therapeutic community and milieu therapy interchangeably; however, others continue to use them to evoke distinctly different philosophies with accordingly different implications for treatment. The therapeutic community and milieu therapy, however, address the therapeutic potential of the treatment setting. In contrast to this, ecological psychology addresses person-environment interactions in *any* setting. Ecological psychology, with its more global perspective, enables a deeper understanding of how the treatment environment can be a beneficial or destructive setting for patients.[21]

The view presented in this chapter is that these approaches naturally complement one another and can be examined together. Once the environment is acknowledged as having an impact on therapy, any treatment setting and its inhabitants can become the subject of examination. Thus, the target population of the various environmental therapies is not limited to a specific diagnostic or age group or a specific locale. Therapeutic communities and milieu therapy programs have been used in prisons, drug rehabilitation settings, and psychiatric hospitals and with children and adults of all ages.

HISTORY AND PURPOSE

Advocates of moral treatment in the late eighteenth and early nineteenth centuries believed that mental illness was directly related to the environment and that, consequently, the role of the psychiatric institution was to provide a milieu in which patients would demonstrate desirable behavior.[26] Concern with the environment was overshadowed in the nineteenth century by the rapid growth of institutions and the rise of the medical organic explanation of mental illness, leading to an increasingly custodial approach to care and the use of whatever somatic and physical therapies were currently popular.[11,19,26]

Psychoanalysis and the two World Wars caused another reconceptualization of theories of mental illness and treatment. In particular, World War I sensitized psychiatrists to an awareness of the relationship between the social environment and mental illness.[19] This growing awareness of the role of the social environment led Sullivan and Menninger, two psychoanalysts with an interpersonal perspective, to begin to deliberately structure the social environment of psychiatric wards as a therapeutic tool, and to explicitly emphasize the therapeutic role of ward personnel.[26]

In the 1950s, the writings of various anthropologists, sociologists, and novelists greatly enhanced the awareness of the connections between patients' behavior, staff interpersonal relationships, and other aspects of the treatment environment (see Additional Readings). At the same time, neo-Freudians (see Chapter 3) and ego psychologists were expanding on Freud's notions of personality development to emphasize the influence of sociocultural contexts on development.[26]

Two landmarks in the development of environmental approaches to therapy were the work of Maxwell Jones, who developed and wrote about therapeutic communities in England,[8] and the work of Cumming and Cumming,[6] whose ideas represented a synthesis and advancement of environmental trends and the new ego psychologies. Recently, ecological and environmental psychologists have added to this body of knowledge by examining the impact of physical factors in the environment—such as lighting, room size, furniture arrangements, and staff-patient ratios—and of the psychosocial atmosphere on patients' behavior, discharge rates, recidivism, and so on.[8,14,16,20,26]

This tradition has been developed by humanitarians, anthropologists, psychoanalysts, social workers, psychologists, and social scientists. It views the social and physical environment as being intimately linked with the behavior of people. It differs from behaviorism in that it does not see the individual as a passive respondent to the environment, and it differs from organic and classic intrapsychic models of mental health in that it does not see the environment as irrelevant to the development of the individual, or locate the cause of disorder primarily within the patient.

VIEW OF ORDER

For those writers who see the therapeutic community only as a context for organizing a variety of treatments, no particular theory base or view of order is espoused. However, writers whose focus is on person-environment interactions, in treatment or other settings, do present a distinct theory and perspective on order. This latter approach, exemplified by the work of the Cummings[6] and of various ecological psychologists, forms the basis of this discussion.

The Cummings pull together a variety of concepts from ego psychology, sociology, and cognitive psychology to present a theory of human development that focuses on the ego and the environment. They begin by conceptualizing the ego as being an affective and cognitive structure that enables the person to meet and respond to the environment. The ego contains certain capacities, such as thought, perception, and the capacity for motor development, that are latent until the right conditions present themselves. These latent capacities represent potentials for responding to future events. When propitious circumstances or developmental crises arise, the ego will synthesize these capacities in order to enable the individual to accommodate to the milieu and to influence it.[6]

Another major concept in the Cummings' theory is that of differentiation. This term is used to refer to two processes. First, the individual occupies a life space that becomes increasingly differentiated, complex, and integrated as the person explores the environment, grows, and learns. Second, the ego as well becomes differentiated throughout the process of interacting with the environment. The growing child begins to organize objects, ideas, events, and values into sets of relationships, or ego sets. These sets might group together feelings and events that the child has come to associate with one another, such as a warm, loving feeling associated with birthday parties. Or they might categorize classes of objects that share common features, such as female adults. Through the acquisition and organization of these sets, the child learns to discriminate between aspects or qualities of an object, and to generalize aspects to other situations.[6] For instance, a little girl might form a set consisting of female adults. From this set she may learn that although teachers and mothers are similar in their tendency to be caring and nurturing, the teacher's concern is limited to behavior and work in school, while a mother's is more apt to include interest in her friends, eating and sleeping habits, and clothes.

Throughout development, losses and additions of sets require reorganization of the ego, to tie up loose ends and replace meanings that are no longer valid. This process of organizing and reorganizing the ego thus requires a certain stability and predictability in the environment. However, too few stimuli and too little variety in the environment might result in an inadequately organized ego and an inability to deal with changes. The environment, therefore, contributes to the process of development through the opportunities, diversity, fluctuations, and organization inherent within it.[6] As a result of this interactive process, the degree of organization and differentiation of the ego and the degree of ambiguity and richness in the environment come to be reflected in a range of responses in the individual, from curiosity and learning to anxiety and incompetence. The Cummings therefore conclude that ego growth, or the development of psychosocial order, reflects an ongoing process of encountering new opportunities in the environment; reorganizing one's responses, associated meanings and feelings to accommodate these new opportunities; and then meeting the environment again (which now appears different, due to the individual's learning) with these changed perceptions.

This view of order in psychological development is compatible with ecological psychologists' view of development as a process of becoming effective in an increasing range of increasingly complex settings.[4] In fact, the emphasis of ecological psychology on overt interrelationships between people and settings clarifies and completes the Cummings' discussion of order.

To begin with, ecological psychology conceives of the physical milieu in dynamic terms. Physical settings both promote certain patterns of behavior and can be recognized by these characteristic behavior patterns. Nevertheless, these settings are dynamic, open systems, characterized simultaneously by change and stability. They may be changed by the actions of individuals or by natural events, and such changes may occur in the physical or social aspects of the setting. When a setting changes so that it is no longer conducive to the behavior originally associated with it, that behavior may reappear in another setting. Finally, settings are continually exerting influence on inhabitants' behavior, whether or not the inhabitants perceive this to be happening.[22] Human order as described in these propositions is a process of recognizing what behaviors are expected in various settings, determining which settings are appropriate for one's goals, performing in a variety of settings, and appropriately adapting settings to meet changing needs.

Taken together, there is a core of beliefs that relate behavior to the physical and social environment in a dynamic, mutually influential process. From the Cummings' view of ego development we obtain the picture of a person who brings certain characteristics and potentials for functioning and learning in various settings. From ecological psychology, we see that environments present and can be organized to provide individuals with options for further learning and growth. As individuals purposefully engage in these settings, they develop acceptable social behavior, learn to exert influence on settings, and organize and reorganize their capacities, values, and feelings for future interactions with the environment.

VIEW OF DISORDER

A parallel view of disorder in this tradition again has two focuses: disorder in terms of ego psychology, and disorder in terms of person/environment interactions. The Cummings delineate four types of pathology. The first is ego poverty, or too few organizational sets in the ego. Ego poverty might result from an environmentally deprived childhood or from the loss of ego sets due to trauma of some sort. A person with too few ego sets would be unable to deal with complex situations, might respond to all situations with one modal response, or might invent inappropriate mechanisms for dealing with the environment. A second type of pathology arises from poor differentiation of ego sets. In this case, because the sets do not clearly identify or classify situations, the individual would not be able to choose the right set for dealing with a particular event. An example might be a person who feels that clothing is the key to his or her identity and therefore dresses in the same way for all occasions. Another form of pathology occurs when the ego sets are not organized in terms of a hierarchy that would enable the person to determine which responses are appropriate for the present and which should be retained for the future. The epitome of this is the person who feels that everything must be changed now and is unable to identify the realistic changes that can be made in the immediate present and those that should be saved for the future. Finally, ego disorganization may arise from severe environmental stress. Although the ego may have organized, differentiated sets, under certain disastrous conditions the individual may be too aroused to draw on them in a meaningful way.[6]

Implicit in this discussion of disorder is the sense that functional behavior is contingent on the individual's having enough previous experiences in different settings to be able to select the most adaptive response to the current setting. The potential in this interaction for the occurrence of maladaptive behavior is made more explicit by ecological psychologists. Their perspective closely parallels that of ego psychology, but they emphasize the importance of the environment, rather than the development of an intrapsychic structure (i.e., the ego). For instance, the individual whose development has been limited to settings that stress highly similar behavior patterns would be ill-equipped to perform and solve problems under novel conditions because he or she has not had opportunities to experience unpredictable or unfamiliar environments. Or the person who is unable to discriminate the different behaviors demanded by various settings might perform inappropriately in settings, or seek out settings unsuited to accomplishing goals. Because people with a wider range of behaviors, experiences, and competencies can more easily adapt to a wide range of settings, disordered behavior becomes a cyclical response in which the individual, lacking competence, avoids or fails in new experiences, making it less likely that the behavioral flexibility necessary to competence will develop.[18]

ACTION IMPLICATIONS

The action implications of the social ecological approaches fall into two groups: (1) strategies primarily concerned with restructuring the social environment so that all interpersonal encounters have therapeutic value; and (2) strategies for redesigning the physical and task environments to communicate expectations for socially competent behavior. Potentially the two approaches can converge in terms of community norms or expectations for behavior.

A critical aspect of the social environment is the role of the patient. Endemic to the creation of a therapeutic environment is the process of "relabeling" the patient from a sick and passive recipient of care to an active community member, capable of assuming responsibility.[2] In the therapeutic milieu the patient is viewed as a responsible manager of his or her affairs.[6] Along with redefinition of the patient role, staff roles are necessarily redefined as well. Thus, decision making and authority are rationally delegated to different community members.[2,6,17] This creates the opportunity for role paralleling, in which the more competent community members—staff and patients—serve as role models for the less competent.[2]

Another social strategy is that of limit setting and containment. These terms refer to the control or limiting of symptomatic behavior so that therapy can progress.[1,12] Behaviors that would be the focus of limit setting are destructiveness, autistic or regressed behaviors, acting out, extreme dependency, and withdrawal from the environment.[1]

The last major social strategy is that of attention saturation or involvement. This strategy consists of the intensive use of social activities that direct the patient's attention away from inner preoccupations and toward the social community.[2,12] Techniques such as intense social contact, ritual activities, and peer pressure are used to communicate this message.[2]

The second group of strategies involves changing expectations for behavior through changes in the task and physical environments. First, the environment must be one in which the patient can orient him- or herself and feel safe enough to investigate and perhaps try out new behaviors.[6] This is achieved through providing continuity with the patient's previous and future environments; using clear, concrete markings to enable the patient to geographically locate him- or herself; identifying staff with name tags; reinforcing the patient's self-identification by allowing access to mirrors, grooming implements, personal artifacts, and street clothes; and orienting patients to time, with clocks and calendars.[6] Similarly, the environment must reduce fears for personal welfare and security through such means as adequate heating and lighting, comfortable sleeping quarters, and tasteful food.[21]

Traditional assumptions about the physical design of treatment environments are also targeted for examination by this strategy. For instance, the traditional assumption that patients should not be alone has been countered by research showing that lack of privacy in patients' bedrooms may actually lead to an increase in passive, isolated behavior,[15] which would not enhance the patient's social involvement or orientation to the overall environment. Similarly, certain furniture arrangements may induce the same isolated behaviors.[14] Thus, opportunities for choice and flexibility in the environment have become increasingly important in treatment settings.

The other major component of this group of interventions is the provision of opportunities for learning and practicing productive behavior.[1,2,6,17] Transforming the environment into a problem-solving arena implies continuity and overlap of the treatment setting with problems and expectations of the external environment. In this sense, the therapeutic environment can be considered a "school for living," in which the coursework consists of situations that parallel the demands of ordinary life.[17] Task expectations for patients therefore range from involvement in ward management to productive occupation and recreation.[6,8]

Ultimately, both groups of strategies merge in the creation of norms and values pertaining to the uniqueness of the community.[2] These values are maintained by the community and serve to inculcate newcomers to its expectations. Mechanisms such as community meetings, support and reinforcement of valued behaviors, and communication networks of individuals help to create and transmit the shared norms and total environmental demands for socially productive behavior.

CRITICISMS AND LIMITATIONS

Criticisms are generally made in reference to therapeutic communities and milieu therapy, and not to the more recent ecological approaches. First, the ambiguity and inconsistency in defining terms cause professionals to have differing expectations and understandings of this tradition. The lack of one conceptual model underlying the therapeutic community or milieu therapy has meant that professionals who support these approaches are more apt to share with one another perceptions of what they are opposed to than what they favor.[3,24] Further, the eclecticism of the framework has contributed to an eclecticism of treatment techniques in some instances; in other instances, there is a tendency to latch on to the more immediately recognizable trappings of a therapeutic community (e.g., community meetings) without truly incorporating the goals that should characterize a therapeutic environment.[5]

The second group of criticisms derives from the changed role definitions of staff and patients. The leveling of hierarchy and concomitant role blurring among staff often create confusion, tension, and dissatisfaction for many staff who may feel that they are not prepared for their new roles and that they are not using skills they have.[13,17] In addition, although one of the basic assumptions of milieu strategies is that patients should take on greater responsibility, in reality their role may continue to be as restricted as it was in a medical or other model of treatment.[25]

Third, criticisms have been levied against milieu therapy and therapeutic communities with regard to their effectiveness. Therapeutic communities, because of the emphasis on involvement in community life, tend to prolong the patient's stay rather than returning the patient to the outside community.[13] However, expediency in discharge has not been linked to tenure in the external community,[8] so this is not an unequivocal criticism. Related to effectiveness is the charge that behaviors valued in the therapeutic milieu may differ from behaviors valued outside of it. For instance, speaking one's mind or sharing anxieties may be appropriate in the hospital but inappropriate at work.[17] Further, there has been a tendency to assume that therapeutic communities and milieu strategies are equally effective for all types of patients.[13] However, because many therapeutic communities are more talk-oriented than activity-oriented, their effectiveness may be limited to an elite population of highly verbal patients. Finally, because of the variations in implementation of therapeutic communities, research and program evaluation is difficult to carry out and difficult to use as a basis for generalization to other programs.[5,17]

COMMENTARY

In the 1960s Reilly described a model occupational therapy program as a total milieu or culture

> which acknowledges competency, arouses curiosity, feeds in universal knowledge, deepens appreciations and demands behavior across the full spectrum of a human's abilities. . . . It presses for the exercising of life skills in a balanced pattern of daily living. (pp. 63–64)[23]

This prescription was virtually a criticism of the fact that milieu therapy and therapeutic communities had become settings where patients and staff sat and talked about problems, smoked cigarettes, and drank coffee, but engaged in no other activity. These were "under-arousing" environments, posing no challenges to the patient. Because the therapeutic community and milieu therapy had deviated from their original conceptions, Reilly felt that there was no place for occupational therapy in such a setting.

Occupational therapy, however, has traditionally espoused the values presumably held by the milieu movement. Early journals of occupational therapy abound with examples of programs in which the occupational therapy department was responsible for directing recreational programs, industrial activities, personal hygiene and beauty care classes, exercise and dance classes, and hobby shops; arranging trips to local community facilities; and planning and supervising informal socialization and leisure.[9] In addition, an awareness of the need for understanding the interrelationships between the physical and psychosocial environments and occupational performance has permeated the writing of occupational therapists.[7,10,16]

Because of these long-held beliefs and practices, occupational therapy is well suited for a leadership role in designing and implementing therapeutic environments. Action principles pertaining to the environment and the role of the occupational therapist as environmental manager will be discussed in the second half of this text.

SUMMARY

History and Purpose	Social ecological approaches have their roots in moral treatment.
	World Wars resensitized psychiatrists to social environmental factors in mental illness.
	Sullivan and Menninger were early proponents of structuring ward social environments.
	Jones developed therapeutic communities in England. Cumming and Cumming synthesized ego psychology and environmental approaches.
	A current growing research tradition in ecological psychology has increased understanding of person-environment interactions.
	The tradition as a whole seeks to understand the potential of the environment as a therapeutic tool.
View of Order	*Ego psychology:*
	Individuals organize patterns of events into sets within ego. These sets enable discrimination between and generalization to future events.
	Development requires continual reorganization of the ego.
	Variety and opportunities in the environment contribute to organization of the ego.
	Ecological psychology:
	Development involves learning to be competent in a variety of settings.
	Settings promote certain behaviors and are subject to change by their inhabitants. Individuals learn to choose settings that are appropriate to their goals and to modify settings.
	Through purposeful engagement in settings, the individual develops acceptable social behavior.

View of Disorder	*Ego psychology:*
	Disorder occurs because the individual with a poorly organized ego cannot respond appropriately to the environment.
	Ecological psychology:
	A lack of experience in varied settings may lead to a lack of behavioral flexibility for functioning in a wide range of environments.
	The individual may choose inappropriate settings for goal attainment or may not know what behaviors are required by the setting.
Action Implications	Restructuring the social environment involves:
	—relabeling "patient" as "member."
	—limit setting on symptomatic behavior.
	—attention saturation.
	—role paralleling.
	Redesigning the physical and task environments includes:
	—orienting the patient to self and surroundings.
	—reassessment of traditional physical design assumptions.
	—opportunities for problem solving and practice of productive behavior.

Criticisms and Limitations	Because of the lack of one clear conceptual model, definitions are ambiguous and inconsistent.
	Practice is often marked by an eclecticism of techniques.
	Role blurring often leads to role strain.
	Excessive emphasis on talk at the expense of action has predominated, making appropriateness dubious for all but the highly verbal.
	Because of program variations, it is difficult to evaluate effectiveness of therapeutic communities in general.
Commentary	Occupational therapy has traditionally held beliefs associated with the milieu movement.
	Disintegration of milieu into a talk environment has meant that occupational therapy has become incompatible with milieu/therapeutic community.
	An awareness of the relationship between occupational performance and the environment and traditional moral treatment values have prepared occupational therapists to assume a leadership role as environmental managers.

TERMS AND CONCEPTS

attention saturation	the intensive use of social activities to direct a patient's attention toward the social environment and away from preoccupations with inner problems.
containment	limit setting on symptomatic behaviors such as acting out.
ego poverty	the existence of too few ego sets, resulting from environmental deprivation, lack of experience, or trauma.
ego set	the organization of objects, ideas, events, and values into a meaningful pattern of relationships.

milieu therapy	a therapeutic environment designed to help patients improve their competence in problem solving and daily living skills.
modal response	the use of one form of behavior to deal with many different situations.
role paralleling	the use of more competent community members as role models for the less competent.
therapeutic community	an environment that uses all staff, patients, and a variety of treatment techniques to help patients achieve insight and emotional control.

REFERENCES

1. Abroms, G. M. Defining milieu therapy. *Archives of General Psychiatry*, 1969, *21*, 553–560.
2. Almond, R. Issues in milieu treatment. *Schizophrenia Bulletin*, Summer 1975, 12–26.
3. Armor, D. J., & Klerman, G. L. Psychiatric treatment orientations and professional ideology. *Journal of Health and Social Behavior*, 1968, *9*, 243–255.
4. Bronfenbrenner, U. *The ecology of human development: Experiments by nature and design*. Cambridge: Harvard University Press, 1979.
5. Cumming, E. "Therapeutic community" and "milieu therapy" strategies can be distinguished. *International Journal of Psychiatry*, 1969, 7, 204–208.
6. Cumming, J., & Cumming, E. *Ego and milieu: Theory and practice of environmental therapy*. New York: Atherton, 1967.
7. Dunning, H. Environmental occupational therapy. *American Journal of Occupational Therapy*, 1972, *26*, 292–298.
8. Ellsworth, R., Maroney, R., Klett, W., Gordon, H., & Gunn, R. Milieu characteristics of successful psychiatric treatment programs. *American Journal of Orthopsychiatry*, 1971, *41*, 427–441.
9. Feuss, C. D., Jr., & Maltby, J. W. Occupational therapy in the therapeutic community. *American Journal of Occupational Therapy*, 1959, *13*, 9–10, 25.
10. Gray, M. Effects of hospitalization on work-play behavior. *American Journal of Occupational Therapy*, 1972, *26*, 180–185.
11. Grob, G. N. *Mental institutions in America: Social policy to 1875*. New York: Free Press, 1973.

12. Gunderson, J. G. Defining the therapeutic processes in psychiatric milieus. *Psychiatry*, 1978, *41*, 327–335.
13. Herz, M. I. The therapeutic community: A critique. *Hospital and Community Psychiatry*, 1972, *23*, 17–20.
14. Holahan, C. J. Environmental psychology in psychiatric hospital settings. In D. Canter & S. Canter (Eds.), *Designing for therapeutic environments: A review of research*. New York: Wiley, 1979.
15. Ittelson, W. H., Proshansky, H. M., & Rivlin, L. G. The environmental psychology of the psychiatric ward. In H. M. Proshansky, W. H. Ittelson, & L. G. Rivlin (Eds.), *Environmental psychology: Man and his physical setting*. New York: Holt, Rinehart & Winston, 1970.
16. Kannegieter, R. B. Environmental interactions in occupational therapy—Some inferences. *American Journal of Occupational Therapy*, 1980, *34*, 715–720.
17. Kraft, A. The therapeutic community. In A. Dean, A. M. Kraft, & B. Pepper (Eds.), *The social setting of mental health*. New York: Basic Books, 1976.
18. Lawton, M. P. *Environment and aging*. Monterey: Brooks/Cole, 1980.
19. Magaro, P., Gripp, R., McDowell, D. J., & Miller, I. W., III. *The mental health industry: A cultural phenomenon*. New York: Wiley, 1978.
20. Moos, R. H. *Evaluating treatment environments: A social ecological approach*. New York: Wiley, 1974.
21. Peterson, C. R. The challenge of the therapeutic milieu in light of human ecology. *Provo Papers*, Winter 1966–67, 11–50.
22. Proshansky, H. M., Ittelson, W. H., & Rivlin, L. G. The influence of the environment on behavior: Some basic assumptions. In H. M. Proshansky, W. H. Ittelson, & L. G. Rivlin (Eds.), *Environmental psychology: Man and his physical setting*. New York: Holt, Rinehart & Winston, 1970.
23. Reilly, M. A psychiatric occupational therapy program as a teaching model. *American Journal of Occupational Therapy*, 1966, *22*, 61–67.
24. Strauss, A., Schatzman, L., Bucher, R., Ehrlich, D., & Sabshin, M. *Psychiatric ideologies and institutions*. London: Collier-Macmillan, 1964.
25. Wilensky, H., & Herzog, M. I. Problem areas in the development of a therapeutic community. *International Journal of Social Psychiatry*, 1966, *22*, 299–308.
26. Wolf, M. S. A review of literature on milieu therapy. *Journal of Psychiatric Nursing and Mental Health Services*, May 1977, 26–33.

ADDITIONAL READINGS

Caudill, W. *The psychiatric hospital as a small society*. Cambridge: Harvard University Press, 1958.

Goffman, E. *Asylums: Essays on the social situation of mental patients and other inmates.* Garden City, N.Y.: Doubleday, 1961.

Gratke, B. E., & Lux, P. A. Psychiatric occupational therapy in a milieu setting. *American Journal of Occupational Therapy*, 1960, *14*, 13–17.

Holahan, C. J., & Saegert, S. Behavioral and attitudinal effects of large-scale variation in the physical environment of psychiatric wards. *Journal of Abnormal Psychology*, 1973, *82*, 454–462.

Jones, M. *The therapeutic community: A new treatment method in psychiatry.* New York: Basic Books, 1953.

Jones, M. *Social psychiatry in the community, in hospitals, and in prisons.* Springfield, Ill.: Charles C Thomas, 1962.

Noshpitz, J. Milieu therapy. *American Journal of Occupational Therapy*, 1960, *14*, 221–222.

Paul, G. L., & Lentz, R. J. *Psychosocial treatment of chronic mental patients: Milieu versus social-learning programs.* Cambridge: Harvard University Press, 1978.

Stanton, A., & Schwartz, M. *The mental hospital.* New York: Basic Books, 1954.

Toch, H. (Ed.). *Therapeutic communities in corrections.* New York: Praeger, 1980.

Ward, M. J. *The snake pit.* New York: Random House, 1946.

10
Community Mental Health

Community mental health is less a distinct body of knowledge than it is a political movement and a commitment to certain beliefs. As a commitment, it reflects a clear dissatisfaction with certain features of more traditional mental health delivery systems, as well as a belief in several alternatives to these features. As a movement with political origins, it has been embraced by psychiatrists, psychologists, social workers, public health scientists, occupational therapists, nurses, and various community special interest groups that are involved in mental health advocacy programs.

Each major characteristic of community mental health arose in reaction to a dominant characteristic of traditional psychiatric practice.[4] In response to the traditional removal of the individual from the home community to a distant institution, community mental health emphasizes service delivery in the community setting. A traditional lack of concern with the population as a whole has led the movement to identify as its target of treatment or change the community and not the individual. In addition, community mental health has sought to emphasize preventive services instead of curative treatment directed at the reduction of pathology in the individual patient. In an effort to correct the lack of systematic organization and social agency liaisons, the community mental health approach emphasizes continuity and comprehensiveness of care, and service to specific social systems—such as particular geographic regions (catchment areas), schools, or other organizations—developed within the context of a community needs assessment process. Belief in the inadequacy of traditional long-term treatment strategies has led to a focus on innovative techniques such as brief psychotherapy and crisis intervention. To circumvent an impending shortage of traditionally trained personnel, community mental health has looked for ways to use paraprofessional and indigenous mental health workers. Finally, despite varying conceptions of etiology, there is a shared belief that the client cannot be viewed as the he late nineteenth century was characterized byional size, and a changing view of rather than environmental causes of mentalossess cures for organically based psy-mbined effect of these two trends was that treatmentbecame largely custodial in nature.[10,16] In the early twentieth century, reformers such as Adoph Meyer and Clifford Beers reacted to this trend by promoting a "citizen's mental hygiene" movement.[4,27] They proposed the establishment of community mental hygiene districts, containing aftercare clinics for follow-up treatment of psychiatric clients, and child guidance clinics, for preventive work with families. Although this movement was overshadowed by the rise of psychoanalysis, the field of psychiatric social work emerged from it.[27]

The mental hygiene movement also foreshadowed a growing awareness of the importance of prevention in mental health. Erikson and Lindemann, both psychologists, had begun to conceptualize psychosocial order as the ability to resolve developmental crises or problems. They postulated that disorder might be prevented in certain individuals if they were helped to acquire coping and problem-solving skills before they were actually faced with particular crises. Following this line of reasoning, Lindemann established a clinic for at-risk populations devoted to preventive techniques and crisis intervention. In his community mental health laboratory, he worked with people facing bereavement and loss, as well as with groups anticipating stressful experiences.[27]

In the 1950s the advent of biochemical treatment for mental illness led to the discharge of large numbers of chronically ill individuals from institutions. At the same time, individual psychotherapy, the form of treatment that had dominated much of the twentieth century, came under substantial attack for lacking effectiveness, social utility, and value.[11]

Finally, the event that most immediately impelled the community mental health movement into existence was the report of a national mental health study, initiated in 1955 and completed in 1961. This report, entitled "Action for Mental Health," recommended that: (1) immediate and intensive care services be provided for acutely psychotic people in outpatient clinics and psychiatric units in general hospitals; (2) that inpatient and outpatient care for chronically mentally ill people be improved; and (3) that public mental health education be implemented to change attitudes toward mental illness.[4] In response to this report, President Kennedy in 1963 proposed a national mental health program, the core of which was the Community Mental Health Centers Act. This act mandated the initial provision of inpatient care, outpatient care, and emergency and education services at community mental health centers. Other services that were eventually required included diagnostic services, rehabilitation, precare and aftercare programs, staff training, and research and evaluation.[4]

VIEW OF ORDER

The community mental health movement does not have a well-articulated view of order. The movement has generally incorporated theories and beliefs from several fields (e.g., social psychology, anthropology, sociology, and environmental psychology) in order to understand psychosocial order and disorder as a social phenomenon.[1] Some of these beliefs delineate a political and psychological view of people and relationships, while others describe a rationale for action implications.

Proponents of community mental health believe that order and disorder are defined by society and culture and that the environment can promote both health and illness.[28] Within this sociocultural environment, interpersonal relationships play a particularly vital role. Community mental health practitioners consider long-term relationships, such as those found within the family, to be a valuable and essential component of psychosocial order.[28]

Theoretically, the cornerstone of the community mental health view of order is a competence, as opposed to a deficit, view of health.[11,26] The competence model is essentially an expansion of the idea that health is the outcome of successful adaptation to the environment.[7] It posits that people have two basic needs: (1) to avoid or adjust to traumatic events, and (2) to engage in positive experiences in order to derive a sense of competence and well-being.

What this suggests is that the disruptive stress of life events can be mitigated when a person evaluates these events positively. Because of the need to feel competence and well-being, people will seek the skills that enable them to successfully cope with stress, in other words, to achieve or maintain mental health.[26]

Because health is viewed in relationship to the environment, the community mental health movement to a large degree shares its theory base with the social ecological approaches (see Chapter 9). In fact, it is reasonable to depict this movement as an extension of therapeutic community/milieu therapy concepts to the larger community outside the institution or treatment setting.

While the theory base of community mental health is not clearly defined, the core of the movement's view of human order is the individual's ability to positively and meaningfully adapt to life events and the environment. For most community mental health workers, the concept of adaptation to the environment implicitly connotes an ability to develop skills and resources to competently interact with the setting, as well as an ability to recognize when the environment needs changing. This view of health stresses the importance of identifying social support systems that maintain or promote health.

VIEW OF DISORDER

The community mental health view of disorder is largely a multifactorial perspective in that it assumes that many factors—genetic, constitutional, developmental, and environmental—contribute differentially to pathology.[11] This model, however, lends itself more to identifying risk factors than to describing disordered behavior.

A major target of the model is the prevailing social structure. Various writers point to the dehumanization that accrues from our consumer-oriented industrial society as being a major risk factor. Excessive industrialization is seen as leading to the dehumanization of work and the loss of a sense of personal identity and competence.[2] These writers contend that present-day community life has contributed to a prevalent feeling of helplessness, leading in turn to alienation and anomie (a feeling of not belonging to society), a lack of faith and trust in service delivery systems, a feeling of lack of control, and the loss of a psychological sense of community.[9]

The social structure also poses risk through its unequal valuation of roles. Certain roles are less valued by society than others, and people in these roles are candidates for psychological problems.[9] This can be further complicated when people fill two or more incompatible roles, or when the roles valued by the whole society conflict with those valued by a subculture.[9] For example, many college students in the early seventies faced a conflict between the alternative, nontraditional life-styles valued by the student subculture and the competitive, economically oriented life-styles valued by their parents and the cultural mainstream.

In addition to the social environment, the physical environment is also considered to be a source of potential stress or risk. Crowding, noise, the fast urban pace of life, and poor lighting conditions are among the many facets of the environment that have been implicated. For instance, crowding has been associated with such deleterious effects as an inability to maintain social relationships, increased aggression, unwillingness to help others, and learned helplessness.[21]

Genetic and organic factors and individual levels of competence are also seen as contributing to disorder. Both order and disorder can therefore be seen as arising from a relationship between organic causes of illness, stressful factors in the environment, individual competence and belief in this competence, and the prevalence and adequacy of social support systems.[2] The ultimate importance of this view lies in its implication that preventing or alleviating stress and improving social support systems will affect a larger number of people and do more to decrease the incidence of mental illness than will the medical emphasis on isolating and treating organic causes.

ACTION IMPLICATIONS

As suggested earlier, community mental health has been more of an action model than a causal or explanatory model. As such, it has led to a variety of interventions, including the development of clubhouse programs for discharged clients; the establishment of short-term, acute care psychiatric units in local general hospitals; preventive and educational services in settings such as libraries, churches, and hospital waiting rooms; screening and early intervention programs in public schools; crisis intervention and telephone hot lines; and greater use of home care.

This range of services is girded by a set of beliefs that reflect a democratic orientation to mental health services and a social systems perspective on change. According to these beliefs, mental health services are a public utility and a civil right, rather than a service available only to those individuals who possess adequate finances or insurance. In addition, individuals for whom these services are intended should retain personal freedom and make decisions regarding the use of resources.[28] Finally, because the *method* of service delivery is believed to be as important as the nature of the service, the community mental health movement maintains that change must be planned for, be systematic, and be aimed at social systems, such as schools, organizations, industry, or families, rather than at individuals,[1,11,28] and that prevention and early intervention are more desirable than later intervention and treatment.[11]

Prevention can occur on three levels. *Primary prevention* aims at the reduction of incidence or occurrence of disorder through two main strategies: modifying environments and strengthening people's coping abilities. Neither of these strategies is carried out on an individual level. The first is accomplished by analyzing social systems and intervening at this level. For example, developing special high school programs that combine community work with academic classes is a social systems intervention directed at the educational environment. The second strategy is achieved through consultation to schools and churches, to programs for at-risk populations (such as children of divorced parents or families of people who are terminally ill), and to individuals who work with large groups of people (the clergy, for instance).[9] *Secondary prevention* involves early detection of problems, through such means as educating the public and ensuring that services are available to and used by individuals. Thus, although the occurrence of the problem is not eliminated by this level of prevention, the problem is minimized by early identification and treatment. Finally, *tertiary prevention* is concerned with eliminating or reducing the impact of problems by returning individuals to productive community roles and preventing further recurrences.[9]

Another emphasis in community mental health is intervention that is directed at groups. Groups are more economical, and through approaches such as family and network therapy, complete social systems within a community can be influenced.[9] Network therapy is an interesting development in community group treatment. The network therapist, labeled "conductor," collects as many different people as possible who know the identified client. These people may range from family members and close friends to persons working in the community with whom the client has contact. This enables examination of the person's problems in all sectors of daily life. All members of the network are then involved in formulating and enacting solutions to the problems.[9]

Community mental health programs have fostered a reconsideration of the traditional role of the professional. In part, the situation has been one of professionals changing their role in *reaction* to the increased use of indigenous and paraprofessional workers. The use of nonprofessionals, such as teachers' aides, childcare workers, psychiatric aides, parents, students, and so on, has been found to have beneficial effects on both the helper and client, because the helper is seen as a competent role model.[12] In addition, social support from a peer may have more immediate and personal value to the recipient than more clinically oriented treatment provided by a professional.[11] Nontraditional work roles have also been seen as providing a way of bringing groups of people who are traditionally outside the cultural mainstream—and thus at risk for disorder—into it.[11] As nonprofessional personnel have been used to provide primary intervention, or direct care, the professional has had to broaden his or her role to encompass staff training, supervision, consulting, program development, and evaluation.[12]

Professional roles have changed *proactively* as well as reactively. An example is the involvement of professionals in the development of mass media programs for radio, television, newspapers, and film designed to educate the public about preventive, healthful life-styles.[12]

Along with alternative work roles and careers, the last major action implication in this movement is the creation of alternative institutions. These new institutions have most commonly been alternatives to traditional schooling, to incarceration of criminals, and to long-term residential treatment of psychosocially disordered people. The purposes of these new settings have generally been to return deviants to mainstream society or, particularly in the case of schools, to maximize the match between a person's needs and what the setting provides.[11] For psychiatric clients these alternatives to hospitalization include board-and-care homes, day programs emphasizing the development of vocational and recreational skills, and halfway houses designed to bridge the transition from institution to community.[11,12,14]

CRITICISMS AND LIMITATIONS

The reality of community mental health is not as innovative or exciting as the ideal picture that has been portrayed. To a great extent, the failures of this movement stem from its inability to separate from traditional American medicine. In a sense, the movement was doomed from the very beginning when the original Community Mental Health Centers Act stated its intent to "return mental health care to the mainstream of American medicine" (p. 185).[12] This immediately tied the movement to the medical model.

The first problem arising from the link to the medical model was that the original services mandated by the government were traditional clinical services, or the things psychiatrists were "good at."[12] Delineating and requiring these traditional services precluded or slowed the development of innovative services and made more difficult the use of nonprofessional workers. When the latter were used, having to fit into the hierarchical structure of the medical model created conflicts around decision making, discrimination, career-advancement opportunities, and working relationships in general. The one nonclinical service that was mandated by the initial act and which did not derive from the medical model—consultation and education—was intended as an adjunct to clinical services, and not to change social institutions.[12] In addition, this service was the least consistently enacted.[4] Through this early medical model dominance, the potential for social innovation that many hoped for from the movement was severely limited.

The original act implicitly designated long-term hospitalization as bad, contributing to a lasting polarization between community mental health personnel and hospital personnel.[4] Further, the act created a need for local, state, and federal governments to work interdependently and for the federal government to assume responsibility for equalizing affluence across states.[4] With hindsight we can see that this has left the poorer states in a vulnerable position as federal monies have become scarcer.

Another problem stemming from the original act is that it derived from a belief in the benevolence of both government and medical professionals. Interestingly, the original enthusiasm and trust in government and professionals' efforts to manipulate the environment in order to promote mental health has changed to distrust and skepticism.[17] The climate of our country currently does not favor a strong governmental role, and individuals seem wary of sociological and legal interpretations of mental illness. Psychiatrists, if not yet wary, may soon be, as they are now becoming frequent victims of violent "patients."[23] Insanity as a legal defense is less popular and has been banned in some states altogether; this too seems to be a reflection of a more generalized dissatisfaction with the role of mental health professionals in the community in its implication that psychiatrists cannot and should not determine when crime is truly the product of insanity.

Recently, criticism of the process of deinstitutionalization has surfaced. Although the overall hospital population has decreased, the number of admissions has not, and it is felt that this is largely because the community centers have not offered support services and follow-up care to discharged clients. Many board-and-care homes and halfway houses, which were presumably created to offer these services, have turned out instead to be back wards in the community where the typical resident spends most "of the day in virtual solitude, either staring vacantly at television . . . or wandering aimlessly around the neighborhood" (pp. 461–462).[25] These residential facilities have frequently become entrepreneurial, profit-making operations that see residents as commodities to be obtained and controlled.[13] Further, many clients have been prematurely "dumped" without adequate preparation for community living.[20] The too-frequent result has been that deinstitutionalized people have not become a part of the community in any real sense.[13,20]

Finally, although the community mental health movement was guided by the belief that the source of disorder was in the community, many critics feel that it actually succeeded only in relabeling social problems as psychiatric problems instead of pinpointing social determinants of psychological problems.[12]

COMMENTARY

Many of the most innovative and exciting programs to be developed in the community have developed, unfortunately, without occupational therapists; yet these programs offer social and daily living skills training, prevocational training, and leisure programs. Occupational therapists who *have* moved along into the community have often too willingly adopted the roles created for them by other mental health workers already there. For instance, Schechter[20] describes a psychiatric day program in which the occupational therapist assumed the role established by the psychiatrist and social worker and became a primary therapist, coordinating treatment for assigned patients, working with families, participating in group therapy, and providing psychodynamically oriented occupational therapy groups. While the role of counselor and case coordinator may be interesting and important, it may not be the one for which the occupational therapist is best suited. On the other hand, Broekema, Danz, and Schloemer[6] describe a more suitable occupational therapy role in a community aftercare program where occupational therapy provided basic living skills and job finding skills groups, and an arts and crafts group in which members were able to experience feelings of competence and pleasure during leisure. Also capitalizing on the strengths of occupational therapy, Auerbach,[3] along with a client from a day treatment center, joined the Bernal Heights Ladies' Club. Becoming a regular member enabled her to help ease the transition for other clients into community groups and to help community members accept psychiatric clients into their group. Working with a psychologist and a management consultant in the early seventies, Dunning[8] presaged an important role for occupational therapists in collaborative job training programs for psychotic people, but the area of consultancy to industry on job adaptation, relocation problems of living, and balancing leisure and work meaningfully and with satisfaction to the individual has yet to be exploited by occupational therapists.[22] Bockoven,[5] a psychiatrist, suggests that the future of the community mental health movement lies with occupational therapists, who must assume the role of occupational developers for the community:

A new era of moral treatment tailored to our times is sorely needed not only by thousands of persons in our communities who are burdened with chronic residues of psychoses, but also by many thousands of others with emotional and physical limitations.

It is fair to say that modern society has a greater need for comprehensive community occupational-recreational programs than it has for mental health centers. . . . Similarly, I would like to suggest that occupational therapy be the wellspring for a sorely needed alternative system of education for individuals of all ages for whom the formal public school system, as we know it today, is inadequate. (pp. 224–225)[5]

As Wiemer,[26] Laukaran,[15] and other writers note, occupational therapists already possess the knowledge and skills to be unique and important participants in the community mental health movement. Whether or not we become successful in this role may yet depend on our willingness to reassess the importance of the disparate strands of knowledge we still claim as vital to our work. The importance of this role, as part of our function as environmental managers, will be further elaborated in the second part of this text.

SUMMARY

History and Purpose	The rapid growth of institutions and an organic view of disorder led to an increasingly custodial emphasis in treatment in late 19th century.
	Various reformers proposed establishment of community mental hygiene districts.
	In the 1950s biochemical treatment led to the discharge of many chronically ill people from large institutions.
	Under President Kennedy, a Community Mental Health Centers Act was proposed to improve inpatient and outpatient services and to change public attitudes toward mental illness.
View of Order	As an interdisciplinary, politically based movement, the view of order is not well articulated.
	Emphases include a belief in the importance of interpersonal relationships (particularly the family unit), a competence view of health, and belief in the necessity for developing social support systems that promote health.
View of Disorder	Disorder arises from a number of factors: genetic, constitutional, developmental, and environmental.
	The present-day social structure has also contributed to disorder, through the alienation of individuals from their work and communities, through conflicting values in modern life, and factors such as crowding and the fast pace of life.

Action Implications	A focus on prevention and early intervention is the cornerstone of the movement.
	Three levels of prevention exist: *primary* concerns modifying environments and people's coping abilities so that the incidence of disorder is reduced; *secondary* involves early detection of problems; and *tertiary* aims to reduce the impact of problems.
	Intervention tends to be directed at groups and social systems rather than individuals.
	The increasing use of nonprofessionals has led to changing roles for professionals.
	Many alternative "institutions" have been created.
Criticisms and Limitations	Community mental health has been dominated by the medical model, which has limited its potential for social innovation.
	The movement created a polarization between mental health workers in hospital settings and those in the community.
	Many of the alternative treatment settings established in the community do no more for their residents than long-term institutions did.
Commentary	Although occupational therapists clearly have a place in community treatment, they have frequently assumed the roles created by other mental health workers instead of capitalizing on their own strengths.
	Bockoven suggests that the future of community mental health lies with occupational therapists.

TERMS AND CONCEPTS

action model of mental illness	a model that emphasizes treatment strategies and courses of intervention.
catchment area	geographically defined region to which a particular community mental health center offers services.

causal model of mental illness	a model concerned with conceptualizing the origins or formation of mental illness.
multifactorial view of disorder	a perspective that identifies many sources (or factors) as contributing to pathology, rather than one cause.
primary prevention	strategies that seek to prevent the occurrence of disorder, e.g., environmental modification and programs for "at-risk" individuals.
proactive	making changes in anticipation of future needs as opposed to changing in response to some event or some need that has already been identified.
secondary prevention	early detection of problems, accomplished through public education and increased availability of services, so that the impact of problems is diminished.
tertiary prevention	minimization of the effects of pathology, by enabling people to return to productive community roles after illness.

REFERENCES

1. Adelson, D. A concept of comprehensive community mental health. In D. Adelson & B. L. Kalis (Eds.), *Community psychology and mental health.* Scranton, Pa.: Chadler, 1970.
2. Albee, G. W. A competency model of health to replace the defect model. In M. S. Gibbs, J. R. Lachenmeyer, & J. Sigal (Eds.), *Community psychology.* New York: Gardner Press, 1980.
3. Auerbach, E. Community involvement: The Bernal Heights Ladies' Club. *American Journal of Occupational Therapy,* 1974, *28,* 272–273.
4. Bloom, B. L. *Community mental health: A general introduction.* Monterey, Calif.: Brooks/Cole, 1977.
5. Bockoven, J. S. *Moral treatment in community mental health.* New York: Springer, 1972.
6. Broekema, M. C., Danz, K. H., & Schloemer, C. U. Occupational therapy in a community aftercare program. *American Journal of Occupational Therapy,* 1975, *28,* 22–27.
7. Cohen, L. D. Health and disease: Observations on strategies for community psychology. In G. Rosenblum (Ed.), *Issues in community psychology and preventive mental health.* New York: Behavioral Publications, 1971.
8. Deacon, S., Dunning, R. E., & Dease, R. A job clinic for psychotic

clients in remission. *American Journal of Occupational Therapy*, 1974, *28*, 144–147.

9. Gottesfeld, H. *Abnormal psychology: A community mental health perspective.* Chicago: Science Research Associates, 1979.

10. Grob, G. N. *Mental institutions in America: Social policy to 1875.* New York: Free Press, 1973.

11. Heller, K., & Monahan, J. *Psychology and community change.* Homewood, Ill.: Dorsey, 1977.

12. Jeger, A. M. Community mental health and environmental design. In L. Krasner (Ed.), *A psychology of the individual in society.* New York: Pergamon Press, 1980.

13. Kielhofner, G. An ethnographic study of deinstitutionalized adults. *Occupational Therapy Journal of Research*, 1981, *1*, 125–142.

14. Lamb, H. R., and associates. *Community survival for long-term patients.* San Francisco: Jossey-Bass, 1976.

15. Laukaran, V. H. Nationally speaking—Toward a model of occupational therapy for community health. *American Journal of Occupational Therapy*, 1977, *31*, 71–74.

16. Magaro, P., Gripp, R., McDowell, D. J., & Miller, I. W. III. *The mental health industry: A cultural phenomenon.* New York: Wiley, 1978.

17. Musto, D. F. The community mental health movement in historical perspective. In W. E. Barton & C. J. Sanborn (Eds.), *An assessment of the community mental health movement.* Lexington, Mass.: Lexington Books, 1975.

18. Ozarin, L. D. Community mental health: Does it work? Review of the evaluation. In W. E. Barton & C. J. Sanborn (Eds.), *An assessment of the community mental health movement.* Lexington, Mass.: Lexington Books, 1975.

19. Panzetta, A. F. *Community mental health: Myth and reality.* Philadelphia: Lea & Febiger, 1971.

20. Schechter, L. Occupational therapy in a psychiatric day hospital. *American Journal of Occupational Therapy*, 1974, *28*, 151–153.

21. Scull, A. T. *Decarceration: Community treatment and the deviant—A radical view.* Englewood Cliffs, N.J.: Prentice-Hall, 1977.

22. Sigal, J. Physical environment stressors. In M. S. Gibbs, J. R. Lachenmeyer, & J. Sigal (Eds.), *Community psychology.* New York: Gardner Press, 1980.

23. Sorenson, J. Nationally speaking—Occupational therapy in business: A new horizon. *American Journal of Occupational Therapy*, 1978, *32*, 287–288.

24. Szasz, T. Shooting the shrink. *New Republic*, June 16, 1982, *186*, pp. 11, 13–14.
25. Van Putten, T., & Spar, J. E. The board-and-care home: Does it deserve bad press? *Hospital and Community Psychiatry*, 1979, *30*, 461–464.
26. Wiemer, R. B. Some concepts of prevention as an aspect of community health. *American Journal of Occupational Therapy*, 1972, *26*, 1–9.
27. Zautra, A., & Simons, L. S. Some effects of positive life events on community mental health. *American Journal of Community Psychology*, 1979, 7, 441–451.
28. Zax, M. History and background of the community mental health movement. In M. S. Gibbs, J. R. Lachenmeyer, & J. Sigal (Eds.), *Community psychology*. New York: Gardner Press, 1980.
29. Zusman, J. The philosophic basis for a community and social psychiatry. In W. E. Barton & C. J. Sanborn (Eds.), *An assessment of the community mental health movement*. Lexington, Mass.: Lexington Books, 1975.

ADDITIONAL READINGS

Barton, W. E., & Sanborn, C. J. (Eds.). *An assessment of the community mental health movement*. Lexington, Mass.: Lexington Books, 1975.
Borus, J. F. Issues critical to the survival of community mental health. *American Journal of Psychiatry*, 1978, *135*, 1029–1034.
Butz, C. W. *A study of the roles of the O.T. in community mental health programs*. Unpublished thesis, University of Nebraska, 1969.
Conte, W. R., & Meuli, A. L. Occupational therapy in community mental health. *American Journal of Occupational Therapy*, 1966, *20*, 147–150.
Howe, M., & Dippy, K. The role of occupational therapy in community mental health. *American Journal of Occupational Therapy*, 1968, *22*, 521–524.
Iscoe, I., Bloom, B. L., & Spielberger, C. D. *Community psychology in transition: Proceedings of the National Conference on Training in Community Psychology*. Washington, D.C.: Hemisphere Publishing Corp., 1977.
Levine, M. *The history and politics of community mental health*. New York: Oxford University Press, 1981.

11
Deviance or Labeling Theory

Deviance or labeling theory, a sociocultural tradition of thought, seeks to explain the social processes that occur when persons deviate from the ordinary ethos of daily life. Erikson[6] defines deviance as:

> conduct which is generally thought to require the attention of social control agencies—that is, conduct about which "something should be done." Deviance is not a property *inherent in* certain forms of behavior; it is a property *conferred upon* these forms by audiences which directly or indirectly witness them. (p. 11)

As this definition illustrates, deviance involves a concatenation of actions and reactions. This tradition argues that persons labeled mentally ill or retarded violate social rules, evoking the judgments and actions of others and creating a situation of social deviance. Psychosocial dysfunction is one of many forms of deviant behavior studied by social scientists.

Deviance theory is of particular interest to the clinician since, unlike many other explanations of psychosocial dysfunction, it does not locate the "problem" entirely within the person who has an emotional or cognitive difficulty. Strictly speaking, it is not a theory of psychosocial dysfunction, but a theory about its underlying social processes.

HISTORY AND PURPOSE

The study of deviance arose within the fields of sociology and anthropology. It reflects their classic concern with the structures and processes of group life. The study of deviant persons, their aberrations, and societal reactions to them provides a perspective for understanding how society maintains its ordered character.[1] Initially, social scientists focused on deviants themselves, detailing their characteristics, practices, and life-styles. However, the topic of more recent work is the interactive process between "normals" and deviants.[1] Concern has shifted from how the deviant transgresses social rules of conduct to how deviance is created not only through rule breaking but by social response. Social scientists study how both everyday cultural members and organized institutions and professionals respond to and act toward the deviant person.[2,3]

According to recent concepts of social groups as integrated systems that maintain their own boundaries, deviance is a process of social self-control.[6] Deviant behavior appears to have a paradoxical relationship to social processes. On the one hand, deviants are threats to the ongoing order since they violate social norms. At the same time, they constitute an important source of information to other members about what behavior is out of bounds. Consequently, it is argued that society needs its deviants as means of demarcating social boundaries. For instance, mentally ill and retarded persons are recognized foremost as individuals who violate social norms. They are, therefore, responded to in predictable ways by everyday cultural members and by socially approved agents and agencies of control. At the same time, they enable society to advertise and maintain its concepts of sanity and appropriate behavior.

VIEW OF ORDER

The social science concepts underlying deviance theory present order as the result of interaction between persons and their social surroundings. Participation by the individual in the ongoing processes of social life yields a view of self and of society.[2,4] This view comprises both the person's and society's beliefs about reality and provides personal guidelines for social actions. It includes such elements as the values and norms of society and recognition of roles and their related behavior. Thus, the social participant, in each encounter with others, is acting out a view of reality that he or she acquires from society. The individual is shaped and defined by social processes to conform to the values, norms, and other expectations of the social group.

At the same time, social life itself consists of individuals interacting with each other, employing their respective views of reality. As they interact, they continually reshape each others' views and, thus, construct ongoing reality.[3] Social life and its patterned order is, then, a system of interacting viewpoints and behaviors. Collectively, social actors constitute and create the reality of everyday life as they participate in it.

Of particular relevance to the situation of deviance is the social science concept that what persons become is a function of complex social interactions. Goode[9] refers to this process as sociogenic identity. By this he means that persons eventually behave as others expect them to and see themselves as others see them. One's identity is thus a function of one's social surroundings. Everyone has experienced this phenomenon in a small way when entering new social situations. Individuals may have thought of themselves, and have been viewed in the past, as having a great sense of humor or the ability to give good personal advice. In a new situation, one may find that it is not so easy to tell a joke or offer advice in the same manner as one did in the old familiar setting. There is typically a "warming up" period in which one slowly and gradually offers such behaviors geared to shape others' impressions toward one's view of self. As one's own and others' views become similar in their expectations, one can more freely and frequently engage in old humorous or advice-giving behaviors. On the other hand, if those in the new setting do not find one funny or wise, one may come to doubt one's own abilities. As the example illustrates, the individual and society (both consciously and automatically) shape each other. The order of social life and the order of the individual's identity and behavior result from this mutually influential process.

VIEW OF DISORDER

Several currents of thought characterize social science explanations of the processes that underlie becoming and being deviant. Classically, social scientists, attempting to counteract the popular cultural notion that deviance was an undesirable property of the individual, portrayed the deviant as reacting to intolerable or troubled social conditions.[6] The deviant person was often romanticized as a folk hero. The image of the mentally ill person as highly sensitive to the insanity of the world at large is an example of this orientation. More recent views of deviance recognize that attributes leading up to the violation of social convention (i.e., emotional and intellectual disturbances) may be properties in the individual, but they emphasize that the recognition or attribution of deviant status (for it is the construction of deviant status which most concerns social scientists) is an interactive process involving both the deviant's behavior and social response.[2]

Thus, the deviant phenomenon is a complementary process of rule breaking by the deviant, and recognition and attribution of deviant status to the rule-breaker by members of society.[1] In this sense, deviant identity (including mental illness) is socially constructed reality. This view stresses that the deviance is not merely a quality inherent in the person, but the result of social processes involving interaction of social members. This has led naturally to an increased focus on those who interact with the deviant, especially those who officially define and attempt to control deviant behavior.

Identifying and Labeling Deviance

Because social reaction to rule infraction is recognized as an essential component of deviance, the problem of differential definition and reaction to behavior is important. For example, since behaviors are labeled and reacted to differently over time, the same act may be labeled or not labeled as a deviant performance.[1] A simple example is society's negative reaction to the long hair worn by males in the 1960s and 1970s by a society whose religious and civil symbols include ample protrayal of men from other eras who also wore long hair.

The particular social institution given responsibility for controlling a form of deviance will define the deviant act according to its own concerns and methods. For example, when religious institutions attempt to control homosexuality, they define it as sin. Several years ago, when psychiatry attempted control of homosexual behavior it defined homosexuality as an illness. When legislative bodies attempt control, they define homosexuality as a crime. Thus, the deviant may be considered immoral, diseased, and/or criminal depending on the institution that attempts to control the deviance.

In addition, societal views may be varied so that social institutions are no longer required to control a behavior once considered deviant. For example, in many communities and among many heterosexuals, homosexuality is now considered a normal life-style option. If such an opinion is accepted by a majority of society, social institutions such as churches, prisons, and mental health professionals will find no reason to condemn, treat, or punish such behavior. What this also illustrates is that deviance is less an inherent property of any behavior than it is a property of the social groups that react to and attempt to control it.

Deviance theory offers an important perspective on the arbitrary nature of current psychiatric practice. It has been pointed out that values embedded in modern psychiatry represent the current ideology of middle class Western society.[17] One important set of observations on the indeterminacy of modern psychiatric procedures demonstrates that the process of identifying or labeling mental illness can be highly inaccurate. Studies have shown that a plethora of elements can influence the outcome of a psychiatric diagnostic procedure, resulting in disagreements between different diagnosticians or changes in a person's view of someone's mental problem over time.[12] In a dramatic study, a group of social scientists and graduate students were admitted covertly to various psychiatric wards as "psychotic patients." None of the mental health personnel detected or even suspected the sanity or true identity of these persons. The fact of their hospitalization and the label of mental illness overruled all other evidence and maintained their social identities as mental patients.[15]

Thus, deviance theory emphasizes that human identities are not only a feature of inherent characteristics, but also are a function of social values, definitions, and expectations that are guiding elements of human interactions in which deviance is created. It stresses the arbitrary nature of many social judgments and, thus, offers a more humanistic perspective of the deviant person.

Intensifying and Perpetuating Deviance

Some sociologists argue that society unnecessarily labels certain kinds of personal traits and behaviors as deviant,[5,7] and that the actions of those charged with managing deviants actually intensify and maintain deviant behavior.[2,18] This concept, often referred to as "labeling theory," stresses the role of societal reaction in augmenting the deviant career of those labeled as mentally ill or mentally retarded. According to this view, the person with psychosocial dysfunction violates social rules, is subsequently recognized as having a problem, and receives the ministrations of persons and institutions (e.g., institutionalization and therapy). As a result of these social responses, the person with psychosocial dysfunction acquires both an internal and external deviant identity. That is, such persons come to view themselves as possessing certain undesirable qualities, they come to view others who are likewise labeled as undesirable, and they are in turn recognized and treated by others as undesirable. This may result in the deviance becoming permanent or more pronounced. For example, a study of retarded persons demonstrated that those labeled intellectually subnormal fared better in the long run if their families rejected the retarded label. Those whose families accepted the label apparently fared worse, since they were more likely to view themselves and to be treated by others as mentally defective.[13]

Goffman[8] documented what he called the "moral career" of the mental patient. He argued that there are effects of social processes separate from any pathological disturbance in the mentally ill person. He points out that, while persons who become mental patients vary widely in their personalities, symptoms, and underlying pathology, they come to have a common deviant identity and exhibit similar deviant behavior. He attributes this to the experience of hospitalization and the treatment of persons labeled as mentally ill. Goffman explains that people who are mentally ill enter into a process of self-redefinition that is directed by the social circumstances of hospitalization and results in many of the apparently asocial features associated with psychosocial disorder. Paradoxically, those institutions whose purpose is to control or eliminate deviance instead yield their own special brand of deviance.

Thus, deviance theories recognize that while the etiology of mental illness or retardation may have biological and psychological roots, it also has an identifiable social genesis. Erikson[6] describes this as follows:

> The community's decision to bring deviant sanctions against an individual is not a simple act of censure. It is a sharp rite of transition, at once moving him out of his normal position in society and transferring him to a distinct deviant role. The ceremonies which accomplish this change of status, ordinarily have three related phases. They provide a formal *confrontation* between the deviant suspect

and representatives of his community (as in the criminal trial or psychiatric case conference); they announce some *judgment* about the nature of his deviancy (a verdict or diagnosis, for example); and they perform an act of social placement, assigning him to a special role (like that of a prisoner or patient) which redefines his position in society. (p. 16)

The process of labeling may intensify deviance through the self-fulfilling prophecy, since deviant persons are typically expected to retain some element of their deviance permanently. For instance, a common expectation is that the person who was once mentally ill will always possess a weak or deficient personality. Such expectations make it difficult for the deviant to reenter society (e.g., to find jobs after having been hospitalized for mental illness). As a result, labels often create the reality they assume. For example, the expectation that people who were once mentally ill are poor job prospects adds to their difficulties in developing sound job histories.[6]

Stigma

Another aspect of deviance theory's contribution to explaining psychosocial problems is the concept of stigma. Goffman[8] borrows the term stigma from the Greek word that referred to individuals marked (by disfigurement) for their offenses against society. Goffman defines stigmatized individuals as persons who bear a psychological or physical trait that makes them stand apart from the average cultural member of any setting. As Goffman[8] notes, the one pervasive law of all social settings is that people must fit in. Those who are different, who do not fit in, who are noticeable by virtue of their nonconforming traits, are stigmatized.

The stigmatized individual is perceived and treated as though he or she were not quite human.[8] Stigmatized persons are viewed as bad, undesirable, dangerous, or weak. According to Goffman there are three different types of stigma: abominations of the body; the tribal stigma of race, nationality, and religion; and blemishes of individual character, which include mental illness and mental retardation.

What is important about stigmatized individuals is that their "virtual social identity" (i.e., that identity imputed to them by virtue of the stigmatizing characteristic) overrides an actual identity. Ordinary human foibles and limitations are often construed as a function of the stigmatizing characteristic. For example, if a "normal" person forgets to take change from a cashier and begins to walk away only to be called back, his or her mistake is recognized as just that—a mistake due to being absentminded or preoccupied at the moment. It is seen as a situational act that does not reflect on the person's real identity. If, however, a retarded person commits the same error, one's tendency is to construe the act as, first, the result of the retardation and, second, evidence of the problematic nature of the retardation. Thought processes related to stigma can thus make pathological mountains out of the molehills of common human error.

In summary, deviance theory illustrates much of the complex social dynamics that accompany and affect psychosocial dysfunction. Deviance or labeling theory is not an attempt to explain the original cause of a person's deviant behavior, rather, it illuminates important social processes that influence the experience, behavior, and identity of the deviant person.[2]

ACTION IMPLICATIONS

Deviance or labeling theory does not provide guidelines for action on an individual basis. Instead, it provides a framework for reexamining traditional assumptions or approaches to therapy. Social scientists have often taken a pessimistic view of therapeutic enterprises, emphasizing that systems and persons charged with care and control of deviants oppress them and augment their deviance. The term "moral entrepreneurs" is used to characterize those who devote their life efforts to pursuing and correcting a certain genre of deviance.[1] Therapy is often looked on as a process more oriented to maintaining social reality at large than to ameliorating individuals' problems, because it attempts to eliminate behaviors that threaten the legitimacy of mainstream values, ideas, practices, and rules.[3,5]

While much of the sociological literature does paint a negative view of therapeutic efforts, some writers stress that positive effects can result when therapeutic endeavors take into consideration the need for positive socialization of the deviant.[16] This means that therapy must offer persons with psychosocial dysfunction access to legitimate roles in society. Further, they must be viewed in terms of their commonality with others instead of being treated as outcasts.

Deviance or labeling theories should not be seen as nihilistic statements on therapy, but as providing useful guidelines for avoiding processes that unwittingly socialize patients into permanent deviant roles or intensify deviance. In general, deviance theory suggests that therapy should not remove the mentally ill person from mainstream society and that all therapeutic efforts that necessarily involve removal should focus on maintaining ties with and roles in social life. A final theme is that social change must accompany more humanistic approaches to psychosocial problems. More enlightened attitudes and greater tolerance and understanding of deviant behavior will be needed to avoid the negative effects that can occur from social reaction to the deviant person.

CRITICISMS AND LIMITATIONS

Criticisms of deviant perspectives come from two opposite directions.[2] On the one hand, critics propose that deviance perspectives have often overlooked the undesirability or pathology of the deviant act. Others propose that deviant perspectives have not fully accounted for the oppression that social systems impose on their members as manifest in reactions to deviants. Becker[2] argues that the purpose of social science views of deviance was to accomplish neither of these objectives, but rather to document the processes involved in the deviant status.

It remains that deviance perspectives offer only partial accounts of what happens to mentally ill people or what constitutes psychosocial disorder. This is offered not as a criticism but as a statement on the scope of deviance theory and its relationship to the problem of psychosocial disorder. While biological or psychological etiology and processes are not accounted for in this perspective, it does offer important insights into the social processes surrounding reaction to and management of those who have a psychosocial dysfunction.

COMMENTARY

The deviance perspective enhances understanding of how the processes of therapy can affect the career of the hospitalized person. Reilly[14] acknowledged the theme that hospitalization can intensify the deviant pattern by negatively affecting the occupational skills and roles that individuals need for community life. She suggested organizing occupational therapy as a socializing process that assumes responsibility for maintaining these occupational roles and skills. In therapy, the person should be treated in terms of social expectations and rewards for performance of normal life tasks.[10,11]

Goode[9] has pointed out how, in occupational therapy as in other health disciplines, clinical evaluation procedures can be unnecessarily fault-finding in their orientation. Such assessment does more to stigmatize people's identities than to suggest any clear directions for treatment. He argues that assessment procedures must meet deviant people on their own terms and reflect the ways in which individuals would view their own behaviors and life circumstances.

The deviance perspective is instructive in pointing out how treatment or therapy is always a process of negotiating between viewpoints and over what is proper, acceptable, and worthy of learning. For occupational therapists to socialize individuals into those perspectives and practices that are deemed more competent from the dominant cultural perspective, they must be sensitive to the person's own viewpoints and common sense. Therapy should be a way of bridging the gap, of making the desired social behavior acceptable and meaningful to the person.

Occupational therapy is particularly suited to this process since it has a long tradition of providing action contexts in which individuals can opt to try out and experience socially approved behaviors in various situations. Thus, while therapy does serve the purpose of reducing or controlling deviance, it can do so in a manner that gives the deviant person a reason to choose and enact adaptive behavior.

SUMMARY

History and Purpose	Deviance or labeling theory is part of the social science concern for the structures and processes of group life.
	Early studies romanticized the deviant as a martyr of a disturbed society.
	Current views focus on the interactions between the deviant and society and the role of the deviant in maintaining the boundaries of society.
View of Order	Order results from the interaction of the person and social environment.
	The individual's view of reality and behavior is shaped by the values and norms that society provides.
	Society is maintained and created through the interactions of its members.
View of Disorder	Psychosocial disorder is recognized as deviance—a situation in which people violate rules of society and are identified and responded to as rule-breakers.
	Social control agents and agencies may intensify and perpetuate deviance.
	Because of societal reaction, the deviant's identity (as a deviant) undergoes a transformation (e.g., the moral career of mental patients, acquisition of stigma).
Action Implications	Some social scientists are pessimistic about therapeutic efforts, but others recognize that when therapists are sensitive to the deviance process and seek positive socialization experiences, therapy can benefit people.

Criticisms and Limitations	Deviance theory has been criticized for underrating either the deviant's pathological behavior or the degree to which society oppresses the deviant. Actually, deviance theory seeks to describe the interactions between the deviant person and society without creating blame for either.
Commentary	Therapists should be sensitive to their own attitudes and actions toward the deviant person, taking care to focus on healthy aspects of behavior and the deviant's humanity.
	Positive socialization experiences can be developed so that occupational therapy is an arena where social expectations and individual perspectives can profitably be brought into interaction.

TERMS AND CONCEPTS

asocial	showing no awareness or regard for society's definitions of appropriate behavior.
moral career	a process of self-redefinition in which the institutionalized person receives a new identity as a subhuman entity and learns to behave as a chronic patient.
moral entrepreneur	a person who takes it upon him- or herself to identify people with a type of deviance and who seeks to control it.
norms	implicit and explicit expectations of society for how its members should behave; norms generally pertain to one's age, life, role, and the particular subgroup to which one belongs.
social control	any process that seeks to limit or change behavior of those who violate social rules.
social rules	a process whereby people interacting with a social group come to take on its attitudes and beliefs and to conform their behavior to the rules and norm of the group.

| sociogenic | arising from or caused by social factors. |
| stigma | a physical, mental, and/or emotional trait that is identified by others as being inferior, bad, flawed, or otherwise undesirable. A person with a stigma is identified through the stigma (e.g., one is a "cripple," a "crazy"). |

REFERENCES

1. Becker, H. S. (Ed.). *The other side: Perspectives on deviance.* New York: Free Press, 1964.
2. Becker, H. S. *Outsiders: Studies in the sociology of deviance.* New York: Free Press, 1973.
3. Berger, P. L., & Luckman, T. *The social construction of reality.* New York: Anchor Books, 1967.
4. Blumer, H. *Symbolic interactionism: Perspective and method.* Englewood Cliffs, N.J.: Prentice-Hall, 1969.
5. Dexter, L. A. On the politics and sociology of stupidity in our society. In H. S. Becker (Ed.), *The other side: Perspectives on deviance.* New York: Free Press, 1964.
6. Erikson, K. T. Notes on the sociology of deviance. In H. S. Becker (Ed.), *The other side: Perspectives on deviance.* New York: Free Press, 1973.
7. Freidson, E. Disability as social deviance. In E. Freidson & J. Lorber (Eds.), *Medical men and their work: A sociological reader.* Chicago: Aldine-Atherton, 1972.
8. Goffman, E. *Asylums.* New York: Anchor Books, 1961.
9. Goode, D. Who is Bobby? Ideology and method in the discovery of a Down's Syndrome person's competence. In G. Kielhofner (Ed.), *Health through occupation: Theory and practice in occupational therapy.* Philadelphia: F. A. Davis, 1983.
10. Kielhofner, G. The temporal dimension in the lives of retarded adults. *American Journal of Occupational Therapy*, 1979, *33*, 161–168.
11. Kielhofner, G., & Takata, N. A study of mentally retarded persons: Applied research in occupational therapy. *American Journal of Occupational Therapy*, 1980, *34*, 252–258.
12. Mehan, H., & Wood, H. *The reality of ethnomethology.* New York: John Wiley and Sons, 1975.
13. Mercer, J. Career patterns of persons labeled as mentally retarded. In E. Freidson & J. Lorber (Eds.), *Medical men and their work: A sociological reader.* Chicago: Aldine-Atherton, 1972.

14. Reilly, M. A psychiatric occupational therapy program as a teaching model. *American Journal of Occupational Therapy*, 1966, *20*, 61–67.
15. Rosenhan, On being sane in insane places. In T. J. Scheff (Ed.), *Labeling madness*. Englewood Cliffs, N.J.: Prentice-Hall, 1975.
16. Samson, H., & Messinger, S. The mental hospital and marital family ties. In H. S. Becker (Ed.), *The other side: Perspectives on deviance*. New York: Free Press, 1964.
17. Scheff, T. J. *Labeling madness*. Englewood Cliffs, N.J.: Prentice-Hall, 1975.
18. Zusman, J. Some explanations of the changing appearance of psychotic patients. In R. H. Price & B. Denner (Eds.), *The making of a mental patient*. New York: Holt, Rinehart & Winston, 1973.

Part Two

**Toward A Unified Identity
And Practice In
Occupational Therapy**

12
The History and Purpose of Occupational Therapy

Although the field of occupational therapy formally came into existence only three-quarters of a century ago, the use of occupation as a form of treatment has a long and colorful history dating from the mid-eighteenth century. Quite remarkably, some fundamental concepts that emerged at that time have been preserved in occupational therapy and still constitute the core of its relevance and efficacy for those with psychosocial dysfunction. This is not to suggest that there has been a smooth progression of ideas and techniques over the past three centuries. On the contrary, the use of occupation as therapy for psychosocial problems died for a period of time and was reborn in this century.

Historical shifts and changes in psychosocial occupational therapy have been chronicled elsewhere.[2,3,9,14] The present purpose is to illuminate and order those central themes and practices that have endured. The underlying assumption is that those perennial elements that have survived are the core elements of psychosocial occupational therapy. Thus, this and the following chapters are not only descriptive but also prescriptive. That is, they offer a picture of how occupational therapy practice developed, and they propose a way of viewing and enacting occupational therapy in psychosocial practice.

The ideas and techniques that today are referred to as occupational therapy were stimulated in the past by concerns with the limitations of predominant methods of treatment. The earliest form of occupational therapy, referred to as moral treatment, emerged in the mid-eighteenth century as an alternative to the predominant abusive and punitive methods of responding to the insane. This moral treatment movement eventually died out. It was replaced with a medical model approach, which viewed mental illness as largely incurable and resulted in a custodial system of care. Modern occupational therapy emerged from the impetus of a few enlightened physicians and others as an alternative to the pessimism and inaction of the medical model.

MORAL TREATMENT: THE FIRST OCCUPATIONAL THERAPY

During the Middle Ages, persons with psychosocial dysfunction were largely neglected and abused. By the eighteenth century, it was common to incarcerate the mentally ill along with other problematic and indigent people. The dominant ideology of treatment was that the mentally ill needed to be imbued with fear. Thus, they were often frightened and tortured, albeit with therapeutic intentions.[10]

In reaction to these deplorable conditions, a number of reformers set out to turn the insane asylum into a place of genuine care. Moral treatment became the name for their movement. Moral treatment included not only the belief that patients needed kind and compassionate care but also the assertion that they should be engaged in the normal occupations of everyday life.

Moral treatment flourished because it worked, but also because the political and ideological climates of Western culture supported it. There was a growing optimism at the time that science would provide new answers and new hope for humanistic goals. The lawfulness of human behavior was stressed with a concomitant assertion that it could be systematically influenced. This led to the belief that those with psychosocial problems could be helped.[11] The optimistic belief that people had the potential for normal behavior also included the idea that some element of "normality" always remained within the person and that this remaining healthy aspect could be nurtured through moral treatment. In fact, the assumption that those with psychosocial problems possessed some degree of control and awareness was the basis for the proposal that they could be positively influenced by normal surroundings and routines of behavior.[1]

Bockoven[2] described moral treatment as an endeavor to awaken feelings of communality (a sense of belonging to a social group) in the mentally ill. This could be achieved through occupations "which required the patient to invest interest in something outside himself in cooperation with others, namely manual work, intellectual work, recreation, and religious worship" (pp. 75–76).[2] Bockoven went on to describe moral treatment as:

> organized group-living in which the integration and continuity of work, play and social activities produce a meaningful total life experience in which growth of individual capacity to enjoy life has maximum opportunity. (p. 76)[2]

Moral treatment was more than a reform and a method; it was also a philosophy of human nature and a theory of mental disorder that provided a rationale for treatment. Bockoven's discussion of the fourfold meaning of the term "moral" is especially instructive for understanding what have always been the main themes of occupational therapy.[2] One meaning was close to what is meant by "morale," and it implied such emotions as enthusiasm, hope, confidence, and related feelings of well-being. Thinking about emotional disturbance, on the other hand, implied the opposite feelings of despair, lethargy, ennui, helplessness, and the like.

"Moral" also referred to mores or folkways, the ethos of normal conduct, and the meanings attached to a way of living. Thus, it connoted the confident and enthusiastic embracing of some recognizable external order (i.e., some cultural way of life) that had meaning for the person and resulted in a sense of well-being.

The third connotation was that the mentally ill were not responsible for their problems or culpable for their undesirable actions. This was an important step away from earlier interpretations that construed mental illness as moral degeneration and demonic possession. The fourth meaning was that society had an ethical obligation to care for less fortunate individuals.

One of the most interesting aspects of moral treatment is its view of the human mind and emotions. It was believed that all human thought was organized by the same underlying laws.[2] Thus, there was commonality in the human experience. In addition, the mind and the brain were seen as highly malleable and greatly influenced by physical and social surroundings.[11] The thrust of the occupations that filled the days of mental patients in moral treatment was to bring their thoughts and emotions into congruence with those of the larger community. This was to be accomplished not by force but by the gentle persuasion of participation in the occupations of a community.

In addition, there was also a perspective on how the mind worked and could be influenced by occupation. Licht quotes a discussion by Jarvis, a moral treatment writer:

> As no two particles of matter can occupy the same point in space at the same moment, so no two absorbing thoughts or emotions can occupy the mind or heart at the same instant of time. So long then, as those, whose minds are prone to wander in delusions, are engaged in mechanical or other employments, their thoughts must be given exclusively to the conduct and succession of natural events and real processes; and as the mind can not admit or be possessed by both the sane and the insane idea, the insane one must be excluded, and the sane one reign paramount; all the mental powers of the worker which are in action for the moment are sane, and the mental disorder is for the moment, or that succession of moments, suspended. The sanity may be, and probably is, in most cases, broken and interrupted by insane thoughts and emotions. The attention to work may be, and undoubtedly often is, uncertain and fitful, and

interspersed with sudden temporary alternations of order and disorder. The man may look at and think of his shoe, his awl and his hammer, and bring them together for a second, and let his crazed imagination carry his thoughts away into his delusions, or permit his morbid feeling to take possession of his soul, and absorb him in grief, or hate, or passion, or exuberant joy—but during that time, however short or long it may be, in which he is applying his awl to the leather, and lifting the hammer and striking the blow in the right place and with the intended effect, his mind must be given to the observation of those processes to see that they are conducted according to his plan; and, of course, his thought is sane, his hands are perfoming a sane act, the cerebral as well as the muscular movements are of the same character, and so much sanity is thereby developed and manifested. (pp. 11–12)[10]

This eloquent passage sums up the fundamental assertion of moral treatment that occupation brings the person into the order of the external world, which becomes imprinted on the mind and body.

The Demise of Moral Treatment

A number of interrelated changes in science, society, and medicine contributed to the decline of moral treatment. By the middle of the nineteenth century, American attitudes were rapidly changing. A massive influx of immigrants, many of whom were poor and indigent, resulted in growing prejudice, and asylums became overcrowded with what came to be known as the "insane foreign pauper."[2] With the emergence of Social Darwinism, the belief in a survival-of-the-fittest social dynamic and the concomitant conviction that people are not equal, the notion of a moral obligation for the care of the insane made less and less sense.

Science was also rapidly changing. In the previous era, scientific and humanistic goals had been united.[11] Science was now pursued for its own sake, and human problems often had to conform to its views and methods. Medicine's view of mental illness changed accordingly. Causes of mental illness were no longer ascribed to environmental pressures; rather, the new scientific perspective was that insanity was a disease with identifiable symptoms and a discoverable neurological cause.[11] Discovery of brain lesions in some patients gave impetus to the argument that mental illness was caused by brain disease. Because no cure for the faulty brain was known, this perspective led to growing pessimism about the curability of insanity.[2]

The crowding of hospitals and the economic concerns they posed also constrained the practice of moral treatment, which required an optimal ratio of patients to staff and pleasant surroundings. With growing pessimism about curability, it seemed unnecessary to allocate funds for the "superfluous" methods of moral treatment. Large asylums simply became warehouses for the hopelessly incurable. These alterations in social values, in economics, and in the population, combined with internal changes in medicine, led to a demise of moral treatment, and a period of custodialism ensued.

THE EMERGENCE OF OCCUPATIONAL THERAPY: A SECOND MORAL TREATMENT

In the first decades of this century, a number of persons reestablished moral treatment principles and techniques, labeling them occupational therapy. Several factors appear to have been instrumental in this reemergence. The study of psychological phenomena reawakened interest in emotional and cognitive factors in psychosocial problems, and the mental hygiene movement precipitated reforms in custodial care.[16] The most instrumental factor was the discontent of several physicians with the dominant medical model approach to psychiatry. Such physicians as Herbert Hall,[7] William Rush Dunton,[4] and Adolph Meyer[12] sought an alternate approach to the problems of mental illness. Their enthusiasm for and their theoretical and practical support of the occupational therapy movement was essential to its growth. In addition, a number of other leaders of varied backgrounds contributed to the early development of occupational therapy in psychosocial practice. Susan Tracy,[17] Louis Haas,[6] Eleanor Clarke Slagle,[15,16] Thomas Kidner,[8] and others represented such diverse interests and backgrounds as nursing, architecture, industrial arts, and social welfare.

The Thought of Early Occupational Therapy

Early occupational therapy was organized around the premise that human beings were complex creatures who required occupation in order to maintain their health:

> The whole of the human organization has its shape in a kind of rhythm. It is not enough that our hearts should be in a useful rhythm, always kept up to a standard at which it can meet rest as well as wholesome *strain* without upset. There are many other rhythms which we must be attuned to: the *larger* rhythms of night and day, of sleep and waking hours, of hunger and its gratification, and finally the big four—work and play and rest and sleep, which our organism must be able to balance even under difficulty. The only way to attain this balance in this is *actual doing, actual practice*, a program of wholesome living as the *basis* of wholesome feeling and thinking and fancy and interests. (p. 6)[12]

This statement embodies several fundamental tenets. First, human organisms are complex, and their organization is represented as a balance or rhythm. Second, that organization is dependent on the organism's occupation. Last, healthy mental states are the result of healthy occupational life-styles, and, by implication, disturbed mental states can result from a breakdown of occupational life. Conversely, because of the importance of occupation in human life, it could be used to remediate loss of health:

> The development of the human brain is the result of man's struggle with the forces of nature throughout countless centuries and a continuous effort to adapt himself to his environment and provide for his own needs. Therefore, no more wholesome condition can be chosen for man than an environment of work, which when properly prescribed and controlled, can be of great value in restoring health. (p. 15)[6]

An Alternative View of Mental Illness

Early occupational therapists for the most part did not view mental illness through the medical model. Rather, they embraced a view of mental illness articulated by Adolph Meyer, in which habits, modes of adjustment, and environments were major factors.[13] Meyer's perspective came from many years of research with mentally ill patients. He discovered that the universal feature of their problems was a disorganization of habit.[2] He decried the medical model view that mental illness was a disease caused by some organic entity, and noted that "many formidable diseases are largely problems of adaptation and not some mysterious devil in disguise to be exorcised" (p. 1).[12] Meyer's theme of habit deterioration was echoed by Slagle, who noted that mental illness was largely a process of disorganized habits learned from exposure to disruptive environments.[15,16]

Dunton[4] and Kidner[8] emphasized the importance of habits balancing work, play, rest, and sleep and noted that a lack of leisure interests and pursuits, fatigue from overwork, exposure to monotonous and disinteresting work, and idleness could be sources of psychosocial problems.

Mental illness was viewed as a breakdown not only of patterns of behavior but also of the patterns of healthy emotion. This was generally expressed as a disruption of morale or demoralization. Those with mental problems were recognized as having lost interest, confidence, and hope, becoming isolated from their communities—all components of the process of demoralization.

The Rationale and Role of Occupation as a Remediative Measure

Quite naturally, the overall approach to remediation in early occupational therapy was to expose patients to tasks and pastimes in the context of normal daily and weekly routines. Dunton[4] was instrumental in developing much of the rationale for the mechanism of recovery or improvement from psychosocial problems through occupation. In his view, an important part of occupation for those with psychosocial problems was simply to maintain functional capacity and to prevent depression and other problems that result from inactivity.

A second important role of occupation was to correct faulty patterns of attention and behavior; activity acted as an antidote, drawing the patient into a state of mind and action opposite to the problematic one toward which he or she had a tendency. The following passage illustrates such an approach:

> In a case of dementia praecox where the subject is given to daydreaming or so-called mental rumination, occupation is given to keep the patient's train of thought in more healthy channels. In a case of mild excitement occupation will keep the patient's mind more continuously on one subject than is possible if he has not this stimulus to control his attention. (p. 25)[4]

A third aspect of occupation's influence on those with psychosocial problems was termed "substitution." It was generally accepted that mental illness involved the fusion of morbid and obsessive thoughts into the train of everyday consciousness. Occupation served as a means of replacing such thoughts with healthier ones generated in the course of interesting pastimes and tasks. This rationale was based on a continuation of the moral treatment idea that the mind could be occupied with only one dominant thought. Continued application to life tasks and interesting activities would eventually train the mind in patterns of healthy thought.

A fourth role of therapy was habit training.[15] Since people with psychosocial problems suffered from disorganized habit patterns, therapy would have to retrain them into adaptive patterns of living. Habits were thought to be acquired through practice and shaped by the social, temporal, and physical surroundings. Thus, patients would learn a healthy pattern of living only if they were exposed to a normal timetable of work, rest, play, and sleep; if they engaged in communal and cooperative tasks; and if they lived in pleasant surroundings that provided stimulation and opportunities for a variety of pursuits.[4,12,15]

A fifth aspect of occupational therapy was the restoration of morale, a social-psychological phenomenon.[4,16] Morale was the person's enthusiasm for a way of life. It was maintained through participation in a community's everyday life tasks and events. That is, morale was a feeling of interest, commitment, hope, and well-being supported by cultural and social meaning. It was thus reasoned that by exposing patients to meaningful pursuits of the culture, their morale could be restored.

Principles of Treatment

The roles of therapy implied several principles of treatment. The first principle found consistently in descriptions of occupational therapy was that it must arouse interest, courage, and confidence.[4,6,15,17] Methods of accomplishing this were the introduction of novel occupations that aroused curiosity, the personal interest of the therapist in the activity, the skillful presentation of activities to create arousal, and careful matching of the occupation to the patient's capacities and needs. This required the availability of a wide range of opportunities for action.

A second principle was that occupations should be applied with system and with precision.[4,8,16] This meant that the therapist had to pay careful attention to mental and physical limitations and abilities and to dispositions of the patient in order to choose and apply the proper occupations.[5] Similarly, consideration had to be given to the nature of the patient's problems and to the carefully planned presentation of occupations to counteract these problems.

A third treatment principle was that of gradation of occupations according to the increasing capacity of patients. Slagle articulates this principle as "grading the occupation from simple to complex, passing from the known to the unknown, increasing interest and requiring an increasing degree of concentration" (p. 15).[15] Gradation could be accomplished by varying a single activity or it might be embodied in a total program in which patients moved through phases of therapy.[6] For the most regressed patients in early occupational therapy, the first phase, habit training, was used to restore the basic skills and habits of self-care, giving the patient some degree of control over his or her immediate surroundings and over attention and action.[15] After habit training, patients progressed to work in an occupational therapy shop, which allowed them greater freedom to act and use skills.[8] The final phase of treatment was the pre-industrial or industrial therapy stage. Here patients worked in various industries of the hospital or in cottage industries maintained by the hospital under the supervision of lay workers. Occupational therapists served as consultants to those who supervised the patients in these work experiences. This progression from ward life to hospital industry helped assure the smooth transition of the patient from hospital to community life. It graded demands for performance so that the patient was gradually reorganized and gained increasing capacity, resulting in the ability to return to a more normal life.

A fourth principle was that occupational therapy focused on the health of patients rather than pathology and that it emphasized the expression of healthy emotions and attitudes.[4,6,16] This meant that occupation was not seen as a prescribed "remedy" but as something to be:

> followed for its own sake, . . . so that instead of being a medicine that can be dropped when the patient is cured, it has become rather a part of the restored individual's life, to be retained in some form as long as health exists. (p. 2)[5]

In order for occupational therapy to accomplish this goal, the ethos of the clinic had to differ from that of the ward and other therapies, where focus on pathology was more likely. One way of accomplishing this was that:

> A rigid rule against the discussion of symptoms or any matters relating to illness or treatment was enforced and the room became at once a cheery and attractive place. The atmosphere of interested activity prevailed. The work became the source of new purposes, of changed avenues of thought and of stimulated ambitions. . . . The evils of the idle association of nervous invalids were in a measure remedied, and a more positively wholesome spirit pervaded the institution. (p. 7.)[5]

In addition, the importance of having an esprit de corps, an atmosphere of cheerfulness, hope, industriousness, and order, was deemed critical. Haas[6] was especially articulate in this regard. He specified the details of both a physical plant and a social atmosphere that would positively influence patients. Haas,[6] Dunton,[4] and Hall[7] also stressed the importance of qualities such as craftsmanship and sportsmanship in the therapist and in the therapeutic occupations. If the occupations did not embody these wholesome and uplifting characteristics, they would not be therapeutic. Similarly, the therapist had to be patient, cheerful, enthusiastic, and resourceful in solving problems.[15,17]

A fifth principle was that occupational therapy had to be a total program of care. One of the most important facets of treatment in early occupational therapy was the recognition that it could not be limited to a few short sessions a week. Because most humans live in a balance of daily life occupations, total programs involving the activities of the patient's entire day were necessary for adequate treatment. It was further reasoned that without proper exposure to a total physical, social, and temporal environment the effects of occupational therapy on the patient would not be substantial. In order to effect such comprehensive programs, occupational therapists often had to assume roles as supervisors, consultants, and planners working with other disciplines and with laymen in the institution.

The knowledge and technology of early occupational therapy psychosocial practice appears more sophisticated than one would expect of a fledgling profession. However, if one considers that early occupational therapy was an extension of moral treatment—a long-standing approach to mental health— then it is not surprising that the field possessed a well-formulated tradition of knowledge. Despite its apparent coherence and viability, the early occupational therapy perspective came to be questioned deeply during the middle of this century. Eventually, it was largely dropped in favor of a more psychodynamically based version of occupational therapy.[9] When this happened, the view of mental illness, the rationale and role of occupations in therapy, and the principles of treatment changed in large measure. Psychoanalytic concepts promoted by psychiatrists as the most sophisticated and acceptable view of mental illness became the new conceptual foundation of psychosocial occupational therapy. Thus, humans were viewed primarily as tension-reducing organisms driven by unconscious forces. Problems of mental illness were seen as anxiety states and failures of ego maturation. Therapy focused on the expression of feelings through activity and the gratification of primitive needs. Occupation was no longer viewed as an important force in maintaining the organization of human behavior, but rather as one of several vehicles (talk being the predominant one) through which patients could therapeutically fulfill needs and express feelings. Some therapists came to see occupations as only secondary to the process of establishing a verbal relationship with clients, and eventually some therapists abandoned occupation altogether in favor of purely verbal methods of treatment.

Occupational therapists soon recognized that this shift in psychosocial practice had taken the field away from its original purpose, knowledge, and practice. This resulted in a new series of efforts to articulate and shape theory and practice in a manner consistent with the moral treatment and early occupational therapy traditions. Thus, modern occupational therapy in psychosocial practice is once again returning to its core concepts and practice. The remaining chapters illustrate the elements of theory and practice that reflect this continuity.

SUMMARY

Moral Treatment

The history of using occupation as therapy began with the moral treatment movement of the mid-18th to mid-19th centuries.

Moral treatment was a humanistic treatment of mentally ill persons that stressed compassion and the commonality of the human condition.

Moral treatment was based on the scientific view that human behavior was subject to certain discoverable laws and that the environment influenced the mind and body. Thus, the possibility of remediating problems of mental illness was viewed with optimism.

Moral treatment had four connotations:

1. morale, or the enthusiasm, hope, confidence, and well-being that supported and resulted from involvement in one's everyday world;
2. the ethos of normal conduct—that is, mores or folkways reflecting the order and meanings of the culture;

3. the lack of culpability of mentally ill persons for their actions and their right to compassion; and
4. society's moral obligation to care for the mentally ill.

Occupation was used in moral treatment to bring persons into interaction with their environments so that the order of the external world was imprinted on the mind and body.

Moral treatment subsided despite its empirical success because of changes in science, medicine, and social values.

Early Occupational Therapy

Early occupational therapy was a reemergence of moral treatment ideas and practices.

The thought of early occupational therapy stressed that:
1. humans were complex beings whose bodies and minds were organized into a balance or rhythm;
2. occupation (i.e., doing the tasks of daily life provided by one's culture) was necessary to maintain the organization and balance of humans; and
3. the organization of behavior is reflected in human habits.

Early occupational therapy viewed mental illness as:
1. a reaction to the environment and a disorganization of rhythm and balance instead of a disease caused by some germ or trauma;
2. a manifestation of disrupted or maladaptive habits; and
3. a form of demoralization that resulted from poor occupational life-styles or disruption of occupation.

The rationale and role of occupation as a remediative measure was:
1. to maintain functional capacity and prevent depression and other problems that resulted from inactivity;
2. to correct faulty patterns of attention and behavior;
3. to substitute healthy thoughts for pathological thoughts by orienting the patient to life tasks;
4. to train persons in correct habits of behavior needed for competence; and
5. to restore morale for living.

Principles of treatment were:
1. that occupation should arouse interest, courage, and confidence through the qualities of the occupation and the therapist's skill and interest in the occupation;
2. that occupation must be applied with precision to match the strengths and weaknesses and the personal dispositions of the patient;

3. that occupation should be graded from simple to complex to provide a continuum of reorganization of behavior;
4. that therapy should focus on health rather than pathology and that the clinic should reflect concern with the normal life of the culture; and
5. that occupational therapy was a total program of care that organized the patient's entire daily activity.

Early occupational therapy was drastically changed because of pressure from medicine, and it became largely a psychoanalytic treatment for a period of time.

Current efforts seek to return occupational therapy to its traditional role and practices

REFERENCES

1. Bing, R. Occupational therapy revisited: A paraphrasic journey. *American Journal of Occupational Therapy*, 1981, *35*, 499–518.
2. Bockoven, J. S. *Moral treatment in community mental health*. New York: Springer, 1972.
3. Diasio, K. Psychiatric occupational therapy: Search for a conceptual framework in light of psychoanalytic ego psychology and learning theory. *American Journal of Occupational Therapy*, 1968, *22*, 400–414.
4. Dunton, W. R. *Occupational therapy: A manual for nurses*. Philadelphia: W. B. Saunders, 1915.
5. Fuller, D. The need of instruction for nurses in occupations for the sick. In S. Tracy (Ed.), *Studies in invalid occupation*. Boston: Whitcomb & Barrows, 1912.
6. Haas, L. *Practical occupational therapy*. Milwaukee: Bruce Publishing Co., 1944.
7. Hall, H. *Occupational therapy: A new profession*. Concord: Rumford Press, 1923.
8. Kidner, T. B. *Occupational therapy: The science of prescribed work for invalids*. Stuttgart: W. Kohlhammer, 1930.
9. Kielhofner, G., & Burke, J. P. The evolution of knowledge and practice in occupational therapy: Past, present and future. In G. Kielhofner (Ed.), *Health through occupation: Theory and practice in occupational therapy*. Philadelphia: F. A. Davis, 1983.
10. Licht, S. *Occupational therapy sourcebook*. Baltimore: Williams & Wilkins, 1948.
11. Magaro, P., Gripp, R., & McDowell, D. *The mental health industry: A cultural phenomenon*. New York: John Wiley & Sons, 1978.

12. Meyer, A. The philosophy of occupational therapy. *Archives of Occupational Therapy*, 1922, *1*, 1–10.
13. Mora, G. Theories of personality and psychopathology: III. Other psychoanalytic and related schools. Adolph Meyer. In Freedman, Kaplan, & Sadock (Eds.), *Comprehensive textbook of psychiatry II* (Vol. 1) (2nd ed.). Baltimore: Williams & Wilkins, 1975.
14. Mosey, A. C. Involvement in the rehabilitation movement—1942–1960. *American Journal of Occupational Therapy*, 1971, *25*, 234–236.
15. Slagle, E. C. Training aides for mental patients. *Archives of Occupational Therapy*, 1922, *1*, 11–17.
16. Slagle, E. C., & Robeson, H. *Syllabus for training of nurses in occupational therapy* (2nd ed.). Utica, N.Y.: State Hospitals Press, 1941.
17. Tracy, S. *Studies in invalid occupation*. Boston: Whitcomb & Barrows, 1912.

13
The View of Order in Occupational Therapy

Order is viewed in occupational therapy as the individual's ability to competently perform the everyday tasks and behaviors of life and to gain satisfaction from this performance.[25,43] Work, play, and self-care have been identified as the major areas of daily life performance. Collectively they are referred to as occupational behavior[32] or occupational performance.[48] Thus, the view of order in occupational therapy can be described as focusing on people's ability for occupational behavior or performance.

In occupational therapy, a person can be recognized as having a disease process (e.g., Down's syndrome) and still exhibit order, since the capacity for occupational behavior can exist concurrently with certain diseases. Similarly, people may simultaneously exhibit some pathological symptoms (e.g., hallucinations or anxiety) and still be able to function adequately and, thus, be considered in a state of order. Conversely, occupational therapists do not assume that because a pathological state or symptom is removed that order automatically follows. There is a tendency in psychiatry to assume that once a patient's symptoms are allayed with medication or when anxiety is reduced through verbal therapy, that competence will be a natural sequel. This is not the case. Order is a state of organization for productive and playful functioning that requires the integrity and interrelationship of many components of the human being.

Several major themes generated in occupational therapy to explain and describe order can be delineated: (1) humans as open systems, (2) intrinsic motivation, (3) humans as decision makers, (4) roles as organizers of behavior, (5) temporal adaptation, (6) person-environment interaction, and (7) occupational performance components.

In this chapter, we will examine each of these themes and the ways in which they illuminate order in human occupational behavior. These themes overlap and collectively constitute an overall view of order.

HUMAN BEINGS AS OPEN SYSTEMS

Open system concepts represent an interdisciplinary movement in the sciences aimed at generating a more adequate conceptualization of living phenomena.[5,50] Open systems concepts attempt to go beyond thinking of living systems as machine-like, to acknowledge that they are more complex than inanimate, closed systems. Open system concepts have been identified by several occupational therapy writers as being relevant to explaining order in the occupational behavior of humans.[10,13,16,20,25,39,52] This section provides an overview of systems concepts and how they are being used to conceptualize order in occupational therapy.

Self-Maintaining Systems

The fundamental property of the open system is the capacity for self-maintenance and self-change through the system's own action. An open system, to use the Fidlers' phrase, can become through doing.[13] This property is present in all living systems.

The way in which an open system maintains and changes itself through doing or action is explained by the concept of a cycle. In the open system, the cycle is a self-repeating process, involving four interrelated stages.[20,25] *Intake** is the importation of energy and information from the environment. *Throughput* is the transformation of the energy or information into some other form and its incorporation into the system's structure and process. In the throughput phase, the system often changes itself to accommodate incoming information. *Output* is the behavior or action of the system. In the final stage, *feedback*, information concerning the progress and consequences of action (output), is returned to the system. It then becomes part of the intake of the system. As this feedback enters the system, it is used in the throughput stage to adjust and rearrange internal components.

This cycle is an ongoing process. The system takes in information, transforms the information and itself, acts, generates feedback, incorporates it, and so on. Because of the nature of this cycle, the open system's action (output) is critical for maintaining and changing its structures. Open system processes permeate all of human existence and behavior. The act of reading this book is a process of taking in information; interpreting it and incorporating it into

---

*Intake is used here instead of the more common term *input*. The change is to reflect the active nature of intake. People do not passively receive information from their environments; they seek out and selectively take in information.

one's understanding and memory (throughput); eventually using it in some fashion, such as responding to an exam or designing patient treatment (output); and thus generating consequences that can be used to evaluate the knowledge and how well one has incorporated and used it (feedback). The outcome of one's use of the information (in an exam or in the clinic) will shape further action and decisions for action. Thus, what one does will further influence what one becomes and what one will do in the future.

The importance of the open cycle for maintaining and changing the system can further be appreciated from the perspective of another property of open systems, the primacy of function over structure. Closed systems (i.e., inanimate systems such as machines) function only in ways determined by their structure. For instance, a car engine's functions are totally specified by the internal structure of its parts. In an open system, the relationship is somewhat reversed. Rather than function being totally dependent on structure, structure largely depends on function. Process or function is basic to the open system. Structure is always changing and results from processes underlying the open system. This becomes more apparent if we consider an example such as the development of a human being. The structure of the human from the stage of the fertilized ovum through adulthood is constantly changing. That structure is first determined by the functions of cell division and a plethora of other physiological events that occur in sequence with intricate interrelationships. Later, especially from the period of birth, the function of the human being becomes a determinant of evolving structures in the musculoskeletal, nervous, and personality systems. The action of the child facilitates nervous pathways, increases muscle strength and bone mass, and develops cognitive and perceptual abilities. These are a few of the many facets of the system that must be developed through the system's action.

Particularly relevant to psychosocial practice is the open system concept that a person's life experiences (the ongoing cycles of output, feedback, intake, and throughput) shape and determine abilities, preferences, self-assessment, values, and other variables critical to psychosocial adaptation. This concept parallels the Fidlers' discussion of doing:

> *Doing* is viewed as enabling the development and integration of sensory, motor, cognitive, and psychosocial systems; serving as a socializing agent; and verifying one's efficacy as a competent, contributing member of one's society. (p. 305)[13]

Thus, to say that a human being is an open system is to say that what he or she is and becomes is a function of what he or she does. This not only provides a foundation for understanding order in the human system, but it also spells the basic rationale underlying the therapeutic approach of occupational therapy. Engaging people in purposeful tasks, play, and other occupations is a means of shaping their doing (output) and thereby influencing change. This change may be in the nervous system, in the person's beliefs about self, in the ability to perform some skill, or in a variety of other dimensions.

Hierarchy

Another system concept that is critical to the view of order is hierarchy. In an open system, hierarchy refers to the way in which parts are organized into a gestalt, or meaningful whole.[20,41] The functional components of a system are arranged in different levels with specific relationships between the levels.[22] Higher levels in a hierarchy govern lower levels. Lower levels constrain higher levels; that is, by virtue of their own abilities and limitations, they set limits on what higher levels can command them to do.

We can observe a hierarchy in the functional aspects of the human body. At the lowest level is the musculoskeletal system. This system consists of the structures that enable movement. The next higher level is the nervous system, which commands and governs musculoskeletal action. In turn, the nervous system is constrained from commanding what the musculoskeletal system is not capable of performing.

In the psychosocial practice arena, an important aspect of the hierarchy of human function is the relationship of the musculoskeletal system to the nervous system, of the nervous system to the symbolic or conscious system, and of the latter to the social system. According to hierarchical principles, the nervous system, which governs the musculoskeletal system, is commanded and governed by human consciousness and in turn constrains that consciousness.[21,22,28,41] By the same token, the social system gives commands to the individual through norms and role expectations. The individual and his or her capabilities, in turn, constrain the social system's ability to command behavior. For example, a family may place a high value on academic performance, thus influencing a child's efforts in school. If, however, the child has limited intellectual capacity, the family's expectations for high academic achievement cannot be fulfilled. Levels of function and structure are thus intimately interrelated in the human open system.

Work and Play as Output

Work and play have been conceptualized as the output of the open system.[25] Play contributes to the development of competence. Early childhood play develops sensory motor abilities,[29,33] rules (or internal images) that guide competent action,[41,42] and understanding of various roles and their requirements.[26] Play is an effective learning medium because it is free of overwhelming consequences. In play, the individual has freedom of exploration and can express creative and risk-taking behaviors.[41,49]

In adolescence, play serves as an arena for further developing interactional skills and for socializing with one's peers.[2,41,45] The hobbies of adolescence allow expression of personal mastery. In adulthood, play generally serves as an antidote to work, providing relaxation and recommitting the individual to the realities and demands of the work world.[40] Adult play (especially in the form of such cultural rituals as the celebration of holidays) serves an important function of reaffirming the values of the culture and social group. For example, sports express the American values of competition, teamwork, and giving one's best.

Work is important to the individual as an arena for expressing interests and values and for developing self-esteem.[17,45] Since work is valued by the culture, those who work experience a sense of personal worth through their contribution to the social group. Work begins with childhood chores and self-care and progresses through the paid and unpaid productive tasks of adult life.

Occupational therapy has always recognized the importance of play and work for maintaining health. Open system concepts allow the field to conceptualize how occupation organizes and changes the system. As output, the occupational behaviors of play and work are important for the development of capacities and commitments in childhood and for their maintenance in adulthood. Both work and play must exist in order for the person to be healthy.[45] When robbed of access to these occupations, the basic cycle of the open system is interrupted and degeneration follows.

INTRINSIC MOTIVATION

Early occupational therapy was based on the conviction that humans needed to engage in occupations. The field sought to extend its original concept by incorporating emerging theories of motivation. The major concepts of motivation in the first half of this century were generated by adherents of behaviorism and psychoanalysis. These theories share a view of human beings as passive creatures seeking equilibrium through tension reduction. They also view humans as driven by forces over which they have little control. They are diametrically opposed, however, in that behaviorism considers behavior to be environmentally determined, while psychoanalysis sees it as being psychically or inner-determined. According to both these theories, occupation is not a direct motive or need of humans. Behaviorism resulted in the view that people engage in work and play because it was a means to satisfy drives and thereby was reinforced (e.g., working in order to be able to buy food). Psychoanalysis suggested that occupation was an activity that mediated unconscious drives through symbolism. For instance, hammering could be a way of acting out aggressive drives, or boring a hole in wood might have the symbolic meaning of releasing sexual tension.

While both theories offered plausible explanations for occupational behavior, they suggested that it was extrinsically motivated. That is, it was done not for its own sake but for some ulterior motive. For a period of time, occupational therapists sought to incorporate these theories into the field's view of human behavior and to develop related treatment approaches.

Eventually therapists began to view these theories as unsatisfactory because they offered no direct explanation of the motive for occupation.[11,14] These therapists pointed to new theories that offered better explanations. Theories of intrinsic motivation emerged from the efforts of behavioral scientists to include a drive for action, stimulation, competition, achievement, arousal, and like experiences. Intrinsic motivation theories shared the common themes that humans engaged in action for its own sake without the benefit of extrinsic reinforcement or unconscious motivation. In short, they recognized another major motive in human behavior that complemented and counterbalanced the motive of seeking equilibrium or tension reduction. This motive was one of tension-seeking, leading to change and growth in the organism.

Intrinsic motivation has been identified as the underlying dynamic of occupational behavior and the motivational force best suited to the occupational therapy clinic.[1,14] Recognizing intrinsic motivation as the basis of occupation allowed the field to speak of occupation as a basic human need. Further, it led to a greater understanding of the dynamics of occupation in human life.

Whereas psychoanalytic and behavioral thought show how extrinsic motives are useful to the organism's survival, intrinsic motivation theories point to another major function in human life. By seeking activity for its own sake, organisms encounter new events, objects, and people; generate new experiences for themselves; and, in the course of so doing, learn and change. Intrinsic motivation is thus recognized as the basic force underlying change and growth in the person. In terms of the open system, intrinsic motivation leads systems to produce output and thus energizes the basic cycle of the system, facilitating its maintenance and change.

Intrinsic motivation theory emphasizes the critical nature of childhood play for development. Children engage in play for its own sake.[14] The motive of play is a drive for exploration manifest in an attitude of curiosity in the child. Children develop competence when they curiously explore their environments; that is, through play and exploration they learn to act successfully in and on the human and nonhuman environment by rules of competent behavior.[41,42]

The intrinsic motive also maintains competence in adult life. The exploratory drive of childhood is translated into a drive for competence and later for achievement.[41] As individuals develop and acquire basic abilities, their need for stimulation leads to a search for greater challenge. Finding out how to manipulate the environment leads to being able to perform tasks with a degree of mastery, and finally to the ability to accomplish things according to standards of excellence or in comparison to the accomplishments of others. These motives underlie the productive contributions of people to society. The motive for early play becomes the motive for productive participation in the family and in a succession of social institutions throughout life.

In addition to generating skills that support competence, intrinsic motives also lead to behaviors that generate feelings of accomplishment, satisfaction, and effectiveness. Feelings of efficacy are critical to the ongoing competent behavior of people because they generate a sense of hopefulness.[47] The concept of personal causation elaborates this point.[26] Personal causation refers to the person's drive to be a cause, to have effects. People who are successful in their interactions with the environment develop a sense of personal causation, which leads them to confidently seek out opportunities for action and challenges for behavior.

Intrinsic motivation in the human system is not just a compelling force that drives humans; it is a process of choosing or willing one's course of action.[25] This volitional aspect of humans means that humans are decision makers. The decisions underlying the process of exploring and mastering one's world through occupation are a basic force in the dynamics of the human system and its maintenance of order.[25]

HUMANS AS DECISION MAKERS

A perennial theme in occupational therapy is the importance of personal control and self-determination. In concert with the theme of intrinsic motivation, which directed attention to people's internal and conscious reasons for engaging in occupation, several concepts have been developed which further delineate the dynamics of how and why people make choices about occupation. Included are the concepts of interests and values and the developmental process of occupational choice.

The decision to engage in particular occupations is informed by the meaning these activities have for an individual.[9] Occupations derive their meanings from the culture's view and definition of them and from an individual's values and personal interpretation of past and present experiences. In a culture, certain occupations may be highly central, imbued with the values of the group, and capable of signifying a range of emotions and convictions. For example, Thanksgiving dinner signifies values of family and country, freedom and plenty; it evokes emotions of well-being and gratitude, and it recommits people to these fundamental values. Other activities have meanings that are highly personal and determined from a lifetime of experience. Cynkin[9] points out, for instance, that the simple act of making a pie can signify personal competence, security, a sense of order and calm and productivity. The meanings of other occupations may be largely in their intrinsic pleasure, the satisfaction and interest they generate. Still other meanings of activities lie in their relationship to accomplishing goals. Completing an exam or a semester of courses is all the more significant when it means nearing the goal of completing a degree and entering a chosen profession. Occupational behavior is maintained when the person finds meaning in it. Meaning is thus an important dimension of order in human occupation.

Interests

Interests are affective phenomena that influence one's choices.[31] They are preferences for types of objects, people, or activities because of their ability to afford enjoyment.[4,21]

Matsutsuyu[31] elaborated the meaning of interests in six propositions: (a) interests are influenced by the family through socialization; (b) interests bring forth affective responses to objects, persons, and ideas; (c) interests determine choices for action; (d) interests are important to action that is personally satisfying; (e) interests can maintain persistent action; and (f) interests reflect a person's awareness of his or her areas of ability and identity. As these propositions illustrate, interests are important components of individuals' personalities that influence what action they will choose and why it is likely to be enjoyable.

Interests are important organizers of behavior because the internal priority of interests enables one to choose among alternatives for action and to establish a pattern of behavior for satisfying use of time.[25] Without interests, a person's ability to make consistent choices is obstructed and the individual is less disposed to interact with the environment.

Social approval and personal success influence what likes and dislikes a person will develop.[4] In addition, the development of interests is a function of the individual's participation in activity. The individual who lacks motivation and who fails to explore and experiment will tend to lack interests. Thus, whether people have well-defined interests depends on their initial opportunities to act on an innate tendency to explore and master the environment and receive feedback on various activities.

Values

Individuals possess a value orientation or collection of personal images of what is good, right, or important. This value orientation reflects a person's set of priorities for behavior; these priorities, in turn, guide the formation of operational goals, which influence choices for behavior.[25] Values vary among cultural subgroups[27] and include notions of time use, the importance of types of work, and achievement through competition versus cooperation. Values are intimately related to the meaningfulness of activities and to their significance for security and a sense of worth and importance.

Occupational behavior and, similarly, the collective societal understanding of what constitutes normal or abnormal behavior are culturally determined through the influence of society's value system.[27] For example, societal values, such as the "Protestant work ethic," have had a major impact in determining the way people view and use time.[19] These collectively acknowledged social values are acquired through childhood socialization, the child's observation of or instruction in what characteristic behavior is required by the larger culture. As individuals acknowledge the obligatory nature of values, they come to perceive them as compelling their own behavior.

Because people attach emotions to their values, they generally feel compelled to conform to these values or they experience a personal sense of failure or guilt. On the other hand, values are a source of positive emotion, because they carry the meaning of belonging to a social group and provide a sense of personal identity. When a person operationalizes values in occupational behavior, he or she experiences a feeling of doing the right thing, being a good or valuable person, and meeting social obligations. Thus, values both define and shape behavior.

Occupational Choice

The course of development toward adult life is punctuated by an important process of choosing one's life work.[22,39,52] Occupational choice begins in childhood and typically extends through late adolescence in this culture. Originally thought to be an irreversible process, it is now recognized as something people may do more than once as they make major occupational changes in adult life (e.g., changing a career or preparing for retirement).

The first period of occupational choice, which roughly corresponds to early childhood, is labeled the fantasy period. During this time, choices are not constrained by reality and they are ordinarily made solely on the basis of the perceived pleasure associated with the occupation. For instance, the child may choose to be Superman when he or she grows up because of the "fun" of being able to fly and having superhuman strength. The tentative period, which occurs during the second half of middle childhood and in early adolescence, is a time of making provisional choices based on a clearer assessment of personal interests, capacity, and value. These three considerations are delineated as stages within this period. First, choices are made primarily on the basis of likes or dislikes; then they are considered in terms of one's assessment of personal ability; and finally choices are considered on the basis of social values as the person seeks to have a place in the social group. A final stage in the tentative period is termed the transitional stage. This is when the adolescent begins to take steps toward enacting the choice (e.g., getting a degree or training).

The realistic period, which has three stages, is next. In the exploratory stage, the older adolescent takes a closer look at the chosen occupation and the opportunities it provides for satisfaction and security. During the next step, crystallization, alternative choices are more fully explored and the person narrows the choice down to a particular field. Finally, in the specification stage, the individual delineates any specialization within the chosen occupation. This stage often occurs during or just after the period of actual training for the occupation.

Occupational choice is a complex process by which individuals shape their commitment to a particular kind of work and invest both emotional energy and effort into identification with and preparation for a line of work. Occupational choice is an important determinant of the degree of stability and satisfaction a person is likely to experience in his or her career. This process is very much influenced by a person's successes and failures throughout development, consequent self-perceptions, opportunities to explore alternatives, and the presence of adult role models.[39]

Occupational choice is not altogether a process of free self-determination. The individual must seek to balance and optimize several factors. Economic, personal, and social factors may constrain one's ability to make a given choice. An occupation that maximizes one desirable factor may lack another. Ultimately, the choice reflects a series of compromises and reconsiderations that attempt to fit most of the requirements of the individual and the environment.

ROLE AS AN ORGANIZER OF BEHAVIOR

The concept of role was brought into occupational therapy from the social sciences because it provides a means of explaining much of people's regulated behavior.[7] A role is a "position in society that contains a set of expected responsibilities and privileges" (p. 226).[3] Roles have two components: an internal component, pertaining to how the person experiences and acts on his or her roles, and an external component, consisting of ascribed status and expectations for behavior. The role is at once a status and a set of obligations necessary for the maintenance of some social group. For example, the role of a homemaker has classically been an important position necessary for the maintenance of the family. Roles are also a source of identity and a guide for behavior to the people in the roles. They provide avenues through which people can achieve a sense of competence. Thus, the role helps match the needs of the person to the needs of the social group.

The Internalized Role

The concept of internalized role refers to roles that have been incorporated into one's behavior and self-perception.[25] These internalized roles serve as a frame of reference for people as they act in everyday life, defining what and how they should perform. For example, people generally consider themselves to be in a worker role from 9 a.m. to 5 p.m. during the work week. At other times, they may perceive themselves to be in parent, spouse, volunteer, or other roles. This does not mean that they consciously categorize all their behavior and think specifically of being in a role at any given time. However, subtle perceptions of being in a role do shape ongoing personal experience. For example, many people put on a uniform to signal to themselves and others that they are assuming the worker role. When one comes home from work, a change of clothes may again signal a role change. Behavior also changes as one leaves one role for another; the manner in which one speaks to a spouse, a co-worker, and a child varies quite predictably around the expectations and functions of the respective roles.

Each person has a unique and sometimes changing perception of the requirements of any role. Newly married people often learn that each has different expectations of what they should do as spouses. A new worker often finds that his or her perceptions of what is required on the job must change to accommodate predetermined job requirements. Some people expect more of themselves than others do in a given role; other people expect too little and, thereby, are deemed incompetent in the role. Still others may have inappropriate ideas of what is required of them, causing problems in the social system to which the role belongs. Internalized expectations are thus seen as important determinants of how well a person performs in a given role.

People ordinarily assume several roles at any point in their lives. A child is typically a player, a family member, and a student. An adult may be a worker, spouse, parent, volunteer, and hobbyist. A person must be able to balance these roles and their demands as well as the opportunities they provide for satisfying experiences. Balance includes being able to fit role performance comfortably into one's schedule, having sufficient variety in the types of role activities one performs, and having sufficient roles to fill one's time meaningfully.

Organizing Effects of Role

The organizing effects of role derive from the fact that one's set of roles prescribe time use, normative guides for behavior, and standards of competency. Everyday use of time is, for the most part, structured by a succession of roles.[3,19] For instance, a working woman may find that her succession of roles includes being homemaker, worker, and homemaker again at the end of the day. In daily life, one may often perform two roles simultaneously and may interrupt one role to perform some duty belonging to another role.

Roles also carry with them unique expectations for behavior and demeanor. For instance, work roles may include expectations for how one dresses and talks, what attitudes one exhibits, and how one relates to peers, supervisors, and subordinates. Each role has its own ambience. For instance, some roles require formal behavior while others allow more freedom. The ability to discriminate these fine points of role requirements is important for successful role performance.

Finally, each role has a set of built-in requirements that set minimum standards for competence. Often, these are formalized in job descriptions or made explicit in orientations and other verbal exchanges. At other times, they may be negotiated, as when spouses decide how to share household duties. Failure to live up to these basic demands of the role constitutes role incompetence and invariably evokes negative reactions from others in the social system.

In summary, the roles one possesses organize behavior by determining how time will be used, by influencing subtle demeanor and attitudes, and by specifying what performances are expected. The degree to which roles actually exert this organizing influence is determined by how clear expectations are made in the environment, how accurately the individual has internalized them, and the process of negotiation and compromise that occurs when internalized and external expectations do not match.[15]

Role Careers and Socialization

The course of occupational development has been described as the occupational career.[3] It involves a series of role shifts that is partly socially determined and partly a matter of personal choice. For example, in our society a typical succession of roles over the life span is player, student, worker, and retiree. People are expected to make a transition from one role to the next at fairly specific ages. In some cases, there are even laws to enforce these role transitions (e.g., mandatory education and retirement)

Heard conceptualizes the process of acquiring new roles as an open system process.[15] The intake to the system is the expectations that go with a given role. At this stage, the person negotiates between his or her own expectations for a role and those of the external society that is setting the priorities. The next phase, throughput, occurs when a person begins to sift through and select alternatives for role behavior that suit the role demands. Output is the actual role behavior that the person produces. Through feedback, the person learns about the success of his or her performance in meeting role demands. This results in adjustments in role behavior to better meet role demands.

Through socialization, individuals learn what roles they are expected to assume and what they should do in these roles.[3] Socialization begins with the play of children. During this time, they observe many adult roles and begin to try them out. For example, dramatic play (e.g., playing house) gives the child a chance to see what it might be like to perform adult roles. Later, children find out they are expected to enter school and therein learn a whole new set of demands for performance. Concurrently, children experience an increase in expectations for contributing to their own self-maintenance and to the maintenance of the household through chores. This gradual process prepares the young person for entry into the more demanding roles of adult life.

Socialization does not cease once one has reached adulthood.[15] Each time a person changes jobs, enters into a new role through marriage, joins a church or social group, or becomes a volunteer, there is a period of socialization during which the person learns the particular expectations and requirements of the new role.

Transitions from role to role require reorganization on the part of the individual and can be adaptively challenging.[19] Major role transitions (e.g., from student to worker or from worker to retiree) place demands on the individual to reorganize the use of time in daily life. Often, the individual will be required to learn new skills and to reorganize habits of daily life to find new sources of identity and satisfaction.[25] On the other hand, past role success is viewed as a resource for current role adaptation. The history of role performance tends to influence a person's success in roles.[34]

The Range of Occupational Roles

When role theory was incorporated into occupational therapy, three major classes of roles were identified: personal-sexual, familial, and occupational. The latter were noted as the primary concern of occupational therapy.[34]

It now appears more accurate to suggest that an individual role (e.g., a spouse) might have both personal-sexual and occupational aspects. A spouse must not only relate affectively and sexually to a partner, but also perform certain tasks related to maintaining a common household. To view roles in this way would appear to preserve the intention of earlier writers—that is, to focus on roles that demand performance in life tasks—while providing a more accurate and complete way of describing roles within which a person can engage in occupational behaviors. Following this rationale, Oakley[37] developed the following taxonomy of occupational roles: participant in an organization, hobbiest/amateur, friend, family member, care-giver, home maintainer, student, religious participant, worker, and volunteer.

TEMPORAL ADAPTATION

The theme of time or temporal adaptation is one of the earliest and most central concepts of occupational therapy. Today, occupation is still generally defined in occupational therapy as one's use of time in productive and playful pursuits.

A conceptual framework of temporal adaptation was formulated by Kielhofner[19] as a means of viewing how people ordered their daily and developmental behavior. For human beings, the awareness and experience of time is a reality so fundamental that it influences and directs all action. Temporal adaptation is defined as the organization of daily life behavior on an ongoing basis. Two aspects of human temporality are stressed—the internal image of time and the organization of time use.

Internal Image of Time

Human beings have an internal image of time, a temporal framework shaped by the prevalent culture and personal experiences. Each culture carries with it definitions of time, values concerning time, and prescriptions for the use of time. For instance, Americans tend to view time as a finite commodity that they can compartmentalize and thus schedule, save or waste, spend or sell. This view and valuation of time leads most Americans to feel an obligation to profitably fill time with activity. Further, persons may be judged incompetent when they habitually waste or cannot manage time.

Socialization exposes people to the temporal framework of their culture. If they successfully incorporate cultural attitudes and prescriptions concerning time use, they will be better able to meet the demands of their social environments. Time perspective is also an individual matter. Childhood and later experiences result in a set of individual attitudes about time and a collection of images or rules for how to organize and use time. These rules range from simple learnings about how to sequence behaviors in time, to complex time management practices needed in adult life. Time perspective also includes one's view of self in time. Culturally derived norms specify how a person should progress in his or her lifetime (e.g., from player to student to worker), when such transitions should take place, and how a person should behave at a given age. People generally see themselves as progressing along a time continuum and thereby plan for the future. Future orientation and goals organize present action by placing demands on and setting priorities for how one uses time.

Interrelated with one's temporal perspective are the values and interests that people use as a guide to making decisions. Barring environmental and other constraints, people's healthy use of time reflects the activities that they find interesting or valuable. Thus, it can be seen that the temporal perspective of an individual is a complex network of images that guide how a person plans, organizes, and uses time in everyday life and over the life span.

Organization of Time Use

The second aspect of temporality is the organization of time use. There is a natural order to daily life represented in a balance of work, play, and self-maintenance.[19] This balance consists not only of adequate amounts of each behavioral domain in daily life, but also on the interdependence of each. Work success requires performance of self-maintenance activities such as hygiene and dressing. Play serves to refresh and energize the individual for work. Play is earned through the work of adulthood. Consequently, these behaviors exist in a dynamic balance necessary for healthy existence.[44]

In order to achieve an organization of time that reflects this adaptive balance, a person must develop a routine. The regulator of temporal organization is habit. Kielhofner notes that "habits are instantaneous automatic choices of action made throughout the day . . . organizing temporal behavior to meet societal requirements for competence" (p. 239).[19] Habits serve to organize a person's skills into regular sequences and to order them in the context of the day and week.[24,25] Habits (along with roles) maintain the output or behavior of a person, organizing behavior so that it fulfills both the demands of the external environment and the internal needs of the individual.[24] This is illustrated through the simple routine of activities of daily living. Getting up in the morning, bathing, and dressing may meet individual needs for a sense of orderliness and personal standards for acceptable hygiene and appearance, while meeting environmental expectations that one arrive at work on time and appear neatly dressed to fit the norms of the work setting. These activities occur quite automatically and within a coordinated routine for most people. The skills that are necessary for the motor and mental performances of self-care are organized by habits into a pattern. Thus, a habit functions as collections of performances organized into coherent wholes that serve the larger daily routine.

Habits are developed through a process of mechanization; that is, they become patterned through repetition in consistent environments.[24] Once mechanized, a habit functions as a cybernetic process with the built-in ability to adjust itself within certain parameters. Habits trigger automatic adjustments to allow accomplishment of a goal under varying conditions. As an example, the habit of driving to work allows one to arrive each day although traffic patterns and other factors may vary. Similarly, one can adjust the pace of morning activities of daily living to get to work on time even though one has overslept. Habits of meal preparation allow a homemaker to cook food while simultaneously giving children attention. Habits are like beacons that always return the person to the task at hand and allow it to flow in an organized manner even with a fair amount of variation.

Habits are able to guide behavior in this way because they possess a "canon of rules."[24] These rules, which are not conscious processes, constantly monitor action and make needed adjustments. Thus, the rules must contain information about the goal and about how action can be varied yet still maintain its goal-oriented character. Learned through trial and error, rules eventually become encoded and fade out of consciousness as one practices the behavior. A rough indicator of how much one is functioning in a habitual manner is the degree of attention that must be paid to what one is doing. We all routinely drive to work, dress ourselves, and clean house while engaging in fantasy, thinking about some other activity, or actually doing something else like carrying on a conversation. When we are not consciously in charge of our activities, our habits are.

Habits develop with input from the environment in terms of social expectations and feedback from one's behavior. When these habits no longer suffice to meet the demands of either the environment or the individual's values and roles, then the individual explores new patterns of behavior. As these innovations are adopted by the individual, they become integrated into his or her personal network of habits.[24]

PERSON-ENVIRONMENT INTERACTION

Early occupational therapists asserted that people with emotional problems had succumbed to their stressful environments and that restoration of function was a process of designing and exposing the patient to healthy environments. Modern occupational therapy writers have contributed to a more systematic understanding of how environments influence and shape behavior. Dunning[12] identified three environmental variables as having an important impact on behavior: space, people, and tasks. She notes that an individual's behavior is as much a function of these environmental characteristics as it is of the internal makeup of the individual.[12] Understanding order in the person thus involves understanding how the environment supports and elicits orderly behavior.

Space is a critical dimension of the environment, including both the amount and quality of space available, as well as the placement or arrangement of objects within space. These variables may determine the kinds of behaviors in which a person engages. For instance, a large environment may invite gross motor activity, whereas a smaller one may demand sedentary behavior.

Placement of objects in space can encourage or discourage interaction. People in the environment also use space in recognizable ways and influence others' use of space. Proxemics, or the way people place themselves in respect to each other, includes a culturally learned set of behaviors. For example, different physical distances between people are culturally recognized as appropriate for various types of interactions—thus, one generally stands farther away from a stranger than from an acquaintance and closer to an intimate friend.

The social environment comprises people, the roles they fill, and the network of relationships between them. The social environment therefore influences behavior through the organizing effects of roles, through the collective values of people in the environment, and through the unfilled roles left for newcomers.[1,16,18] Finally, the task environment, which includes demands for task performance, nonhuman objects and their expected patterns of use, and situations that stimulate task performance influences behavior.[1,12,38]

The interaction of humans as open systems with the physical and social environment suggests two stages: a choice or decision to enter a setting and a period of occupying or performing within a setting.[1]

Entering Environments

The decision to enter an environment is influenced by the environment's potential for arousal, interest, and value.[1] Optimal arousal, or excitement, is experienced as pleasurable; thus, environments that provide the right levels of arousal invite one's participation and entry. Three kinds of variables can evoke arousal: psychophysical variables, such as the intensity of color or sound; ecological variables, which refer to the significance of a stimuli to well-being; and collative variables, which are comparisons or discrepancies that arise in the environment or between the environment and the person. The latter category includes complexity, novelty, surprise, incongruity, and ambiguity. As these variables suggest, the impact of the environment is always a function of the person's internal makeup. What is arousing to one person may not be to another person or may not be at a later time when the environmental stimulus is no longer threatening or novel. When the environment provides correct amounts of stimulation, the individual will be motivated to enter, rather than avoid, an environmental setting.

In addition to embodying a potential for arousal, the environment has different capacities to evoke interest.[1] Objects and events within the environment may stimulate interest. Interest exists when the individual sees the potential for engaging in some behavior that he or she knows to be pleasurable or that appears to hold promise of yielding satisfaction. Obviously, different people find different settings more or less interesting.

Environments are also sources of different values.[1] Values can be communicated explicitly through verbal or written messages or implicitly through dress, attitudes, types of interactions, and so on. As with interests, settings tend to attract those people who find the environmental characteristics congruent with their own values. Occupational choice is strongly influenced by a person's tendency to see a match between the interests and values embodied by the occupational setting and his or her own interests and values.

It is critical that people enter settings based on choices motivated by arousal, interest, and value.[1] When people do not choose the settings they enter (e.g., when forced to relocate or to remain in a setting), they suffer adverse psychological and sometimes physical effects. Thus, the process of choosing the environments in which one behaves is important for health.

Interaction with the Environment

Once a person has made the decision to enter environments, the ensuing interaction tends to shape both the environment and the person. Press, population density, and objects are three variables that affect the quality and quantity of interaction.[1] *Press* refers to the demands that the environment places on the individual for behavior. Press may be physical (e.g., tennis courts and theaters invite different behaviors by virtue of their physical arrangement). Press can also be social, as when members in a setting encourage or demand certain behaviors of an individual who wishes to remain in the setting.

Population density affects behavior by determining the ratio of people to tasks in the environment. This characteristic is referred to as the "manning level" of an environment. Environments that are overmanned (too many people and too few tasks) offer less opportunity for active participation, whereas undermanned environments provide more opportunity and will draw people into more central and responsible roles.

Finally, the availability and quality of *objects* in the environment determine what kinds of interactions can take place. This has been demonstrated in studies of childhood play where different amounts and types of objects were shown to have effects on the duration and types of play behavior. Objects can influence behavior both through the potentials for action they represent and through the use-expectations they connote. An example of the latter is that a tricycle invites sitting and pedaling in order to locomote, and a magazine suggests reading. Some objects invite social participation, while others invite solitary activity. Some offer opportunity for prolonged but specific activity, whereas others are open to multiple kinds of behavior.

It was noted earlier that the impact of the environment is influenced by the person's internal makeup. Barris[1] refers to this as resonation; that is, the characteristics of person and environment interact to determine how the environment's qualities will influence the person.

In healthy people, the interaction with the environment involves a trajectory of increasing competency.[1] This means that as a person becomes more capable, he or she increasingly enters more and more environments, requires more stimuli for arousal, and can respond to greater environmental demands. Thus, the interaction between the person and the environment is a dynamic process involving a spiral of change.

OCCUPATIONAL PERFORMANCE COMPONENTS

Occupational therapy has always recognized that competent behavior requires the integrity of certain performance components. However, the ways in which performance components have been delineated has varied. These components, which can include such variables as cognitive functioning and motor performance, are sometimes equated with skills or abilities to accomplish tasks. At other times they are equated with the underlying constitutents of skills, for example, integrity of the nervous system.

A Taxonomy of Skills

Different collections of skills and their components have also been offered in the literature, however, no consistent conceptualization has emerged. Some authors offer a wide range of skills, including derivations from the psychoanalytic tradition[30,35] that are not relevant to occupation. To be consistent with the view of order and disorder that has been identified so far, occupational performance components should focus on the skills and their constituents that are necessary for and developed by occupation in everyday life.

More recent works identify the following as occupational performance components: sensory integration, motor function, cognitive function, psychological function, and social function.[8,36] This taxonomy is more relevant to occupational functioning and helps clarify the field's domain of concern.

A recent taxonomy attempts to differentiate between skills and their underlying constituents.[23] Three types of skills are identified as comprising occupational behavior: communication/interaction skills, process skills, and perceptual-motor skills. Communication/interaction skills are those skills employed when one interacts with others and engages in collaborative and competitive activities. Process skills are skills used for dealing with events and functions in everyday life. They involve planning, problem solving, and similar cognitive performances that organize action in time and space. Perceptual-motor skills refer to abilities to interpret sensory data and move one's body in response to and in order to act on the environment. Perceptual-motor skills range from simple perceptions and movements to complicated tool use abilities. These three areas of skill are intended to delineate the ways in which persons act on their environment and the people, events, and objects within it.

Skills are defined as sets of subroutines or constituents that are organized together and achieve some end under varying conditions.[25,33,41,42,51] Thus, skills are flexible routines of behavior that can respond to environmental variation. They are guided by a purpose or intention, and they involve the organized contributions of subroutines or constituents. The fact that skills are guided by intentions links them to the decision-making and intrinsic motivation characteristics of humans. Humans intend action and its consequences when they choose to act for the pursuit of an interest, value, or goal. In this way, skilled action is always purposeful.

Constituents of Skills

The other dimension of this taxonomy concerns the constituents of skills. Three constituents of skill—symbolic, neurological, and kinesiological—make up a hierarchy with the symbolic as the highest level and the kinesiological as the lowest level.[23] Symbolic constituents of skills refer to the internal images that coordinate and interpret incoming sensory information; formulate internal ideas, intentions and plans of action; and trigger and guide nervous system activity.[22] These symbols are internal maps of external reality that inform the individual about the potential for and the constraints on action.[41,42] Images for how to perform skilled action are generated through experience. Human beings are endowed with very few skills at birth, and they must engage in a long period of activity or doing (an open system process) to generate the symbols that eventually serve as throughput in the human open system. The symbols one has acquired serve as internal guides to interpreting intake and formulating output. Thus, they are critical for all kinds of performance. Images are initially conscious and later become automatic. For instance, in first learning to walk or ride a bicycle, a person must consciously concentrate on the intended performance and the coordination of actions. Once mastered, the activity is accomplished automatically, guided by images that are out of awareness. The same process of conscious learning becoming automatic takes place in both process and communication/interaction skills. Such experiences as learning the rules in a new game or learning to display proper manners in a social gathering are examples of how all skills begin as conscious processes and eventually become automatic.

The neurological constituent of skills is the nervous system and its processes. The nervous system is the infrastructure of the symbolic component.[22] Since the neurological constituent is below the symbolic component in the hierarchy of human function, it is organized by and constrains the symbolic processes.

If the brain is traumatized or lacks proper integration, it limits the symbols that can be learned.[28] By the same token, the brain depends on the formulation of images from experience to guide its process of integrated and coordinated action. The two are thus mutually dependent and influence each other in reciprocal ways.

The musculoskeletal constituent includes the anatomical structures and processes involved in movement. Order in the human being requires the coordinated interface of all three constituents and their integration into various skills. The performance of any skill (interaction/communication, perceptual-motor, or process) generally involves an interplay of all three. For instance, communication involves the symbols that underlie language production as well as the neurological commands that evoke motor behavior for talking and gesturing. Similarly, process skills, such as the ability to bake a cake, call on symbolic constituents for the image of how to sequence steps and on the neurological and musculoskeletal constituents for the perceptions and coordinated movements required.

SUMMARY

Human Beings as Open Systems

Open system concepts are aimed at recognizing the complexity of human beings rather than viewing them as simple machines.

Open systems are self-maintaining and self-changing because of a cycle that involves:

1. intake, or the importation of energy and information from the environment;
2. throughput, or the transformation of energy and information into another form and its incorporation in the system's structure and processes;
3. output, or the behavior of the system; and
4. feedback, or information on the process or consequences of output.

Open systems exhibit a primacy of function over structure; that is, the structures of open systems are secondary to and are maintained by underlying processes.

Primacy of function of structure is embodied in the notion that open systems become what they do.

Open systems consist of heirarchically arranged parts. In human behavior the following simple hierarchy is found:

1. the social system
2. the symbolic system (conscious processes)
3. the nervous system (i.e., brain)

4. the musculoskeletal system

In this hierarchy the highest level—social system—governs the symbolic system, the symbolic governs the nervous system, and so forth. Conversely, the lower level systems constrain the higher ones.

The occupational behavior (play and work) of the human being simultaneously calls into play each of these levels and collates them into an organized gestalt.

Intrinsic Motivation

In contrast to motives that lead the organism to seek homeostasis (e.g., hunger), occupation is motivated by a drive for activity.

The motive for occupation is referred to as intrinsic because it proposes that occupation is engaged in for its own sake rather than for extrinsic or secondary rewards.

Intrinsic motivation is the basic drive leading to growth and change in the person.

Intrinsic motivation begins with the exploratory drive of children, transforms developmentally into a competence urge, and finally into a need for achievement.

Actions based on intrinsic motives generate feelings of competence or effectiveness that support and augment it.

Humans as Decision Makers

Human beings are decision makers who must take personal control and determine their own life courses.

Decision making in human life, as it pertains to occupation, is influenced by interests and values, which give meaning to various occupations.

Interests:
- are affective phenomena; they are predispositions to find various objects and occupations pleasurable;
- are influenced by family socialization and social approval;
- reflect an individual's self-perceptions;
- guide choices for action and maintain persistence in action.

Values:
- reflect the individual's cultural background;
- are learned through socialization;
- determined internal priorities of action and lead to the formation of goals;
- specify what is good, right, or important and determine the meaningfulness of many activities;

- have a strong affective component—that is, they carry a sense of obligation and provide a sense of belonging to a group.

Occupational Choice:

- is the major developmental process of decision making relevant to occupation;
- occurs from childhood to early adulthood in series of fantasy, tentative, and realistic periods;
- is a process of optimizing one's inner desires and abilities against a background of environmental supports and constraints.

Role as an Organizer of Behavior

Roles are positions in society that have both status and expectations for performance.

Roles have an internal component of self-experience and an external component of social status and behavior expectations.

The internalized role is incorporated into the person's self-concept and serves as a framework for action; it includes:

1. perceived incumbency, or the belief that one is in the role;
2. internalized expectations, or the perception of the expected behaviors that go with a personal role;
3. role balance, or the healthy integration of roles.

Roles organize behavior by prescribing time use, norms for behavior, and standards of competency.

Occupational development involves a succession of roles referred to as the occupational career.

Role acquisition is a complex open system process involving an input of expectancies for performance, a throughput process of selecting priorities for role behavior, and an output of role behavior, followed by feedback, which shapes the person toward meeting role demands.

Movement through a succession of roles is guided by socialization or the process of social expectations coming to influence behavior and identity.

Occupational roles were originally identified as work and play roles but have been expanded to include the following roles, which have productive and active aspects:

- participant in an organization
- hobbiest/amateur
- friend
- family member

- care giver
- home maintainer
- student
- religious participant
- worker
- volunteer

Temporal Adaptation

Awareness and experience of time influences and directs all of human actions.

Humans have an internal awareness of time shaped by the culture and by development and socialization processes.

Human adaptation involves a natural order of daily life as reflected in a balance of work, play, and self-maintenance.

Habit is the critical regulator of human temporal organization.

Habits:
- organize skills into coherent wholes for the routine performance of daily behaviors;
- are developed through a process of mechanization whereby they become more consolidated over time through practice;
- are cybernetic functions that self-regulate once they are triggered into action; the canon of rules in the habit guides it toward the achievement of routine performances and allows it to use feedback to guide behaviors.

Person-Environment Interaction

Environments influence and shape behavior through:
- the placement of objects and people in space and the available space;
- the social network;
- the task demands for performance.

Entering environments is influenced by:
- the degree of stimulation or arousal provided by psychophysical, collative, and ecological variables;
- the values inherent in the environment.

Interaction with the environment is affected by:
- press, or the demands that the environment places on the person to behave;
- population density or the ratio of people to tasks;
- availability and quality of objects in the environment.

The environment's influence on behavior and its ability to affect entry and interaction depend on how environmental characteristics interact with internal characteristics of the person.

Occupational Performance Components

Competent behavior requires the integrity of performance components.

Components can include motor, cognitive, psychological, and social aspects and generally refer either to skills or their constituents.

Skill is a set of subroutines or constituents that are organized together to achieve some intended end under varying conditions.

A taxonomy of skills is offered:
- communication/interaction skills or skills for acting with others;
- process skills or skills for dealing with events (e.g., problem solving and planning);
- motor skills or skills for moving self and objects.

Constitutents of skills are:
- symbolic, or the images that serve as an internal map for acting on and in the world;
- neurological;
- musculoskeletal.

REFERENCES

1. Barris, R. Environmental interactions: An extension of the model of human occupation. *American Journal of Occupational Therapy*, 1982, *36*, 637–644.
2. Black, M. Adolescent role assessment. *American Journal of Occupational Therapy*, 1976, *30*, 73–79.
3. Black, M. The occupational career. *American Journal of Occupational Therapy*, 1976, *30*, 225–228.
4. Borys, S. Implications of interest theory for occupational therapy. *American Journal of Occupational Therapy*, 1974, *28*, 35–38.
5. Boulding, K. General systems theory—The skeleton of science. *General Systems Yearbook*, 1956, *1*, 11–17.
6. Burke, J. P. A clinical perspective on motivation: Pawn versus origin. *American Journal of Occupational Therapy*, 1977, *31*, 254–258.
7. Burke, J. P. Defining occupation: Importing and organizing interdisciplinary knowledge. In G. Kielhofner (Ed.), *Health through occupation: Therapy and practice in occupational therapy*. Philadelphia: F. A. Davis, 1983.
8. Clark, P. N. Human development through occupation: Theoretical frameworks in contemporary occupational therapy practice. Part I. *American Journal of Occupational Therapy*, 1979, *33*, 505–514.

9. Cynkin, S. *Occupational therapy: Toward health through activities*. Boston: Little, Brown, 1979.

10. deRenne-Stephan, C. Imitation: A mechanism of play behavior. *American Journal of Occupational Therapy*, 1980, *34*, 95–102.

11. Diasio, K. Psychiatric occupational therapy: Search for a conceptual framework in light of psychoanalytic ego psychology and learning theory. *American Journal of Occupational Therapy*, 1968, *22*, 400–414.

12. Dunning, H. Environmental occupational therapy. *American Journal of Occupational Therapy*, 1972, *26*, 292–298.

13. Fidler, G., & Fidler, J. Doing and becoming: Purposeful action and self-actualization. *American Journal of Occupational Therapy*, 1978, *32*, 305–310.

14. Florey, L. Intrinsic motivation: The dynamics of occupational therapy. *American Journal of Occupational Therapy*, 1969, *23*, 319–322.

15. Heard, C. Occupational role acquisition: A perspective on the chronically disabled. *American Journal of Occupational Therapy*, 1977, *31*, 243–247.

16. Howe, M., & Briggs, A. Ecological systems model for occupational therapy. *American Journal of Occupational Therapy*, 1982, *36*, 322–327.

17. Johnson, J. A. Consideration of work as therapy in the rehabilitation process. *American Journal of Occupational Therapy*, 1971, *25*, 303–308.

18. Kannegieter, R. Environmental interactions in psychiatric occupational therapy—Some inferences. *American Journal of Occupational Therapy*, 1980, *34*, 715–720.

19. Kielhofner, G. Temporal adaptation: A conceptual framework for occupational therapy. *American Journal of Occupational Therapy*, 1977, *31*, 235–238.

20. Kielhofner, G. General systems therapy: Implications for theory and action in occupational therapy. *American Journal of Occupational Therapy*, 1978, *32*, 637–645.

21. Kielhofner, G. A heritage of activity: Development of theory. *American Journal of Occupational Therapy*, 1982, *36*, 723–730.

22. Kielhofner, G. A paradigm for practice: The hierarchical organization of occupational therapy knowledge. In G. Kielhofner (Ed.), *Health through occupation: Theory and practice in occupational therapy*. Philadelphia: F. A. Davis, 1983.

23. Kielhofner, G., & Barris, R. *Measuring variables in the model of human occupation*. Paper presented at the American Occupational Therapy Association Annual Conference, Philadelphia, 1982.

24. Kielhofner, G., Barris, R., & Watts, J. Habits and habit dysfunction: A clinical perspective for psychosocial occupational therapy. *Occupational Therapy in Mental Health*, 1982, *2*, 1–22.

25. Kielhofner, G., & Burke, J. P. A model of human occupation, Part I. Conceptual framework and content. *American Journal of Occupational Therapy*, 1980, *34*, 572–581.

26. Kielhofner, G., & Miyake, S. The therapeutic use of games with mentally retarded adults. *American Journal of Occupational Therapy*, 1981, *35*, 375–382.

27. Klavins, R. Work-play behavior: Cultural influences. *American Journal of Occupational Therapy*, 1972, *26*, 176–179.

28. Lindquist, J., Mack, W., & Parham, D. A synthesis of occupational behavior and sensory integrative concepts in theory and practice, Part 1. Theoretical foundations. *American Journal of Occupational Therapy*, 1982, *36*, 365–374.

29. Lindquist, J., Mack, W., & Parham, D. A synthesis of occupational behavior and sensory integration concepts in theory and practice, Part 2. Clinical applications. *American Journal of Occupational Therapy*, 1982, *36*, 433–437.

30. Llorens, L. Facilitating growth and development: The promise of occupational therapy. *American Journal of Occupational Therapy*, 1970, *24*, 93–101.

31. Matsutsuyu, J. S. The interest checklist. *American Journal of Occupational Therapy*, 1969, *23*, 323–328.

32. Matsutsuyu, J. Occupational behavior—A perspective on work and play. *American Journal of Occupational Therapy*, 1971, *25*, 291–294.

33. Michelman, S. The importance of creative play. *American Journal of Occupational Therapy*, 1972.

34. Moorehead, L. The occupational history. *American Journal of Occupational Therapy*, 1969, *23*, 329–334.

35. Mosey, A. Recapitulation of ontogenesis: A theory for practice of occupational therapy. *American Journal of Occupational Therapy*, 1968, *22*, 426–438.

36. Mosey, A. A model for occupational therapy. *Occupational Therapy in Mental Health*, 1980, *1*, 11–31.

37. Oakley, F. M. *The model of human occupation in psychiatry*. Unpublished master's project, Department of Occupational Therapy, Virginia Commonwealth University, 1982.

38. Parent, L. Effects of a low-stimulus environment on behavior. *American Journal of Occupational Therapy*, 1978, *32*, 19–25.

39. Paulson, C. Juvenile delinquency and occupational choice. *American Journal of Occupational Therapy*, 1980, *34*, 565–571.

40. Reilly, M. Occupational therapy can be one of the great ideas of 20th century medicine. *American Journal of Occupational Therapy*, 1966, *20*, 61–67.

41. Reilly, M. *Play as exploratory learning*. Beverly Hills, Calif.: Sage Publications, 1974.
42. Robinson, A. Play: The arena for acquisition of rules for competent behavior. *American Journal of Occupational Therapy*, 1977, *31*, 248–253.
43. Rogers, J. Order and disorder in medicine and occupational therapy. *American Journal of Occupational Therapy*, 1982, *36*, 29–35.
44. Shannon, P. The work-play model: A basis for occupational therapy programming in psychiatry. *American Journal of Occupational Therapy*, 1970, *24*, 215–218.
45. Shannon, P. D. The adolescent experience. *American Journal of Occupational Therapy*, 1972, *26*, 284–287.
46. Shannon, P. Work-play therapy and the occupational therapy process. *American Journal of Occupational Therapy*, 1972, *26*, 169–172.
47. Smith, M. B. Competence and adaptation. *American Journal of Occupational Therapy*, 1974, *28*, 11–15.
48. Task Force on Target Populations. Report I. *American Journal of Occupational Therapy*, 1974, *28*, 158–163.
49. Vandenberg, B., & Kielhofner, G. Play in evolution, culture and individual adaptation: Implications for therapy. *American Journal of Occupational Therapy*, 1982, *36*, 20–28.
50. von Bertalanffy, L. General system theory and psychiatry. In S. Arietti (Ed.), *American handbook of psychiatry* (Vol. 3). New York: Basic Books, 1969.
51. Watanabe, S. Four concepts basic to the occupational therapy process. *American Journal of Occupational Therapy*, 1968, *22*, 339–444.
52. Webster, P. Occupational role development in the young adult with mild mental retardation. *American Journal of Occupational Therapy*, 1980, *34*, 13–18.

14
The View of Disorder in Occupational Therapy

In occupational therapy order is viewed as the ability to engage in a healthy pattern of occupational behavior; therefore, disorder is recognized when a person does not have such occupational behavior.[43] Two conditions have been proposed as criteria for a lack of healthy occupational behavior.[21] First, if people do not satisfy their urges to explore and master the world in everyday occupation, a dysfunction is recognized. Second, disorder is seen where people cannot meet the requirements of the external world. Healthy occupational behavior represents a balance between inner needs and external requirements. When either or both are not met, disorder is present.

A number of factors may contribute or relate to dysfunctional occupational behavior. For example, people may fail to find meaning or purpose in their work and play; they may lack the performance components necessary for competent behavior; they may have poor habits or values at conflict with society; they may have failed to develop interests or a feeling of personal causation; or they may fail to fulfill role requirements. The source of such problems may be past experiences, poor socialization, environmental stress, or organic factors that affect performance components. In some cases, clinical pathology may have precipitated or contributed to the occupational dysfunction. For example, organic involvement or intellectual limitations may lead to difficulties in occupational performance. The occupational dysfunction may also precipitate a clinical pathology. For example, reactive depressions may have much of their etiology in an imbalanced or purposeless life-style or in the loss of an occupational role. In other cases, it is difficult if not impossible to separate medically defined pathology from the kind of disorder that occupational therapy recognizes. For instance, the schizophrenic person exhibits pathological symptoms such as hallucinations and extreme anxiety and at the same time may show a dearth of interests, poorly formed or contradictory values, a lack of life goals, and disruption of many occupational performance components.

Occupational therapists require a system for classifying dysfunctions of occupational behavior.[22,38,43] Therapists in psychosocial practice typically find that the medical diagnosis gives them some information that is useful to consider in their therapy, but it tells only a limited amount about the status of occupational behavior. Thus, it becomes necessary for the occupational therapist to collect and interpret data that help define occupational dysfunction in a given client. Without a classification system, the data cannot be used to arrive at a delineation of the problem in universal occupational therapy terms.

The present discussion of occupational disorder parallels the categories used to describe order in the previous chapter. Such categories may be a helpful beginning to therapists who want to order their observations of dysfunction and begin to label them in a way that reflects the occupational therapy focus and concern in psychosocial practice.

OPEN SYSTEM DYSFUNCTION

The open system maintains and changes itself through a cycle in which the output or action of the system yields feedback into the cycle. Dysfunction in the open system occurs when the basic cycle is interrupted, especially when the action or output of the system demonstrates extremes of activity or inactivity.

In early occupational therapy, central problems in psychosocial dysfunction were identified as idleness and unbalanced behavior. In open system concepts, idleness is a cessation of the basic cycle of the open system.

The Fidlers[13] summarize this perspective in the statement, "A reduction in doing generates pathology" (p. 309). For example, when "action does not follow thought, perception is distorted and the critical learning that comes from confronting the consequences of an act is precluded" (p. 309).[13] Such a condition is parallel to the dissociation of feeling, thinking, and acting in people with schizophrenia. The passive, sedentary life-style of many people may contribute to a breakdown of perceptual-motor and psychological skills. Common problems of those with psychosocial dysfunction—the failure to differentiate reality from fantasy, the breakdown of mechanized patterns of behavior (habits), and the loss of control over one's decision making—are all examples of such system breakdown. Interaction of the system with its environment results in a trajectory of change that can support or threaten adaptation. Maladaptive cycles occur when the system's action is somehow interrupted or disturbed, resulting in a cessation of positive feedback. This negatively influences the person's own internal organization of throughput, further disrupting output. If the maladaptive cycle continues, the result can be total regression.

Insufficient output of the system, as play or work, precludes opportunities for learning the rules of socially competent behavior. A child who does not play may not learn how to engage in role behavior, may not develop physical or social skills, and may not proceed through the fantasy and exploration stages necessary to developing an occupational identity.[32,40,42] For adults, work is both a source of self-esteem and a means of fulfilling the requirements of society. Those who do not work in some fashion are at risk of devaluing themselves and being devalued by society.[5,22]

Further, because work organizes one's time in adult life, loss of the work role may promote disorganization of everyday behavior. For instance, at retirement, people may suddenly be left without a major life activity to organize their daily routine, and they may develop psychosocial problems. Because occupation is critical to the maintenance of health and function, a lack or distortion of everyday occupational behavior is a serious component, if not an etiological factor, in psychosocial problems.

DISRUPTION OF INTRINSIC MOTIVATION

The urge to explore and master the environment ordinarily leads to involvement is a succession of lifelong occupations in which the individual achieves success and satisfaction. The person who encounters failures may develop doubts about the efficacy of his or her skills and begin to feel controlled by external factors.[7] Without feelings of efficacy, individuals find it difficult to maintain morale or commitment to their occupations. This breakdown of confidence can lead to the kind of maladaptive cycle described in the previous section.

The literature on people who are mentally ill or mentally retarded reveals that feelings of external control, a sense of helplessness, lack of confidence, and belief that one is not an effective cause are common among these populations.[18,35] Such learned helplessness can also be a concomitant of maladaptive aging,[48] or may be induced through the denial of decision-making opportunities that can occur in institutions.[30,39] Individuals who do not believe they can control their lives or perform competently do not enact their urge to explore and master.

When people cannot act on a fundamental drive for exploration and mastery, they experience pain just as they do when their needs for affection are unmet. Further, a poor self-image or belief in helplessness is a source of suffering.

DYSFUNCTION OF DECISION-MAKING CAPACITY

Values and interests influence how one acts on the urge to explore and master by directing decision making. When people engage in activities that conform to their value system, they experience greater life satisfaction. People with psychosocial dysfunction may often value the same things as members of the mainstream culture but find themselves unable to pursue those values because of internal or environmental constraints.[18,20] When this happens, they may experience stress and despair.

In addition to discrepancies between values and action, people may experience a conflict within their own value system. These discrepancies may lead to problems of inaction or faulty decisions. For instance, a young man experienced a series of emotional breakdowns precipitated by his return to college after successful periods of maintaining a job as a laborer. An occupational history revealed a discrepancy between his own valuation and enjoyment of physical labor and his internalization of his parents' valuing of higher education. Basing his decision to return to college on a value system that conflicted with his own caused excessive stress, and the decision to return to school inevitably ended in a series of failures and hospitalization.

People ordinarily experience meaning in their work and play activities.[11] Psychiatric patients, however, often exhibit a sense of meaninglessness in their lives.[35] They do not find satisfaction, worth, and other values in their work and play. When people cease to experience meaning in their lives, they become immobilized and incapable of making decisions. Such people are unable to find meaning in, for example, the cultural celebrations of holidays and in the world of everyday work. Modern trends such as passive consumer-based leisure and the increasing standardization and compartmentalization of work tend to further rob the individual of access to meaningful occupations[22,51] and, thus, contribute to dysfunctional decision making.

Interests are also important determinants of choices for action. An individual's anticipation of satisfaction in certain occupations and the internal priority of these likes and dislikes leads the person to action. Factors of economics, paucity of experiences, and impoverished environments may suppress the development of interests in special groups such as retarded persons;[18,20] in turn, the lack of interests can then lead to the inability to structure time in a meaningful way.

People who are unable to identify interests and values frequently manifest difficulty in making a commitment to a form of life work.[16,33,37] Since the occupational choice process is critical for the adult's ability to competently perform in and gain satisfaction from fulfilling life roles, a delay or failure in occupational choice often leads to entry into a role by default or through external manipulation by family, professionals, or others. In such cases, the person's chances of a successful occupational career are significantly lessened. People in occupations or vocational experiences they did not choose for themselves are often unable to perform and thus develop a sense of failure that further impedes their smooth transition to an occupational role.[50]

ROLE DYSFUNCTION

Role dysfunction may occur either when personal needs are unmet in a role or when others find the person's performance in a role to be deficient.[21] Further, a "loss of or change in valued personal roles can result in role disorders" (p. 610).[47] Such disorders, which may be precipitated by mental or physical impairment, are more disabling than the original pathological condition that led to the role disorder.[21,47] Psychosocially dysfunctional people are commonly denied access to normal life roles and are cast in deviant or "sick" roles.[8,18,35] Often the roles that are available to them do not provide a sufficient outlet for capacity and interest. Further, because such roles are not valued by society, they are not a source of self-esteem.

People are judged mentally ill when they cannot perform their life roles.[5] Failure to perform life roles is often influenced by poor earlier experiences in which the person has acquired an inadequate sense of what is required for a role or has not learned how to engage in reciprocal role behaviors. Poor role performance can have a cumulative effect, eroding a person's confidence.[33] This is especially true where earlier roles serve as preparation for later roles. For example, the child who is a poor player may be more likely to become a poor student and worker.[21,42]

Periods of role change and role loss are times of risk for role disorders.[19,47] Role changes may require that a person develop new skills, organize time differently, and actualize new values and a new sense of self. People who were competent or marginally competent in a role may become maladaptive when role change occurs, as in the transition from student to worker and worker to retiree. The loss of a life role, naturally or traumatically, may also lead to role dysfunction if the individual is unable to replace it with another role. Role loss may occur naturally, as when children leave the home and the parent role ends, or it may be precipitated by disease. Role dysfunctions may occur when people have entered roles that do not sufficiently match their capacities, interests, and values. A clinical example is a schizophrenic woman who entered the homemaker role primarily out of a sense of obligation but did not feel well prepared for this role and did not find it satisfying and interesting. Many of her difficulties in daily performance stemmed from her inability to competently perform the role and from her lack of another life role to provide a balance in her life (i.e., a role that would embody her interests and allow her to perform skills that she had that were more highly developed).[25]

Role dysfunctions may occur when people find themselves in too many roles, or in roles that compete for their time or loyalty or otherwise create disharmony. Such role conflict or role strain can lead to feelings of loss of control, dissatisfaction, and inadequate performance. Most people manage to negotiate and balance role performance in the relevant social systems and to develop schedules of healthy role behavior. However, some people, under the stress of conflicting role expectations, may develop psychosocial problems. A typical example of this is the person who feels that he or she must excel in a professional worker role while continuing to be a model spouse, parent, and homemaker and while maintaining multiple role commitments in neighborhood and community groups. Such people may develop a sense of not performing adequately in any role and experience a lowered self-esteem and feelings of loss of control.

TEMPORAL DYSFUNCTION

Dysfunction of both temporal perspective and temporal organization have been identified in occupational therapy. In some instances, psychosocial pathology may result in a distortion or limitation of temporal perspective. Mental retardation, organic brain lesions, and a diagnosis of schizophrenia have been associated with the inability to perceive and conceive of time.[20,34] Temporal dysfunction among people with psychosocial disorders is primarily a matter of poor socialization, poor learning, and impoverished or deviant life experiences. People who are mentally ill often have a decreased sense of future linked to a sense of hopelessness and associated with lowered present functioning.[34,34] Unlike most cultural members who view themselves as progressing along a temporal continuum, people who are retarded may find themselves either frozen in time or moving backwards to a less satisfying life-style.[20] Lack of success in life careers, overall inactivity, and a dependent status give little reason for or interest in the future.[18,20]

Temporal disorganization is also a typical problem for people with psychosocial dysfunction. Mentally ill patients may demonstrate chaotic patterns of time use, be unable to describe typical days, and be unable to manage their time.[34] Such patients may have failed to develop habits to organize their time use.[19,24]

Another area of temporal dysfunction is the imbalance of life spaces in one's time use.[19,44] People who fail to have either sufficient work or play in their schedules may experience psychosocial problems. Without adequate play, the individual is not relieved from the stress of work and given an opportunity to approach and participate in the cultural value system through celebration and ritual. This may lead to problems of burn-out, alienation, and depression.

How one views time and organizes one's behavior in time is a critical component of adaptation. People whose temporal perspectives and practices do not provide personal satisfaction and meaning or that do not satisfy societal requirements should be recognized as being in a state of temporal dysfunction.

DISORDER IN ENVIRONMENTAL INTERACTIONS

Occupational therapists are concerned with the impact of institutional settings, such as the hospital, as well as community settings on occupational behavior. Hospitalization may contribute to dysfunctional skills and roles, to decreased feelings of personal causation, to a loss of interests, and to disorder in decision making.[14,35,39] The hospital may contribute to the atrophy of work and play skills if the patient is not given an opportunity to practice these skills. In addition, skills that are developed or practiced in a restricted setting such as an institution may become rigidly and inflexibly applied in all situations.[3,23]

A mismatch between an individual's abilities and the demands of the setting will also contribute to maladaptive performance.[3] This mismatch may occur because the environment requires a level of competence that the person does not have, or because the setting demands too little of the person. In either case, the person's affect and performance will be dysfunctional.

Finally, the physical environment, through such factors as the arrangement of chairs, restrictions on activities, or placement of televisions in day rooms, may provide few opportunities for social interaction. Consequently, what is communicated is an expectation for maladaptive behavior rather than for the development of functional occupational behavior.[3]

Other factors that may contribute to a deterioration of role and habit performance include lack of opportunity for patients to engage in work, play, and self-maintenance activities; the lack of appropriate role models, unavailability of suitable peers; disruption from former roles; and lack of sufficient stimulation to perform.[3,14,36,39] Frequently patients are in overmanned situations; that is, there are too few tasks for the number of patients. When this is complicated by the fact that patients' activities may be viewed as inconsequential, patients may feel little or no pressure to perform.[3]

Individual decision making is frequently circumscribed by institutional settings, leading to learned helplessness and decreased feelings of personal causation. The long-term effect of this denial of personal decision making may be increased mortality rates.[15,30,41] Personal causation may be additionally affected by institutions because of their inability to satisfy needs related to the self-esteem of residents.[17,46]

Community settings can also foster dependent behavior, afford little opportunity for decision making, discourage activity and interaction, and lack objects and people that can be resources to residents for work and play activities.[27] Different types of environments have been found to have differential effects on the competence of retarded adults. For example, less structured environments, such as recreation settings, may provide more opportunity for retarded people to assume responsible roles, whereas more structured environments, such as the sheltered workshop, may limit their exercise of capacity.[18]

A study of the environments of mentally ill people found that psychiatric outpatients generally did not choose their residences and that they lived in protected environments characterized by a high degree of conflict. Further, their families were ordinarily not sources of support and affiliation, and economic limitations and personal acquiescence tended to make them vulnerable to environmental conditions.[12]

Environmental variables affecting all types of people with psychosocial disorder are stigma and decreased expectations for performance. Both professionals and others have a tendency to expect trouble and substandard performance from the psychosocially dysfunctional person. These altered expectations often serve as disincentives for normal performance. They communicate that other people lack confidence in the person's ability to perform. The types of performances expected of psychosocially dysfunctional people may be a further source of problems. When tasks are trivial, unstimulating, and undemanding, people are not challenged by their environment. The failure to require behavior of which a person is capable is an important variable in limiting that person's competence. Ultimately, "When a life space is . . . restricted there develops little mastery over one's environment and control over one's life situation" (p. 439).[49]

DISORDERS OF PERFORMANCE COMPONENTS

The most common observation made of those with psychosocial dysfunction is that they lack appropriate skills for interacting with others. Interpersonal relations have long been the major focus of mental health. Occupational therapists are concerned primarily with how inabilities or problems of interacting with others lead to failure or disruption of one's work and play. For instance, Bailey[2] suggests that the primary difficulty of psychiatric patients in work role performance is their inability to produce the social behaviors and interactions that are required as part of job performance. Relating to peers, supervisors, and subordinates, making small talk, and knowing how to dress are types of behaviors that can cause trouble in the work setting. Similarly, retarded people often lack understanding of simple social behaviors, such as taking turns, and they often lack the social skills needed for negotiating interactions in the community.[26]

Both mentally ill and retarded people have also been observed to have deficits in such process skills as problem solving, planning, anticipating consequences, organizing objects in space and sequencing behaviors. Problems in these areas may be exacerbated by impoverished opportunities for learning and by atrophy of skills during periods of disuse (e.g., when people are institutionalized).

Problems in perceptual-motor performance have also been noted among those with psychosocial disorders. Many retarded people have perceptual-motor incapacity associated with brain damage, or more subtle neurological problems such as sensory integrative dysfunctions.[1,28]

Skill deficits are ordinarily accompanied by deficiencies or dysfunctions in the underlying symbolic, neurological, and musculoskeletal constituents. In psychosocial dysfunction the major problems are found in the first of these constituents. Symbols or images underlie all skills, from the simplest motor acts through sophisticated social interactions.[31,40,42] They are internalized maps for how to act in the external world. When the individual has poor play, foiling life experiences, or inadequate socialization, the process of symbol formation may be adversely affected. For example, retarded children may not have learned the images of motion needed for game behavior, adults with psychosocial disorder may have learned inadequate rules of social interaction, and delinquent adolescents may lack acceptable rules for moral conduct.[9,26]

Dysfunction in the neurological component may be structural, such as a chemical imbalance or lesion, or it may be a processing disorder. Occupational therapists have been particularly concerned with the latter since the work of Ayres concerning sensory integrative dysfunction in learning disabled children.[1] Interest in this constituent of performance has grown with King's[28] application to adult schizophrenics. Abnormal postural and movement patterns in chronic schizophrenics are seen as possibly indicating underlying neurological disorder and as a possible manifestation of the inactivity of chronically ill people, especially those who are institutionalized.[4,28,29] Given the hierarchical and open system nature of constituents of performance, it is probable that many factors are involved in the musculoskeletal and motor manifestations found in this group. Occupational therapists have also explored the relationship of sensory integrative dysfunction to retarded people.[6,10,45] Again, the possible contributions of inactivity cannot be discounted as an important potential cause and as a covariate of any neurological dysfunction.

The particular areas of skill dysfunction or of deficits in constituents of skills will, of course, vary with the particular kind of psychosocial dysfunction. Additionally, dysfunction in performance components may or may not be a part of psychosocial dysfunction in a given patient or client. Therapists must avoid focusing only on the performance components and/or their constituents

226 PSYCHOSOCIAL OCCUPATIONAL THERAPY

while ignoring other potential problems such as decision-making deficits, temporal dysfunction, and role disorder.

SUMMARY

Open System Dysfunction

Dysfunction occurs in the open system when the basic cycle is disrupted by a reduction or cessation of doing (output).

A lack or reduction of doing can result in:
- breakdown of perceptual-motor and psychological skills;
- disturbance of self-image;
- failure to differentiate reality from fantasy;
- breakdown of habits;
- loss of control over decision making.

When the action of the system (output) ceases or is reduced, feedback becomes negative or stops and throughput is disturbed, leading to a cycle that results in maladaptation and regression.

When play is disrupted, the symbols that guide competent action are not generated.

When work is disrupted, self-esteem and social approval for productivity are negatively affected.

Disruption of Intrinsic Motivation

Failures of performance can lead to feelings and images of self as controlled by external factors, without efficacy, and of the future as hopeless.

Negative feelings and images concerning personal effectiveness thwart the urge to explore and master.

Suffering occurs when people do not operationalize their urge to explore and master and when they feel helpless.

Dysfunction of Decision-Making Capacity

People with psychosocial dysfunction may:
- hold mainstream values but find themselves unable to fulfill them;
- have value conflicts (i.e., hold inconsistent values) and oscillate in their decision making;
- fail to find meaning in their work and play and thus become immobilized.

People with psychosocial dysfunction may have deficit discrimination and pursuit of interests because:

- they have been hospitalized and institutionalized and thus robbed of access to interests;
- they have had deficit life experiences and failed to develop interests;
- they may have economic constraints that prevent pursuing interests.

People with psychosocial dysfunction often have difficulty making an occupational choice because:
- choices are forced on them before they can sufficiently develop their own interests, skills, and aspirations;
- they come from deficit environments with limited past experiences.

In the absence of making a good occupational choice, role failure and dissatisfaction are likely.

Role Dysfunction

Role dysfunction:
- occurs when a person fails to meet personal needs or performs the role in a deficit fashion;
- may result from loss or change of roles or when a person is in a deviant role;
- may occur when people are in roles that do not match their interests, values, and capacities.

People with psychosocial dysfunction:
- are often cast in passive or deviant roles;
- are judged mentally ill when they fail to perform their roles.

Temporal Dysfunction

Psychosocial pathology may involve a distortion or limitation of temporal perspective, such as:
- the ability to perceive and conceive of time;
- a decreased sense of the future;
- a lack of self-perception as progressing in time.

Psychosocial pathology may involve a disruption of temporal organization of time use, such as:
- a disorganization of habits of time use;
- an imbalance of work, rest, play, and sleep.

Disorder in Environmental Interactions

Hospitalization may contribute to:
- dysfunctional roles and skills;
- reduced personal causation;
- disorders of decision making.

The physical arrangement of environments may reduce social interaction.

Lack of opportunity to engage in occupational behaviors, lack of role models and suitable peers, and lack of stimulation can lead to reduced performance.

Disruption of roles with institutionalization can lead to further dysfunction.

Institutions tend to take away autonomous decision making and sources of self-esteem.

Environments of people with psychosocial dysfunction are often overprotected, conflictual, and removed from family and the community at large.

Environmental expectations may anticipate poor or deviant behavior from people with psychosocial dysfunction, creating a self-fulfilling prophecy.

Disorders of Performance Components

People with psychosocial dysfunctions typically lack appropriate skills for interacting/communicating with others.

People with psychosocial dysfunctions often have deficits in process skills due to impoverished opportunities for learning.

Problems with perceptual-motor skills may be present in people with psychosocial dysfunction.

The symbolic constituents of skills are images that guide behavior, and they may be deficit in people with psychosocial dysfunction because of inadequate or poor past experience.

There may be deficits or disorganization in the neurological component of skill.

Problems in the musculoskeletal component are fewer and secondary to symbolic and neurological problems.

REFERENCES

1. Ayres, J. *Sensory integration and learning disorders*. Los Angeles: Western Psychological Services, 1972.
2. Bailey, D. A work program in psychiatry. *American Journal of Occupational Therapy*, 1968, *22*, 311–318.
3. Barris, R. Environmental interactions: An extension of the model of human occupation. *American Journal of Occupational Therapy*, 1982, *36*, 637–644.
4. Beck, M. A., & Callahan, D. K. Impact of institutionalization on the posture of chronic schizophrenic patients. *American Journal of Occupational Therapy*, 1980, *34*, 332–335.

5. Black, M. The occupational career. *American Journal of Occupational Therapy*, 1976, *30*, 225–228.
6. Bright, T., Bittick, K., & Fleeman, B. Reduction of self-injurious behavior using sensory integrative techniques. *American Journal of Occupational Therapy*, 1981, *35*, 167–172.
7. Burke, J. P. A clinical perspective on motivation: Pawn versus origin. *American Journal of Occupational Therapy*, 1977, *31*, 254–258.
8. Burke, J. P., Miyake, S., Kielhofner, G., & Barris, R. The demystification of health care and demise of the sick role: Implications for occupational therapy. In G. Kielhofner (Ed.), *Health through occupation: Theory and practice in occupational therapy*. Philadelphia: F. A. Davis, 1983.
9. Carey, C. *Games: An occupational therapy treatment mode for juvenile delinquent boys*. Unpublished master's project, Department of Occupational Therapy, Virginia Commonwealth University, 1981.
10. Clark, F. A., Miller, L. R., Thomas, J. A., Kucherawy, D. A., & Azen, S. P. A comparison of operant and sensory integrative methods on developmental parameters in profoundly retarded adults. *American Journal of Occupational Therapy*, 1978, *32*, 86–92.
11. Cynkin, S. *Occupational therapy: Toward health through activities*. Boston: Little, Brown, 1979.
12. Dunning, H. Environmental occupational therapy. *American Journal of Occupational Therapy*, 1972, *26*, 292–298.
13. Fidler, G., & Fidler, J. Doing and becoming: Purposeful action and self-actualization. *American Journal of Occupational Therapy*, 1978, *32*, 305–310.
14. Gray, M. Effects of hospitalization on work-play behavior. *American Journal of Occupational Therapy*, 1972, *26*, 180–185.
15. Hasselkus, B. R. Relocation stress and the elderly. *American Journal of Occupational Therapy*, 1978, *32*, 631–636.
16. Heard, C. Occupational role acquisition: A perspective on the chronically disabled. *American Journal of Occupational Therapy*, 1977, *31*, 243–247.
17. Kannegieter, R. Environmental interactions in psychiatric occupational therapy—Some inferences. *American Journal of Occupational Therapy*, 1980, *34*, 714–720.
18. Kavanagh, M. *Person-environment interaction: The model of human occupation applied to mentally retarded adults*. Unpublished master's project, Department of Occupational Therapy, Virginia Commonwealth University, 1982.
19. Kielhofner, G. Temporal adaptation: A conceptual framework for oc-

cupational therapy. *American Journal of Occupational Therapy*, 1977, *31*, 235–238.

20. Kielhofner, G. The temporal dimension in the lives of retarded adults: A problem of interaction and intervention. *American Journal of Occupational Therapy*, 1979, *33*, 161–168.

21. Kielhofner, G. A model of human occupation, Part 3. Benign and vicious cycles. *American Journal of Occupational Therapy*, 1980, *34*, 731–737.

22. Kielhofner, G. A paradigm for practice: The hierarchical organization of occupational therapy knowledge. In G. Kielhofner (Ed.), *Health through occupation: Theory and practice in occupational therapy*. Philadelphia: F. A. Davis, 1983.

23. Kielhofner, G., Barris, R., Bauer, D., Shoestock, B., & Walker, L. The play of hospitalized and non-hospitalized children. *American Journal of Occupational Therapy*, in press.

24. Kielhofner, G., Barris, R., & Watts, J. Habits and habit dysfunction: A clinical perspective for psychosocial occupational therapy. *Occupational Therapy in Mental Health*, 1982, *2*, 1–22.

25. Kielhofner, G., Burke, J. P., & Igi, C. H. A model of human occupation, Part 4. Assessment and intervention. *American Journal of Occupational Therapy*, 1980, *34*, 777–788.

26. Kielhofner, G., & Miyake, S. The therapeutic use of games with mentally retarded adults. *American Journal of Occupational Therapy*, 1981, *35*, 375–382.

27. Kielhofner, G., & Miyake, S. Rose-colored lenses for clinical practice: From a deficit to a competence model in assessment and intervention. In G. Kielhofner (Ed.), *Health through occupation: Theory and practice in occupational therapy*. Philadelphia: F. A. Davis, 1983.

28. King, L. J. A sensory-integrative approach to schizophrenia. *American Journal of Occupational Therapy*, 1974, *28*, 529–536.

29. Lindquist, J. Activity and vestibular function in chronic schizophrenia. *Occupational Therapy Journal of Research*, 1981, *1*, 56–69.

30. Magill, J., & Vargo, J. Helplessness, hope and the occupational therapist. *Canadian Journal of Occupational Therapy*, 1977, *44*, 65–69.

31. Matsutsuyu, J. Occupational behavior—A perspective on work and play. *American Journal of Occupational Therapy*, 1971, *25*, 291–294.

32. Michelman, S. Play and the deficit child. In M. Reilly (Ed.), *Play as exploratory learning*. Beverly Hills, Calif.: Sage Publications, 1974.

33. Moorehead, L. The occupational history. *American Journal of Occupational Therapy*, 1969, *23*, 329–334.

34. Neville, A. Temporal adaptation: Application with short-term psychiatric patients. *American Journal of Occupational Therapy*, 1980, *34*, 328–331.

THE VIEW OF DISORDER IN OCCUPATIONAL THERAPY 231

35. Oakley, F. M. *The model of human occupation in psychiatry.* Unpublished master's project, Department of Occupational Therapy, Virginia Commonwealth University, 1982.
36. Parent, L. Effects of low-stimulus environment on behavior. *American Journal of Occupational Therapy,* 1978, *32,* 19–25.
37. Paulson, C. Juvenile delinquency and occupational choice. *American Journal of Occupational Therapy,* 1980, *34,* 565–571.
38. Reilly, M. Occupational therapy can be one of the great ideas of 20th century medicine. *American Journal of Occupational Therapy,* 1962, *16,* 1–9.
39. Reilly, M. A psychiatric occupational therapy program as a teaching model. *American Journal of Occupational Therapy,* 1966, *20,* 61–67.
40. Reilly, M. *Play as exploratory learning.* Beverly Hills, Calif.: Sage Publications, 1974.
41. Riopel, N. J. *An examination of the occupational behavior and life satisfaction of the elderly.* Unpublished master's thesis, Medical College of Virginia, Virginia Commonwealth University, 1982.
42. Robinson, A. Play: The arena for acquisition of rules for competent behavior. *American Journal of Occupational Therapy,* 1977, *31,* 248–253.
43. Rogers, J. Order and disorder in medicine and occupational therapy. *American Journal of Occupational Therapy,* 1982, *36,* 29–35.
44. Shannon, P. Work-play theory and the occupational therapy process. *American Journal of Occupational Therapy,* 1972, *26,* 169–172.
45. Shuer, J., Clark, F., & Azen, S. P. Vestibular function in mildly mentally retarded adults. *American Journal of Occupational Therapy,* 1980, *34,* 664–670.
46. Tickle, L. S., & Yerxa, E. J. Need satisfaction of older persons living in the community and in institutions, Part I. The environment. *American Journal of Occupational Therapy,* 1981, *35,* 644–649.
47. Versluys, H. P. The remediation of role disorders through focused group work. *American Journal of Occupational Therapy,* 1980, *34,* 609–614.
48. Watts, J., & Barris, R. *Aging, the environment, and the model of human occupation.* Richmond: Virginia Commonwealth University, 1981. (Audiovisual presentation)
49. Watanabe, S. Four concepts basic to the occupational therapy process. *American Journal of Occupational Therapy,* 1968, *22,* 339–444.
50. Webster, P. Occupational role development in the young adult with mild mental retardation. *American Journal of Occupational Therapy,* 1980, *34,* 13–18.
51. Yerxa, E. Occupational therapy's role in creating a future climate of caring. *American Journal of Occupational Therapy,* 1980, *34,* 529–534.

15
Action Implications: The Process of Restoring Order in Occupational Therapy

The action implications of occupational therapy are multifaceted. However, they focus on a singular process of restoring and/or maintaining order in occupational behavior through facilitating people's engagement in occupation. This discussion of action implications is divided into four sections. The first section describes the occupational therapy process; the second section provides a list of principles of practice; the third examines evaluation; and the fourth highlights the treatment approaches used in psychosocial occupational therapy.

THE OCCUPATIONAL THERAPY PROCESS

Occupational therapy is a process of gathering information about people and situations, analyzing and interpreting that information, and formulating a rational course of action and a means of evaluating its outcomes. Each of these activities can be delineated as separate phases of therapy: screening and evaluation, treatment planning, treatment implementation, and monitoring progress. Although they are described here as a sequence of activities, it should be remembered that they often overlap. For instance, while evaluation generally precedes treatment, it may take place during a treatment session as a therapist observes the person engaging in an activity in order to ascertain strengths and weaknesses.

Screening

While the most traditional route for entry into occupational therapy services is the physician referral, there are many reasons why occupational therapists may need to screen people in order to identify whether they require occupational therapy services. The most notable reason is that not all patients with medical conditions have an occupational dysfunction and not all occupationally dysfunctional persons have medical problems.[114] Thus, the potential routes to occupational therapy in the future may be much more varied than in the past. Already therapists in such nontraditional settings as the school system, residential facilities, and community centers may take responsibility for assessing a person's need for services.

Evaluation

Once a need for occupational therapy has been determined, the therapist engages in an evaluation process. Evaluation has two aspects: (1) the selection and use of appropriate instruments and procedures for gathering data on a person's strengths and weaknesses; and (2) the organization of this data collection under a conceptual framework that guides interpretation of the data and its translation into a treatment plan. Evaluation seeks to determine areas of order and disorder in occupational functioning. By identifying both, the therapist can plan the person's engagement in therapeutic occupations.

While the therapist's conceptual expertise is critical to guiding the formulation of valid and reliable conclusions about areas of function and dysfunction, it is also important that the person be involved as much as possible in this process. When both the therapist and the person being treated agree on the latter's strengths and weaknesses, the therapeutic process is greatly enhanced.

Treatment Planning

The evaluation process is directly connected to the next phase, treatment planning. Based on the identification of areas of function and dysfunction, the therapist draws up a plan of treatment that includes: (1) expected outcomes or goals of therapy; (2) the occupations and other processes to be used as therapy; and (3) the means for monitoring progress toward outcomes or goals. Both long-term and short-term treatment plans are helpful. Long-term plans may include the most global objectives for maintaining function, restoring lost function, and eliciting new areas of function in occupational behavior. Short-term plans may delineate daily or weekly activities in detail. The latter allow for modification of treatment as the person progresses or otherwise changes while still addressing the long-term plans.

Implementation

Implementation of treatment is, of course, the core of occupational therapy. The focus of treatment in occupational therapy is the facilitation or provision of occupations. Engaging in occupation is an open system process that allows generation or restoration of capacity.

Monitoring Progress

Monitoring progress in therapy has two goals. The first is to examine the effectiveness of the therapeutic program in achieving goals. The second is to determine the readiness of an individual for a new phase of therapy, for a change of settings (e.g., discharge), and finally for termination of the occupational therapy service.

Termination

Termination of occupational therapy should reflect the occupational therapist's judgment that the individual has reached the treatment goals or benefited maximally from available therapeutic services. Too often, termination of service is tied to discharge in an acute-oriented health care system, and patients and clients cease to receive services when they most need and can benefit from them. Availability of occupational therapy services in the community is growing, and this should eventually allow for continuity of care beyond periods of hospitalization. This will require a network of therapists in different types of agencies and a system of referral from one occupational therapy service or practitioner to another.

In sum, the occupational therapy process is an interrelated set of activities (see Figure 1) that the therapist carries out to determine and offer the most relevant services and to monitor their effectiveness.

PRINCIPLES OF RESTORING ORDER

Whether or not they are consciously aware of it, therapists employ certain principles in their practice. While there have been attempts to codify principles of practice, they have generally been in the format of concrete guidelines. Our purpose here is to identify principles that link concepts to action.

Principles are guidelines that are logically derived from some philosophical or conceptual framework and that specify general strategies for therapy rather than representing stepwise recipes for action. Thus, they require thoughtful and creative operationalization and application. To emphasize the continuity of these principles with the field's view of order and disorder, they are arranged in the same categories used in previous discussions. Table 1 summarizes these principles (see page 245).

Open System Principles

The fundamental dynamic of the open system is its ability to maintain itself and transform itself through a cycle of processes in which the output or action

Figure 1
The Occupational Therapy Process

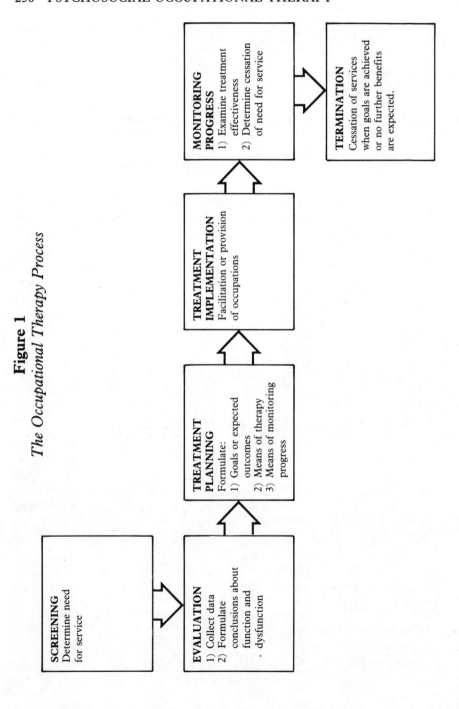

of the system is critical. The open system *becomes* through what it *does*. Occupational therapy is a process of facilitating the action or "doing" of a human system so that it can reorganize, maintain function, and become. The following principles specify how this process is operationalized.

Therapy should seek to increase the patient's productive and playful action.[37,66] A lack or reduction of action signals disruption of the open system cycle. Thus a person's inactivity or passive behavior should always be replaced with action, whether it be simple movement or complex productive activity.

The action elicited should be commensurate with the patient's state of organization or disorganization.[37,66,72] A system's output is limited by the status of the system's internal organization. A severely regressed, disorganized person is not capable of complex behavior and, therefore, should be engaged in activity of which he or she is capable. The therapist should ask what would be a good performance for a person given his or her limitations. For one person it may be the ability to imitate simple motor movements, for another, volunteer work in the community.

Therapeutic occupations should embody the characteristics of normal occupation.[37,72] Occupation is the output of the system and, thus, part of the open system cycle that maintains and changes the system. The kinds of occupations in which a person engages determine the kind of feedback received and eventually what the system becomes. Consequently, occupations used as therapy must represent healthy participation in the culture. When occupations are trivialized or contrived, the person is similarly affected.

Persons must receive adequate feedback on output and its effects.[39,72] Feedback is most meaningful when a person has first determined the goal or purpose of action as a standard to evaluate outcomes. The therapist should carefully monitor people's reactions and verbalizations about performance to make sure they are adequately assessing performance and its consequences.

Increasing levels of performance should be facilitated in therapy.[3,39,62] Reorganization of behavior proceeds from simple to more complex actions. Occupational therapy should provide graded opportunities and demands for increasingly organized behavior. It is especially critical that the environment increase demands as a person's skills increase if new competencies are to be maintained. For instance, one may first learn the method of a craft, later be responsible for managing the supplies and cleanup, and finally teach others the craft.

The reorganizational requirements of the system should determine the kinds of occupations chosen as therapy.[37,68] Disorganization in the human system is manifest in a variety of ways. For a skilled individual whose difficulty is seeing the meaning or worth of his or her behavior, a different course of therapy is indicated from that of the person who lacks basic skills. The output or action of the individual should be aimed at remediating or changing the targeted problem area. In this case, the first person might more profitably engage in values clarification and examination of typical time use, while the second would best benefit from concrete opportunities to learn some new performance or productive act.

Intrinsic Motivation Principles

According to theories of intrinsic motivation, humans have an urge to explore and master the environment. This urge is modified and elaborated through images that people develop of their abilities. People who appear unmotivated do not believe themselves to be effective actors. Restoring intrinsic motivation involves restoring the belief in personal ability and the expectancy of success.

Occupations must be chosen for their intrinsically motivating properties.[16,27,39,71,80] Occupations are intrinsically motivating when the patient engages in the activity for its own sake. The intrinsic value of occupations derives from their relevance to an individual's life situation. A depressed architect plagued with the feeling that she lacks creativity will likely not find a tile trivet particularly meaningful. The housewife who believes she is not a good mother and spouse may not benefit from making something with clay. Individuals' concerns for competence generally revolve around their life roles, and therapy should reflect an appreciation of the demands of these roles.

When people do not initiate action of their own accord, the therapist should exhort them to action.[91] The apathy and hopelessness associated with a loss of belief in personal ability and efficacy can make it impossible for people to initiate action on their own. In such cases, therapists should see to it that they do "get on their feet and do something." Such action coerces the person into a position whereby he or she may "become hopeful by forced exposure to the fact that responding produces reward" (p. 66).[91] Importantly, the message that one is expected to perform also communicates others' belief in one's ability to perform.

People receiving therapy should participate in the process of determining problems and goals for therapy.[3,17,129] A passive, compliant attitude and an expectation of being helped by the ministrations of professionals can reinforce the feeling of external control. People can gain control by participating in the process of designing their own therapy. This is especially important as they progress toward community independence.

The possibility, required efforts, and criteria for success should always be made evident.[16,39] People who chronically expect failure can only begin to expect success if they are shown what steps are necessary and how they can accomplish those steps. Further, by specifying what will constitute criteria of success, the person is enabled to recognize it.

The duration of an activity should be commensurate with the person's ability to maintain a hopeful expectancy of success.[91] People haunted by fear of failure are not able to maintain efforts over long periods. They require immediate feedback on their efforts. Only after a person has generated a series of successful experiences can he or she begin to build on them and generalize an expectation of success to long-term goals and projects.

Occupations should incorporate a moderate degree of risk.[16] Fail-safe projects do not yield a sense of efficacy. Unless the person is aware that a lack of effort or ability would have led to failure, accomplishment has limited significance. The impact of personal effort and skill should be evident.

Decision-Making Principles

The decision to engage in occupations is influenced by an individual's interests and values. Interests are preferences for certain objects, people, and occupations, and values are one's beliefs about what is right and good to do. The ability to recognize personal interests and values is critical to healthy occupational choices throughout life. Therapy often involves a process of enabling people to discover or consolidate their own priorities so that they can become more effective decision makers in their own lives.

Occupational therapy should provide people with the opportunity to discover and develop interests.[12,89,94] Many people come to occupational therapy with deficit past experiences leading to few well-developed interests. Other people come with narrow interest patterns as a result of imbalanced life-styles. Interests arise out of exposure to and participation in situations and occupations. Thus, the action-oriented nature of occupational therapy makes it an ideal setting for generating interests. Further, when people begin to develop interests, they are typically motivated to pursue these interests throughout the day. If the scheduled occupational therapy session is the only time someone can pursue an interest, he or she may be prevented from making natural and healthy choices in the course of the day. Thus, supplies and opportunities for engaging in occupations outside of the clinic space and time should be available.

People should be directed and enabled to develop interests and values that might facilitate correction of past faulty patterns of occupational behavior.[37,80] Sometimes a person's choices for occupation lead to unhealthy patterns of existence. For instance, people may develop only solitary interests, reinforcing a maladaptive pattern of withdrawal from others. Interest and value patterns may reflect imbalanced life-styles such as solely competitive or achievement-oriented interests and values. For example, a group of overachieving, depressed men would need to develop interests and values oriented to leisure and relaxation.

Interests and values consistent with people's everyday settings should be fostered.[3,23,57,68] The development of interests and values serves no purpose if people are unable to pursue them in their life situations. Successful participation in a setting requires that the person assimilate its interests and values. Occupational therapy can increase people's awareness of the values and interests within different kinds of settings. Ultimately, this may lead either to a change in personal interests and values or in the selection of more consistent settings. In either case, when a match is present, competent functioning follows more easily.

People should have an opportunity to discover personally meaningful values by being exposed to a value system in occupational therapy.[6,57,105] People who have been unsuccessful in developing personally meaningful activities and/or a value system that orients them to choices for occupation may come to therapy with a need to develop values. While therapists cannot prescribe or coerce values, they can purposefully embody a set of values in the occupational therapy setting.

Individuals' personal and culturally derived values should be recognized and respected in the treatment process.[38,64,74] People who have been unsuccessful in developing personally meaningful activities and/or a value system that orients them to choices for occupation may come to therapy with a need to develop values. While therapists cannot prescribe or coerce values, they can embody a set of values in the occupational therapy setting. Such values are then present for patients to experience and to make their own choices.

People should be helped to identify ways that they can actualize interests, values, and goals in their lives.[18,23,68,74,102] Some people's problems derive from their difficulty in operationalizing interests, values, and goals in their everyday lives. For example, a lack of skills may prevent someone from pursuing personal interests, values, and goals. Occupational therapy should help individuals to better manage and allocate their time and provide opportunities to develop necessary skills.

Patients should have the opportunity to identify and assess their own occupational choices and to pursue new choices.[68,98,107,131] People may fail to make a realistic occupational choice in the course of development, leading to dissatisfaction and a lack of commitment to major occupational roles. Others may be forced into choices through external pressures or unanticipated changes in life circumstances. Such people may be aided by the opportunity to examine the routes through which they have entered various occupations and careers. If a new or first choice is necessary, occupational therapy can offer an arena in which people begin to match their interests, values, and aptitudes to avenues for productive and satisfying participation in society.

Principles of Role Behavior

Roles are positions in and necessary functions of social groups. When people fill roles, their behavior is influenced by the expectations of the role. They develop an identity that the role provides, and they contribute to the maintenance and development of the social group. Because of their organizing influence on behavior and their importance for personal identity, roles can be used in therapy to influence the process of reorganizing behavior. Roles are acquired through a socialization process that can occur in therapy.

People should have opportunities to enter responsible, active, and productive roles in occupational therapy.[17,127] The "sick" role disenfranchises patients at the risk of making them more helpless. An alternative role in occupational therapy allows people to become responsible contributors to their own self-maintenance and to the maintenance of the ward, clinic, or residential facility.

Occupational therapy should be organized as a socialization process in which expectations for performance are conveyed.[64,110,114] Occupational therapy should be a milieu that embodies the expectation of the culture for productive participation of its members. By participating in this milieu, people become familiar with those expectations and have an opportunity to practice and acquire the role behaviors necessary to fulfill them.

Role behavior is facilitated by participation in groups where roles can be differentiated.[29,37,127] Since roles are the natural components of groups, participation in ongoing groups facilitates their formation and enactment. Groups can also provide an opportunity for people to try on a variety of roles and engage in reciprocal role behaviors. By so doing, they learn the attitudes and responsibilities of members in different roles and how to collaborate with those in other role positions. Enactment of group roles is enhanced when people can identify with a set of tasks and a status that accompany the role position.

Role transition may be precipitated or facilitated in therapy.[52,127] Development involves a succession of life roles. Occupational therapy can facilitate the process of role transition by allowing people opportunities to try out the skills and tasks associated with new roles and to develop confidence that they can fulfill new role demands. In other instances, the occupational therapist may assist people in the process of identifying the need for role change in the present or in the immediate future. Preparing people for the choices that must be made also facilitates role change.

Principles of Temporal Adaptation

Temporality includes an inner sense, perspective, and valuation of time and one's organization of behavior in time. Occupational therapy enables people to achieve temporal adaptation, that is, the organization of daily life behaviors to satisfy one's internal needs and the external expectations of society.

The hospital or other institution should have a schedule of daily activity that approaches or replicates that of the larger culture.[61,110] People who live in care-taking organizations that expose them to schedules at variance with what the adaptive person of the same age would be doing run the risk of losing healthy patterns of adaptive behavior. Effort should be made to establish temporal order that orients residents to the demands of daily life in the community. This includes a time for productivity, a discretionary or leisure period when people can choose behavior, and a time for rest or sleep. At one time, occupational therapists assumed responsibility for scheduling the 24-hour day of the patient. Where that is still feasible, it is certainly within the role of the therapist.

People should be enabled to acquire the temporal perspective of the settings in which they participate.[61,110] Faulty learning, deficient past experiences, and other factors can cause individuals' temporal orientations to be at variance with the settings in which they participate. Some people have not acquired an orientation to the necessity for promptness, organizing behavior in sequences, and discriminating work time from rest time. Consequently, they may not fulfill the demands of various settings. By incorporating the temporal order of the larger culture and the work world, occupational therapy workshops can provide opportunities for people to acquire these perspectives.

People whose past time use has been disorganized or otherwise maladaptive should have an opportunity to examine their temporal behavior, identify areas of needed change, and try out new schedules of time use.[61,79,102,121] This can be accomplished by having people identify how they spend time outside the hospital; classify it according to work, play, or rest; and identify areas of needed change in order to link their schedule to future goals, achieve a balance of time use, and establish a pattern of temporal behavior. This may include a counseling process for people still living in the community who need assistance in planning their time, or it can be a function of discharge planning when people are prepared for return to the community.

People should have opportunities to implement and practice new routines (habits) of time use.[49,65,121] Reorganization of temporal behavior does not occur as a simple function of planning a new schedule. Rather, skills must be developed and skilled behavior must become habituated. Habit change involves four stages: invalidation, or rejection of maladaptive habits; exploration of alternative patterns; innovation, or adopting new routines; and habituation, the integration of a new routine into an individual's existing habit network. Therapy can identify maladaptive habit patterns (invalidation), and provide people with opportunities to try new routines (exploration) and to integrate those routines into a life situation (innovation and habituation). Providing people with opportunities to practice schedules in the treatment context or supporting the practice of these routines in the community are part of the continuum of services that assist temporal adaptation.

Principles of the Environmental Management

The environment consists of people, tasks, and space. Environmental management includes modifications of the task, such as work simplification; modifications to the person (e.g., the use of adaptive equipment); changes in the physical environment, such as the removal or modification of architectural barriers; and structuring or altering the psychosocial climate, particularly through changes in arousal levels and demands for performance.

The environment should provide appropriate levels of arousal (challenge) throughout the treatment process.[3,49,60,64,72,97,110,115] Arousal or challenge is a function of the person's internal status; thus, there is an optimal level of arousal for any person at a given time. When there is too much or too little challenge, a person will not be optimally aroused. As people improve (e.g., as their skills increase), environmental challenges should be increased so that the demands of the environment are commensurate with their abilities.

Opportunities for decision making should be offered in the environment.[3,49,110,128] Denial of opportunities to make choices can lead to learned helplessness and feelings of decreased personal causation. If the overall choice of a setting cannot be made by the person, participation in program decisions, control over one's living space, and optional activities are ways in which the sense of personal efficacy can be enhanced.

The psychosocial atmosphere and the physical environment must be consistent with other expectations for performance.[3,64,97,100] The therapist's actions as a role model, beliefs about the importance of activities used, the physical setting, and objects within a setting all contribute to the psychosocial atmosphere. The accumulated impact of these environmental components communicates certain expectations for behavior. Therapists need to be cognizant of potential inconsistencies between stated therapeutic goals and the environment. For instance, a television set in the day room communicates an expectation for passive, solitary behavior. This may not be congruent, however, with an overall goal of encouraging patients to increase active, social uses of leisure time.

Understaffing the treatment setting can be used as a deliberate strategy to increase individuals' involvement and responsibility.[3,60] People with marginal abilities are more likely to take on passive observer roles when a setting is adequately staffed or overstaffed. In addition, elderly adults are more likely to allow younger or middle-aged adults to fill leadership roles when they are in mixed-age settings. When activities are understaffed, however, individuals feel more personal pressure to assume responsibility and fill positions of leadership.

Individuals must have the opportunity to become involved in a range of settings that increase in their dissimilarity to one another.[3,24,110,113,129] Practice in sequenced, graded settings facilitates the transfer of behavior from one setting to another. However, if these settings remain too similar, the person will be unprepared for the incongruity and unpredictability that occurs in daily life settings. To be truly competent, the person must be effectively involved in a variety of settings.

Principles of Regenerating Performance Components

The components of human performance are one's repertoire of interaction/communication, perceptual-motor, and process skills. They enable one to deal with people, objects, and events. The skills are composed of symbolic, neurological, and musculoskeletal constituents.

Skills are learned best when they have a relationship and relevance to a larger environment.[71,126] Skills are learned in the natural sequence and contexts of daily life where real contingencies and consequences are present. Learning skills out of such contexts can result in rigid or splintered skills, with little ability to generalize outside the learning situation. Further, the development of skills should be attached to a sense of meaning and purpose. Without context, the meaning of skills can be lost. For example, an adolescent hygiene class in which young women put on makeup is more effective if they are dressing up for an occasion such as a dance or outing.

Skills have a developmental sequence that must be acknowledged in therapy.[61,72,90,99,113,125] This principle holds true for all three areas of skills. For instance, play interaction skills develop from parallel, to associative, to cooperative.[86] Process skills develop from the learning of simple sequencing and physical arrangement of action to achieve a task to the complex organization of events in time and space. Perceptual-motor skills begin with simple movement behaviors and proceed toward the more complex performances involved in arts and crafts. An individual must begin with the simpler skills and proceed toward those more complex ones that presume and build on the lower ones.

Skill training should reflect an individual's life roles, interests, and values.[23,66,121] Programs whose aim is to regenerate skills or train people in new skills should recognize that each individual has his or her own skill requirements. These should be ascertained through examination of the individual's life roles and desires for performance. The motivation to learn skills is more readily elicited when this aspect of the person's need for skills is recognized and incorporated into treatment.

All skill training should simultaneously take into consideration the three constituents of skills.[64,72,113] This principle has many implications and applications. First of all, it works both ways in the hierarchy (i.e., recognizing that lower levels constrain and higher levels organize). For instance, if one wanted a patient to organize a skill that involved symbolic awareness, such as planning and executing a craft, it should be ascertained whether the person's neurological and musculoskeletal constituents are sufficiently organized to allow the learning. By the same token, if one wished to achieve better sensory integration at the neurological level, one must stay attuned to the symbolic processes by incorporating motor and sensory experiences into meaningful activities.

Table 1

PRINCIPLES OF RESTORING ORDER

Open System
—Seek to increase playful and productive action.
—Elicit action commensurate with the patient's state of organization/disorganization.
—Use occupations that embody characteristics of normal occupation.
—Provide adequate feedback on output and its effects.
—Facilitate increasing levels of performance.
—Use occupations suited to the person's reorganizational requirements.

Intrinsic Motivation
—Choose intrinsically motivating occupations relevant to people's life situations.
—Allow patients to participate in determining problems and goals for therapy.
—Exhort passive patients to action.
—Make evident the required efforts and criteria for success.
—Choose activities of a duration commensurate with the person's ability to maintain a hopeful expectancy of success.
—Use occupations with a moderate degree of risk.

(Continued)

Table 1

PRINCIPLES OF RESTORING ORDER

Decision Making
—Provide opportunity to discover and develop interests.
—Facilitate development of new interests and values to correct faulty patterns of occupational behavior.
—Foster interests and values consistent with the person's everyday settings.
—Enable discovery of values by providing a value system in occupational therapy.
—Help people to identify ways to actualize interests, values, and goals in their lives.
—Provide opportunity to identify and assess occupational choices and to pursue new choices.

Role
—Provide opportunities to enter responsible active and productive roles.
—Make expectations for performance clear to facilitate socialization.
—Use groups as a context for performing various roles.
—Use therapy to precipitate or facilitate role transition as appropriate.

Temporal Adaptation
—Provide schedules that replicate time use in the larger culture.
—Enable people to acquire the temporal perspective of their settings.
—Guide people with maladaptive patterns of time use to identify change needs and to develop schedules of time use.
—Provide opportunities to implement and practice new routines (habits) of time use.

Environment
—Provide appropriate levels of arousal (challenge).
—Opportunities for decision making should be present.
—The atmosphere and physical environment must be consistent with expectations for performance.
—Understaff settings to evoke performance.
—Allow performance in a range of settings to increase flexibility of performance.

Table 1

PRINCIPLES OF RESTORING ORDER

Performance —Provide skill training relevant to the contexts of
Components daily life.
—Follow a developmental sequence in skill train-
ing.
—Acknowledge roles, interests, and values in
choosing skills to be learned.
—Consider the symbolic, neurological, and mus-
culoskeletal constituents in regenerating skills.

EVALUATING ORDER AND DISORDER

Occupational therapy begins with careful evaluation of both order and disorder so that therapy can build on a person's strengths and abilities and use these directly in remediating areas of disorder.[114] This aspect of evaluation is critical, since occupational therapy is a treatment process with participation at its core. Without an appreciation of a person's abilities, appropriate therapy cannot be chosen. Further, acknowledging ability as well as disability increases people's feelings of competence.[70]

This section first discusses a number of assessments and evaluation procedures developed in occupational therapy that are appropriate for use with people with psychosocial disorders. Then it examines the process of synthesizing assessment data into a complete evaluation. Problems and issues related to constructing an evaluation battery are discussed and several approaches that have been used in the area of psychosocial dysfunction are described.

Individual assessments yield only pieces of a total picture. Total evaluation enables interpretation of the person's order and disorder. The therapist must engage in a cognitive problem-solving process (often in concert with the patient) to arrive at an explanation of order and disorder. When such an explanation is forthcoming from the evaluation process, treatment can be systematically planned and applied.

Assessments for Data Collection in Occupational Therapy

This section includes a range of published and unpublished instruments, chosen for their compatibility with the view of order and disorder presented in previous chapters. Each instrument is discussed in terms of its relationship to order and disorder (see Table 2, page 255). Presentation of each instrument is brief and designed to help readers decide the potential relevance of the instrument to their practice.

Activity Indices. Nystrom[104] and Gregory[50] developed activity indices applicable to adult populations with psychosocial dysfunction. Nystrom developed a descriptive interview with 61 questions concerning participation in leisure activity and the meaning of leisure. Gregory modified this procedure, constructing a paper-and-pencil self-report in which people indicated their participation in a list of activities and rated them in terms of interest, enjoyability, autonomy, and competence. Both procedures offer data about the degree of activity and positive feelings associated with it. Reliability for these procedures is reasonably good, and both instruments are based on a thorough literature review. Gregory found an association between his instrument and life satisfaction, suggesting that it is a valid measure of activity and the positive emotions associated with it.

Adolescent Role Assessment. Black[7] developed an interview-based rating tool from the literature on child and adolescent behavior. The assessment focuses on role development in the family, at school, and with peers. It includes sections on play experiences, socialization in the family, school performance, peer interactions, occupational choice, and work goals and fantasy. The assessment yields a wide range of data, providing an overview of the individual's occupational development. The instrument has some claim to validity since it was developed from the literature; reliability has not been assessed. Black's own use of the instrument suggests that it can be used to identify patterns of dysfunction in adolescents.

Bay Area Functional Performance Evaluation. Bloomer and Williams[9] developed a standardized instrument to assess the skills that underlie daily living activities. The evaluation consists of a preassessment interview, a task-oriented assessment (sorting shells, bank deposit slip, house floor plan, block design, and draw-a-person) and a social interaction scale. It allows determination of a wide variety of functional parameters, from perceptual-motor behaviors through social interaction. It also yields information on such variables as self-esteem and frustration tolerance. This instrument is supported by substantial research, suggesting good reliability and construct validity. The authors also provide normative data, which enables interpretation of the scores.

Comprehensive Occupational Therapy Evaluation Scale. Brayman, Kirby, Misenheimer, and Short[13] reported an occupational therapy evaluation designed to assess skills in a variety of areas. The 24-item scale is divided into three broad areas: interpersonal behavior, task behavior, and general behavior. The latter category refers to such behaviors as activity level, responsibility, punctuality, and reality orientation. The scale was devised to assess behaviors relevant to and frequently observed in occupational therapy. Each item is rated on a 4-point scale with criteria defined for each rating. The scale was developed to permit efficient evaluation in a short-term setting and to be a means of monitoring progress in therapy. Limited research data support the conclusion that the scale can be a reliable and valid assessment of skills.

Comprehensive Evaluation of Basic Living Skills. Casanova and Ferber[20] developed an evaluation for three groups of basic living skills: (a) personal hygiene; (b) ability for meal preparation, telephone use, and transportation use; and (c) reading, writing, understanding time, math ability, and money management. Each item is rated from 1 to 4 with 4 indicating the highest level of independence. The authors provide no reliability and validity data on the instrument. The range of items appears to make this a comprehensive evaluation, suitable primarily for chronic patients with rather severe skill deficits. However, the evaluation is lengthy and time consuming to administer.

Decision-Making Inventory. Westphal[133] developed an observational inventory for assessing the problem-solving ability of psychiatric patients based on observations of their decision making when they encountered problems in arts and crafts. Therapists observing people in an activity make ratings on a 4-point scale in the areas of finding information, organizing information, and selecting a solution. The items within these areas are based on a theory of the sequences of steps for successful problem solving. The inventory yields an overall score of decision-making (problem-solving) ability and an indication of where in the process the person has the most difficulty.

The advantage of this instrument is that it is one of the few available ways to assess process skills. Further, the therapist observes the person in an actual performance situation rather than at a simulated task. Although it appears to have good interrater reliability, it may have poor test-retest reliability.[28,84] Thus, the user must be cautious not to infer problem-solving capacity from a single observation and should note other possible factors influencing performance, such as the nature of problems, the kind of occupational activity observed, and the individual's motivation. The validity of the instrument rests on Westphal's original assumption that problem solving in arts and crafts is representative of the individual's overall problem-solving abilities. Since this remains to be demonstrated, the main use of the instrument would appear to be as a tool for locating potential problems or strengths in problem solving that could be further observed and evaluated through additional data collection.

Environmental Questionnaire. Dunning[30] developed a semistructured interview designed to assess physical, social, and task environments. The questionnaire yields a wide range of data about the physical environment, such as safety and privacy, autonomy of action permissible, and other related features of the environment. No reliability data are reported. Dunning claims face validity and reports that a pilot study supported the clinical utility of the instrument for assessing the residential environment and identifying areas of needed change.

Home Life Survey. Kavanagh[60] developed the home life survey as part of a study of mentally retarded adults. This survey is based on the concept of behavior settings and assesses the degree of responsibility a person has in the home setting (family or residential setting). It includes four sections: meals, dressing, family activities, and chores. Each section has six statements representing varying levels of responsibility and involvement. The instrument can be filled out by anyone who routinely interacts with the person in the setting; thus, it would be a useful way to assess the individual's home environment and behavior in lieu of a home visit. Although developed for a mentally retarded population, it appears to have wider application in the area of psychosocial dysfunction. Kavanagh reports no reliability data; her approach to validity was to carefully base the instrument on the literature concerning behavior settings.

Interest Checklist. Matsutsuyu[93] introduced an interest checklist in which respondents noted which of 80 items were of casual, strong, or no interest. This paper-and-pencil checklist was originally devised to give information on people's patterns of interests and their ability to discriminate interests. In clinical use, the instrument is often accompanied by an interview to validate responses, discover reasons for interests or their lack, and other relevant information. The instrument can be scored by noting the numbers of strong and casual interests in several categories.

Many modifications of the interest checklist exist; they seek to accomplish a variety of purposes, such as including a better range of interests for certain groups of people and gathering data on past and future interests as well as present ones. Rogers, Weinstein and Figone[16] modified the instrument to yield a more discriminative scoring procedure. Their study indicated that the instrument yields reliable findings, but they questioned the validity of Matsutsuyu's categories as domains of interest. Scaffa[119] developed an alternate form of the interest checklist that asks people to indicate strong, some, or no interest in an activity in the past 10 years and the past month, to note whether or not they currently participate in the activity, and whether they would like to in the future. This version offers a wider range of clinically useful information: patterns of interest lost or gained, the degree to which people act on their interests, and their desires for future participation in interests. Retest reliability of the modified instrument is not known.

Inventory of Depersonalization and Occupational Skill Loss During Hospitalization. Grey[49] developed an observational inventory for assessing the hospital and ward environment and its potential impact on the occupational dysfunction of patients. The instrument examines the impact of hospital or other environments on security, privacy, self-identity, self-esteem, contact with the outside world, and occupational skills. Criteria of hospital conditions and practices that negatively affect these dimensions were used to construct the instrument. The most advantageous use of this instrument would probably be for therapists who are involved in consulting and/or modifying the hospital environment. The instrument also can be modified slightly to be used in residential facilities and other total institutions. Grey reports no reliability or validity data. The instrument was developed from a review of the literature and, thus, has a claim to content validity.

Inventory of Occupational Choice Skills. Shannon[122] developed an inventory of occupational choice skills, a paper-and-pencil self-report of play and chore activities. The instrument is designed for adolescents who are in the first occupational choice development stage. The 29-page item inventory is scored to give an indication of a person's self-discovery, decision making, and work-role experimentation experiences. No normative scores are given; the user is to compare the three scores, looking for potential areas of weakness. No reliability data are available. Shannon used expert judgments of occupational therapists to select and weight the items on this inventory. While both validity and reliability remain to be demonstrated for this tool, it appears to be useful as a means of exploring past experiences with adolescents who are experiencing difficulty in making an occupational choice.

Leisure History. Potts[108] developed an interview for evaluating the historical leisure patterns of emotionally disturbed adults. It is based on a theory of leisure development and employs a semistructured interview format. The instrument yields a developmental profile of a person's leisure experiences and information about present leisure. Potts includes a series of cases that are helpful in illustrating the evaluation and treatment potential of the instrument. She reports no reliability; the instrument is based on a thorough literature review and appears to have content validity. As a clinical tool, it would be most helpful when screening data indicate that a person is experiencing special difficulty in the leisure aspects of adult life.

Occupational History and Occupational Role History. Gathering historical data on a person's occupational behavior over the life span offers information about the history of output and the individual's adaptive or maladaptive cycles. Two instruments have been developed to systematically collect historical data on occupational behavior. Moorhead[98] devised the occupational history, a semistructured interview. It has alternate forms for different major life roles (e.g., worker, housewife, and student, and separate sections for work and play). Analysis of the occupational history involves categorizing data from the interview into the areas of childhood learning and socialization, occupational choice process, experiences of success and failure and their environmental concomitants, and the direction of change over the life span and whether it has contributed to solidification of occupational roles. Thus, the instrument gives data on several of the categories of order and disorder.

Florey and Michelman[41] developed an abbreviated historical interview called the occupational role history. While the content is generally the same, this instrument combines the work and play questions and uses a single format for all interviewees. The instrument is analyzed by examining responses and determining whether the subject is in one of four categories: (a) currently dysfunctional in occupational roles, (b) at risk for future role dysfunction, (c) without occupational dysfunction, or (d) having an imbalance of work and leisure. Their instrument examines the sequence and content of occupational roles, the respondent's awareness of interest and satisfaction in occupational behavior, the organization of occupational roles into a life pattern, weaknesses and strengths in skills, and the balance of occupations.

Published descriptions of both instruments are accompanied by cases that are helpful in illustrating data analysis. As the authors note, understanding of order and disorder in occupation is important background for the therapist using the instruments. Both instruments are accompanied by guidelines that enhance their reliability and validity, although no studies have examined these properties of the instruments.

Occupational Questionnaire. Riopel[112] and Kielhofner developed a tool similar to many existing activity configurations, but with the goal of assessing daily behavior in terms of a theoretical model. The occupational questionnaire asks respondents to report a typical day, noting for each half hour period of waking hours what they are doing. Respondents then rate each activity according to its interest and value, the degree of competence they have for performing the activity, and whether they view it as work, play, or rest. The instrument is based on the model of human occupation (i.e., as a measure of the degree to which the volition subsystem[66] was operationalized in daily life). It indicates the degree to which people do things they like, value, and do well. It also gives information about the balance of work, play, and rest from the respondent's perspective. Data can be analyzed to determine which activities yield the most interest, value, and feeling of competence. It can indicate trouble periods during the day, degree of temporal organization, and other information about daily behavior.

In a preliminary study, the instrument yielded acceptable test-retest reliability and concurrent validity. The advantage of this activity configuration over others is its close link to a theoretical model. This allows a clearer interpretation of the findings of the instrument and facilitates developing treatment plans.

Play History. Takata[125] developed a history interview to ascertain a child's developmental play experiences. The history gathers data in four categories: materials, action, people, and settings relevant to the child's play. It allows the therapist to ascertain the level of the child's most recent play experiences (play development is divided into five epochs from childhood through adolescence) and the quality and quantity of play experiences in past epochs. Menarchek[96] and Behnke[6] revised the play history, developing a more standardized protocol, a scoring procedure, and a guide explaining the purpose of questions and their intended yield. They examined the reliability and validity of the instrument and found good interrater reliability, fair test-retest reliability, and strong evidence to support the validity of the instrument. The play history is a source of information about deficits in these play experiences and settings, thereby indicating areas of needed intervention.

Preschool Play Scale. Knox[76,77] developed this observational tool for assessing the developmental level of children's free play. The scale consists of four dimensions: space management, imitation, participation, and material management. Each of these dimensions is divided into four categories, producing 16 areas of play. The instrument yields scores for each category and dimension and an overall score referred to as the play age. Bledsoe and Shepherd[8] revised the scale and studied its reliability and validity; their findings support the conclusion that the scale offers a stable and valid assessment of the child's developmental level of play.

Prevocational Assessment. Ethridge[33] reported on a prevocational evaluation for psychiatric patients. This rating scale includes three major areas: (a) work skills, habits, and tolerance; (b) socialization and attitude toward others; and (c) personality characteristics. Each item within these categories is rated on a 4-point scale from very poor to excellent. Ethridge studied the scale and found that it was a stable tool (yielding comparable ratings in both occupational therapy and work therapy) and that it was a valid predictor of success in work placement. In addition to its usefulness as a placement and referral tool, research with the scale demonstrated that the occupational therapy setting was just as suitable as work placement to be an observational arena to predict job placement success.

Role Checklist. Oakley[105] developed a paper-and-pencil questionnaire in which people respond to questions about 11 life roles. The respondents indicate whether they have been in, are currently in, or plan to enter each of these roles, and the degree to which they value these roles. Oakley developed the instrument as part of a study of adult psychiatric inpatients, and she examined its reliability in a pilot study, which indicated good test-retest reliability. The instrument has a reasonable claim to face validity since Oakley provides clear definitions on the questionnaire for each role.

This instrument promises to be quite useful in clinical practice as a source of information about the continuity of life roles, future plans for roles, disruption of role behavior, and overall role balance. Oakley described the instrument as useful for creating problem-solving dialogues with patients concerning their own occupational performance.

Sensory Integration Assessments. An assessment of sensory integrative functioning for adult psychiatric patients was reported by Schroeder, Block, Trottier, and Stowell.[124] The assessment consists of a number of motor performances and reflex testing. The goal of the instrument is to provide a comprehensive evaluation of perceptual motor ability. Preliminary data suggest good interrater reliability. Since the authors base the battery on a review of neurological literature and employ many procedures that have already been standardized, it has a reasonable claim to content validity; the authors acknowledge the need for further research to establish construct validity of the measures. The assessment of sensory integrative functioning in children has been widely documented. The Southern California Sensory Integration battery developed by Ayres is supported by considerable research.[1]

Because the sensory integration batteries (both for children and adults) seek to measure underlying neurological deficits, these tests require users to have substantial skills and knowledge. Further, because they are designed to detect and delineate the presence of neurological deficits, they are not appropriate for all populations of psychosocially dysfunctional people. Eventually, further guidelines will have to be developed for screening individuals who merit indepth sensory motor evaluation.

Summary. In this section, a number of occupational therapy evaluations were presented. These evaluations yield various types of information related to the areas of order and disorder discussed earlier which Table 2 summarizes. This section is a general guide to the scope and purpose of the instruments. Determination of how well an instrument evaluates function and dysfunction

Table 2

Occupational Therapy Assessments and Their Relationships to Categories of Order and Disorder

	Occupational Performance Components	Environmental Impact	Temporal Adaptation	Occupational Therapy	Decision Making	Intrinsic Motivation	Open System Functions
Activity Indices							
Adolescent Role Assessment				X	X	X	X
Bay Area Functional Performance Evaluation	X						
Comprehensive Occupational Therapy Evaluation Scale	X						
Comprehensive Evaluation of Basic Living Skills	X						
Decision-Making Inventory	X						
Environmental Questionnaire		X					
Home Life Survey		X					X
Interest Checklist					X	X	
Inventory of Depersonalization and Occupational Skill Loss During Hospitalization		X					
Inventory of Occupational Choice Skills					X	X	
Leisure History							X
Occupational History and Occupational Role History		X	X	X	X	X	X
Occupational Questionnaire			X		X	X	X
Play History	X	X				X	X
Preschool Play Scale	X						X
Prevocational Assessment	X		X			X	
Role Checklist			X		X		X
Sensory Integration Assessment	X						

is ultimately a matter of therapists' responsibility and judgment in any particular treatment setting.

The Evaluation Process: Selecting, Organizing, and Interpreting Instruments

While it is important to know what assessments are available, developing a useful, coherent, and meaningful evaluation process requires use of an organizing framework that guides how one selects instruments, organizes data from them, and interprets the findings. Two types of decisions enter into the organization of an evaluation process: logistic decisions and conceptual decisions. Logistic decisions involve consideration of such factors as case load, the average length of time in the treatment program, the age of the typical patient or client, the ratio of therapists to patients or clients, the scope of the program, and so forth. The therapist must attempt to gather as much data as possible in the framework of available time and energy, while at the same time considering what data are necessary and useful to guide the treatment process.

Conceptual decisions that guide development of an evaluation process involve consideration of the nature of the disorders exhibited by the treatment population. One then selects or constructs a model or some other organizing framework that offers a coherent way of viewing both disorder and the processes of restoring order. By carefully linking assessment data to the variables in the conceptual framework, one discerns the meaning of the data (i.e., what it tells one about order and disorder) and the treatment strategies implied by different findings. There are several ways that this process can be accomplished. The following discussion provides a few examples.

A Case Analysis Method. Cubie and Kaplan[22] developed a system for organizing data on psychiatric patients. The process is guided by 10 analytic questions (see Figure 2) that are based on the model of human occupation.[62,63,66,68] The model incorporates three subsystems: the volition subsystem, which includes values, goals, personal causation, and interests; the habituation subsystem, which includes internalized roles and habits; and the performance subsystem, which includes skills and their constituents. The model provides a coherent schema for explaining order and disorder. Cubie and Kaplan translated components of this model into a sequence of questions that guide both data gathering and assessment. Each question orients the therapist to a variable or process described in the model, and a response indicates function or dysfunction in that aspect of the person's occupational behavior. Attached to each negative response is a treatment strategy. Positive responses direct the therapist to the next analytic question. Thus, as the therapist gathers data

Figure 2

Data Analysis Sequence and Related Treatment Implications*

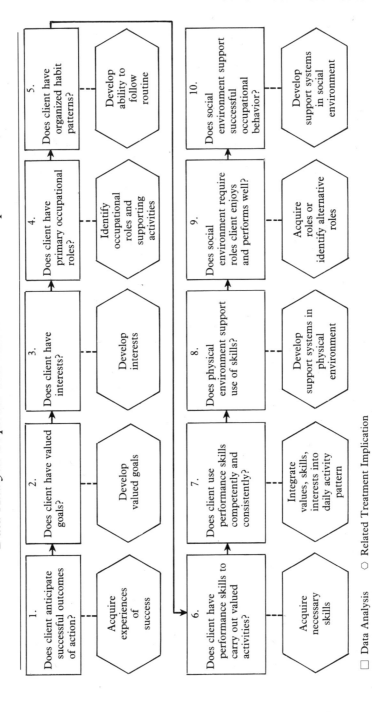

□ Data Analysis   ◇ Related Treatment Implication

A Case Analysis Method for the Model of Human Occupation, AJOT, S H Cubie, K Kaplan.

to answer each analytic question, any problem areas that are found are immediately linked to an intervention.

The case analysis process is designed so that it not only allows the therapist to identify areas of function and dysfunction and related treatment, but it also results in determination of the optimal level of treatment. Levels of treatment are based on the model's delineation of levels of motivation and organization in the human system.[62] The lowest exploratory level is for systems at a minimally organized state, and it is aimed at generating skills; the next level, competence, presents greater demands for performance and thus develops habits. At the final level, achievement, the person is prepared for and enters occupational roles. Cubie and Kaplan also identified properties of different treatment groups that qualified them as exploratory, competence, or achievement level groups. By determining the patient's level of organization, one makes systematic decisions about placement in groups. This case analysis method developed by Cubie and Kaplan is an excellent example of linking theory to assessment and assessment to intervention. It provides a coherent approach to clinical reasoning.

A Psychiatric Assessment Battery. Oakley[105] developed an assessment battery based on the same model of human occupation (see Table 3). She reviewed the literature on mental illness to determine which areas of function and dysfunction identified in the model would be critical to assess in psychiatric patients. Based on this, she chose to analyze data on locus of control (one dimension of personal causation), valued goals, temporal orientation, interests, internalized roles, and skills. She assessed locus of control with the Rotter[118] internal-external locus of control scale. Goals were assessed through a questionnaire adapted from Farnham-Diggory.[34] Temporal orientation was determined through the Time Reference Inventory.[117] For the remaining variables, instruments developed by occupational therapists were used. Interests were measured with the Interest Checklist,[93] roles with the Role Checklist developed by Oakley,[105] and skills with portions of the Bay Area Functional Performance Evaluation.[9]

Oakley synthesized the data from these evaluations into an ordinal ranking that reflected the degree of organization or order in the human system. This 5-point scale ranged from very organized to very disorganized, with each level of organization or disorganization carefully defined. In preliminary research the scale turned out to be an excellent index of patients' level of adaptive functioning.

Assessment of Occupational Role Development. Webster[131] developed an assessment battery based on her proposed model of occupational role development. Her model was designed to explain the process of occupational choice

Table 3
Variables and Their Measures

Variable	Operational Definition	Instrument
Locus of control	Self-report of internal versus external sense of control	Rotter Internal-External Locus of Control Scale[118]
Goals	Number of reported goals; number of goals in content areas	Adapted Expectancy Questionnaire[34]
Temporal orientation	Self-report of average number of years projected into the future and into the past	Time Reference Inventory-Shortened Form[117]
Interests	Self-report of intensity of interests	Adapted Interest Checklist[93]
Internalized roles	Self-report of role performance along temporal continuum	Role Checklist[105]
Skills	Observed ability to perform specific tasks	Bay Area Functional Performance Evaluation[9] (shell sort, deposit slip, and house floor plan subtasks)

in retarded young adults. From this model a measurement grid was developed which served as a profile of the person's occupational role development.

The grid profile indicates the status of a person's possession and awareness of abilities, skills and habits, time concepts, values, awareness of values and satisfactions related to occupational roles, interests, leisure activities, peer interaction, family, culture, economic conditions, social status, and social organizations. These variables are identified as critical for the occupational choice process. The instruments Webster used were the Adaptive Behavior Scale[103] (skills); Time Practices Inventory and Temporal Attitude Scale[81] (subtests of a temporal battery used to assess attitudes toward time); the value orientations inventory[75] (awareness of values); the Interest Checklist;[93] the occupational history;[98] the occupational choice questionnaire and pre-work questionnaire[131] (to assess attitudes toward work and how they were learned); and the Work Satisfaction Questionnaire[131] (to assess whether a person can identify job satisfiers). Webster presents a case history to illustrate the use of this battery and how it generated implications for intervention. Her approach is a good example of an evaluation process designed with a particular population in mind.

An Evaluation of Imitation and Play in Children. DeRenne-Stephan[26] developed an evaluation process based on a framework of play and imitation in children. From the literature, she identified critical characteristics of the child, role models, family organization, and physical environment that influence the imitative process in childhood play. Her aim was to examine the young child with psychosocial problems in terms of his or her relationship to the family and relevant environments. She conceptualizes imitation within play as a systems process, influenced both by the internal characteristics of the child (system) and the child's family and home settings (system environment).

The assessment battery (see Table 4) yields data on the child's characteristics and role models, family organization, and physical environment. Each of these dimensions is defined in terms of unsatisfactory, marginal, or satisfactory status, providing criteria for interpreting data from instruments. The overall data collection and analysis process yields a profile of the child's play/imitation status. She illustrates how the determination of the status leads to intervention strategies through the presentation of a case. As with the previous evaluation battery, this one is an example of taking a particular process critical to occupational development in a defined population and developing a conceptual framework and related assessment process.

Assessing the Developmental Level of Play. Lindquist, Mack, and Parham[86,87] developed a model to synthesize the sensory integration performance constituent of skill and play output of the child. They explained how sensory

Table 4

Summary of Relationships Between Imitation
Factors and the Instruments

Characteristics of the Child	Instrument
1. Vision	1. Play Scale[76,77] Play History[125]
2. Visual Imagery	2. Imaginative Play Scale[76,77]
3. Skill	3. Play Scale[76,77] Play History[125]

Characteristics of Models	Instrument
1. Degree of competence, status, and control over resources	1. Play History[125] Social Competence Interview
2. Nurturing, rewarding behaviors	2. Child/Parent Observation[26]
3. Contagious, major sources of support and control of resources	3. Social Competence Interview Time Analysis[81]
4. Similarity of model to child	4. Child/Parent Observation[26]
5. Number of models having similar behavior and values	5. Time Analysis[81] Play History[125]
6. Similarity of model to dominant values of mainstream culture	6. Value Orientation Inventory[75] Social Competence Interview Internal-External Scale[118] Play History[125]
7. Observation of consequences for model	7. Child/Parent Observation[26]

Characteristics of Family Organization	Instrument
1. Status	1. Social Competence Interview
2. Value	2. Internal-External Scale[118] Value Orientation Inventory
3. Psychological Outcome	3. Social Competence Interview Time Analysis[81]

Characteristics of Physical Environment	Instrument
1. Play Environment	1. Play Agenda[97] Play History[125]

Imitation: A Mechanism of Play Behavior, AJOT, C deRenne-Stephen.

motor processes intermesh with childhood play and the hierarchical organization of play behavior in development. Like the previous authors, they used a systems framework to organize their concepts of play and sensory integration. Assessment plans were developed for the input and throughput processes at three developmental/hierarchical levels: sensory motor, constructive, and social (see Table 5). The authors identified appropriate historical, observational, and standardized occupational therapy instruments and other measures of play behaviors and underlying sensory motor performance capacity. The meaning and interpretations of the assessments are derived from their hierarchical systems model.

This evaluation procedure is especially significant because it represents a synthesis of both occupational performance components and a concern for the child's role as a player. Both are seen as integrated facets of the child. Their schema is a cogent alternative to assessment approaches that focus on only one element or dimension of childhood function while ignoring other important processes. Further, their assessment battery reflects an appreciation for the hierarchical nature of human order.

Summary

This discussion provided an overview of five approaches to organizing the evaluation process. These approaches provide insight into the importance of systematically constructing evaluation procedures and the care that goes into a well-constructed evaluation battery. Each of these batteries proceeded from an examination of occupational therapy themes relevant to a particular setting or population and a type of occupational behavior. This enabled the identification of useful instruments, as well as a meaningful framework for their interpretation.

THE FUNCTIONS AND PROCESSES OF THE OCCUPATIONAL THERAPIST IN PSYCHOSOCIAL DYSFUNCTION

Occupational therapy facilitates participation in adaptive patterns of occupations to elicit, maintain, or restore order. There are three broad ways in which occupational therapists accomplish this. First, occupational therapists directly engage people in occupations (see Figure 3). Second, occupational therapists collaborate with people to enable them to understand their own maladaptive occupational patterns and to alter them through problem solving, planning, and practice. Third, occupational therapists facilitate engagement in occupations by creating a better match between people and their environments. This can be accomplished by effecting changes in the person (e.g.,

Table 5

Assessments of Play Development Considering Environmental (Input) Factors and Internal Processing (Throughput) Factors*

Development Level of Play

Assessment	Sensory Motor		Constructive		Social	
	Input	Throughput	Input	Throughput	Input	Throughput
History	Play history[125]	Sensory history Play history[125]	Play history[125]	Play history[125]	Play history[125]	Play history[125]
Observation	Play agenda[97]	Play scale[16,77] Reflex, range of motion, spasticity, and muscle testing. Clinical observations	Play agenda[97]	Play scale[76,77] Play observation	Play agenda[97]	Observation of social participation Observation of sociodramatic play—Smilansky
Standardized Test	Home observation of the environment (HOME)	Bayley infant scales Bruininks-Oseretsky Test of Motor Proficiency Gesell test Southern California Sensory Integration Test—Ayres Uzgiris-Hunt scales	HOME	Portions of Bayley, Gesell, Uzgiris-Hunt		

A Synthesis of Occupational Behavior and Sensory Integration Concepts in Theory and Practice, Part 2: Clinical Applications, AJOT, JE Lindquist, W Mack, LD Parham.

The American Occupational Therapy Association, Inc., Copyright holder, Copyright 1982, Vol. 36, No. 7, page 435, Table 1.

Figure 3

*The Means by which Occupational Therapists Facilitate Healthy Occupation to Elicit,
Restore or Maintain Order*

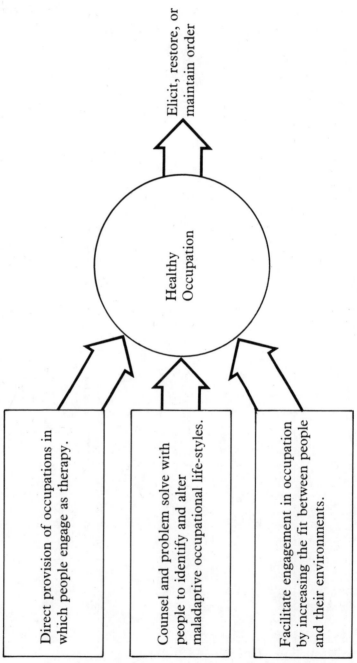

clarifying values, learning new skills) or by altering the environment (e.g., reducing demands, providing structure, increasing resources).

These three broad approaches can be organized into a number of roles and functions of occupational therapists: (1) the therapist as environmental manager, (2) the therapist as mutual problem solver and co-planner, (3) the therapeutic use of self, (4) the use of occupations as therapy, and (5) the use of task-oriented groups. Each of these roles and functions employs concepts of order and disorder.

The Occupational Therapist as Environmental Manager

In moral treatment, the primary therapeutic approach was the arrangement of a healthy environment. The role of the occupational therapist as environmental manager has evolved from this approach.[11] In early occupational therapy, when all patients were treated in the context of the institution, the role was primarily one of making the hospital a healthy place to work and play. With the advent of community-based care and deinstitutionalization, the role of environmental manager became more complex and expanded to include the community. This section first examines the role of the occupational therapist in creating a health-inducing environment, and then discusses the occupational therapist's increasing involvement in community settings.

Creating a Context for Treatment. Early occupational therapists paid considerable attention to the psychosocial environment. In describing occupational therapy programs, writers referred to the mood of cheerfulness and hope, the esprit de corps, the sense of purpose and industry, the feeling of order and rhythm, and other aesthetic and psychosocial properties that exerted a positive influence on the attitudes, conscious processes, and eventual recovery of patients.[67] Bateson[4] argued that occupational therapists must recognize this psychosocial dimension as an essential part of the treatment process. Patient participation in activities is a function of the way in which the environment is organized, the messages given off by the therapist concerning the activity, and the therapist's own attitudes toward the activity. If the activity does not matter a great deal to the therapist, and if the environment does not communicate this concern, the activity becomes a contrivance rather than a genuine human endeavor for the patient. Engelhardt[32] suggested that occupational therapy has as its foundation an appreciation of the value of human achievement and human commerce with the environment and with fellow humans.

Through the communication of such values, occupational therapy has a role in the construction or reconstruction of reality for patients.[123] By becoming a context for action (with certain psychosocial parameters), the occupational therapy setting defines what the patient does and thereby influences how that patient experiences the reality of his or her action and existence. A context is a setting or framework that communicates certain messages and expectations for behavior. The idea of a context or frame is borrowed from our understanding of how such phenomena occur in daily life. For instance, as one enters a church, a classroom, a concert hall, or a romantic French restaurant, it is altogether common to be "moved" by the feeling or tone of the setting and its members, and to feel a compulsion to act in accordance with the implicit rules of conduct. The occupational therapy clinic is not a church or a concert hall, but it is a human context in which the participants will experience and participate in something. By consciously recognizing this fact and carefully arranging the psychosocial climate of the clinic, the therapist has an important impact on what the person will experience and do. Occupational therapists employ identifiable psychosocial contexts derived from the larger culture, such as festivity and ritual, sport, craft, school, and work. Each has its own internal definition and messages, its own mood and meaning, its rules of conduct, and its particular way of influencing the actors within it. Ultimately, occupational therapy provides a context of caring, one that values work and play and signifies hope and the possibility of positive change in the human condition.[134]

A number of sport and game contexts have been used in occupational therapy.[37,56,69] Puzzles provide a sense of mastery over the environment, while games of chance offer events in which one has no such control over outcomes. Games of strategy add a human factor of competition, overt action, and careful attention to others. With each type of game or sport, different behaviors, moods, and values emerge. For example, in games of strategy, fast action and risk in uncertainty may be important values and behaviors. Another type of context that has been used in occupational therapy is that of an educational or school setting.[85] In this context, learning and study are the expected client behaviors. To this end, clients are referred to as students and therapy groups as classes.

The physical and architectural properties of a setting and the dress, behavior, values, and ideals of other people in the setting all help to shape the context. For example, the hospital cafeteria under usual conditions will convey a context of mealtime activities. Transforming the cafeteria with streamers, music, and people in dress clothes who are socializing or dancing communicates a completely different context—that of a party or dance. Work-oriented programs frequently rely on the artifacts and rituals of the real work world to create a simulated work context for clients.[55] For instance, recording members' hours on daily payroll sheets and giving out checks once a week communicate expectations for work behavior similar to that in a real work setting.

Verbal and nonverbal communication also shape the context. When a therapist invites a hospitalized child to "pretend," enjoins a retarded adolescent to take a chance in some game, or joins a group of adult patients in a volunteer program, important messages are given about the expectations, the value, and the possibilities of an activity. Thus, what the therapist communicates by virtue of both talk and action can serve to reinforce or initiate a particular context that is being evoked for therapy.

Anything done to "physically" structure the environment will affect the psychosocial context. Similarly, creating a particular psychosocial atmosphere necessitates corresponding physical changes in the setting. In the previous example of the hospital cafeteria, the context of a holiday dance was enhanced by the use of decorations and other cosmetic changes in the setting. Structuring an activity in a certain way will also influence the psychosocial climate. Providing each member of a group with individual materials and tools communicates expectations for social behavior that are quite different from those communicated by placing a limited number of supplies in the center of a table.[100]

Many occupational therapy interventions contribute to the creation of a general context of competence. One principle for structuring the environment previously noted is that the demands for performance should match the patient's abilities. Essentially, this is the traditional occupational therapy rule of "grading" activities. For instance, in a program of sports with retarded men, sessions progressed from catch to football as the men's athletic prowess increased.[69] In this transition, the environmental demands associated with the games were for increasingly complex levels of skill.

A context for competence is maintained when individuals' feelings of being in control are not undermined by the setting. Involuntary relocation to an institutional setting may infringe on people's sense of control. However, visiting the setting in advance of the actual move, knowing that one's room is a place of privacy, being able to bring one's own possessions and decorations into the room, and continuing contact with friends and activities in the community are environmental interventions that can alleviate the potential feeling of loss of control.[51,128]

Structuring the environment for competence also entails an understanding of which physical conditions are most likely to promote adaptive performance for particular clients. For example, emotionally disturbed children's performance may be enhanced in a distraction-free room with structured activity.[78] For other people, the hospital environment may be understimulating and a more arousing setting may be necessary to induce individuals to give up the passive sick role and resume more active roles.[106]

Managing the environment to create frames for adaptive occupational performance is an intricate and complex process. Everything the therapist says, does, and provides—from interactions with the client to the physical setting, to the choice of activity—is predicated on and contributes to the shaping of the context.

Managing the Community Environment. In the 1950s and 1960s, there was a reverse of the practice of committing psychiatric patients to long-term hospitalization. The community mental health movement has had implications for all mental health workers. In particular, occupational therapists have found themselves modifying and redefining their roles to include more comprehensive responsibility for managing client treatment, to accommodate the changing roles of other disciplines, and to shape a more equal, nonmedical client/ therapist relationships.

The role of the occupational therapist as an environmental manager is one that naturally and meaningfully extends into the community.[71,89] Bockoven[10,11] and Ethridge[33] promote the movement of occupational therapists into responsible leadership positions in community mental health programming. They argue that occupational therapists should establish themselves in roles as community organizers, program developers, and administrators.

The nature of work in the community is quite different from that in hospital clinics.[33] The latter is secure and structured, with limited physical borders, familiar administrative structures and co-worker relationships, a degree of orderliness and domination by the medical profession. The community, a nontraditional work setting for occupational therapists, is characterized by less structure, no physical boundaries, new administrative and co-worker relationships, and a relatively nonmedical orientation. In the hospital setting, the therapeutic relationship tends to be more vertical, with the therapist as helper and the client in a dependent patient role. The community is more conducive to horizontal relationships, in which the therapist is a friendly collaborator in guiding the client and enabling greater client independence.

In the community the therapist needs to be familiar with local standards; to work with a wide range of key support people and agencies such as teachers, neighbors, family and friends, and government and social-recreational groups; and to be familiar with work or volunteer opportunities and the range of productive and play activities available in the community. In addition, the community demands a broader understanding of the life situation, culture, history, and environments in which clients exist and act in order to provide optimally meaningful intervention.[71]

Occupational therapists may be found working in residential programs such as group homes for the mentally retarded, halfway houses, club house rehabilitation programs for deinstitutionalized psychiatric patients, and day treatment programs.[25,53,55,88,89] Programs that have been developed to bridge the gap between the hospital and the community and to prevent rehospitalization include quarterway house programs, partial hospitalization, and other transitional programs.[79,80,92,130] Community programs for the well elderly population have been developed as a prevention strategy.[18,73] In these community programs occupational therapists have worked to promote adjustment and independence in their clients through intervention that focuses on the development of a range of life skills, from grooming to job seeking. For example, a work-oriented day care program with a strong occupational therapy component and a temporary employment program emphasized the value of work in terms of the opportunity it offers for meaningful participation in society.[55] Members attending the work component were found to be more self-directed, more active in directing their treatment program, and more hopeful regarding goal achievement than were clients in the general activity program component. The clubhouse model developed by Fountain House in New York City has influenced the design of many community treatment programs for the long-term psychiatric patient. This is a psychosocial rehabilitation model that requires maximal member involvement in maintaining the clubhouse operation. It offers members the opportunity to be either temporary or full-time workers in competitive employment. The program includes a clubhouse, temporary employment program, apartment program, and various other components. Members' attendance at the clubhouse is wanted, expected, and needed for clubhouse functioning. The model is based on the beliefs that even the most severely psychosocially dysfunctional person can be productive, that work is a worthwhile "regenerative and reintegrative" goal, and that recreational and social activities have value in the normal daily routine.[5]

Transitional programs are designed to ease the move from hospital to community. One task-oriented daily living group available to predischarge patients focused on the use of leisure time, learning about community resources, and general problem solving related to the discharge process.[53] Another, a quarterway house program developed by occupational therapists on the grounds of a state hospital, allowed patients to take increased responsibility in preparation for their return to the community.[92]

A program called neighborhood extension of activity therapy was designed to aid in transition to the community by promoting use of existing community leisure resources.[79] This program emphasized the exploration and matching of interests and resources to promote client involvement in the community. A different type of community program was developed as a preventive strategy for well elderly participants.[73] Elderly clients attending a nutrition program were given avocational and recreational activities, physical exercises, and educational sessions for the purpose of increasing life satisfaction. Positive changes were noted in clients' levels of socialization, general affect, and life satisfaction.

These programs demonstrate the therapist's role as environmental manager and the variety of uses of the community setting for promoting mental health and life satisfaction and providing meaningful, responsible, and productive roles for people in the community.

Therapist as Co-Problem Solver and Co-Planner

Earlier discussions implied that occupational therapists do not function as one-to-one or group psychotherapists. This issue is often confused with that of the appropriateness of occupational therapists offering counseling as part of therapy. This confusion arises over the mistaken notion that counseling implies a psychotherapeutic approach along with its typical goals of achieving emotional catharsis and insight into intrapsychic dynamics. Quite the contrary, counseling is a process that can have very different goals and purposes and that may be used as part of occupational therapy.

The counseling process should be viewed in light of its intended functions in occupational therapy—that is, facilitating the person's participation in a pattern of healthy occupation. This goal can be addressed in the counseling process when the therapist engages in mutual problem solving and planning with individuals. For instance, people often have problems managing their time, relating activities to goals, and identifying problem areas in their daily life occupations. By helping such individuals achieve new directions, decisions, life plans, and time schedules, the occupational therapist facilitates occupation and health.

Three broad areas of occupational counseling can be differentiated: time management planning and problem solving, leisure counseling, and occupational choice counseling. All aim to actively involve the consumer in identifying problem areas and strengths, goal setting, and planning a course of action.[94]

In occupational therapy, counseling results in action through the setting of a goal for performance, be it a full week's schedule or a single hour of activity. Client performance is thus an essential part of this counseling process. For instance, a therapist offering leisure counseling may have established with a client the goal of attending a dance. In the following session, the therapist and client would explore together what had happened, whether the client's actions were adaptive or maladaptive, and decide whether it is time to go on to another activity, if more practice in the same activity is needed, or some other option. Thus, new goals for task performance are set as an outcome of ongoing performance evaluation.

The goal setting process is essential for all occupational therapy counseling regardless of its focus or whether it occurs in an inpatient or outpatient setting. In time, the client should internalize the process and continue it independently. Thus, the person should eventually be able to get information, make well-informed decisions about personal changes and goals, decide on the appropriate tasks related to those goals, set about doing the tasks, and evaluate their outcomes.

Time Management Planning and Problem Solving. Counseling regarding the healthy use of time is a role of occupational therapists. A framework of temporal adaptation[61] can serve as a guide to time management planning and problem solving. Using it the therapist seeks to gather data on several relevant aspects of the person's temporal adaptation. The therapist initially explores the degree of balance in the person's daily life through a diary self-report of time use, a report of a typical day, or an interview aimed at reconstructing the person's usual daily behavior. Lack of leisure time, insufficient work time, lack of rest or sleep, and disorganized time use can be identified. Importantly, the balance of work, play, rest, and sleep includes not only the amounts of time devoted to each activity but also a qualitative dimension. For instance, a person with a smaller percentage of time devoted to recreation may have a more balanced life-style than someone else who has more time for recreation but who replicates the competitive and achievement oriented nature of work in recreation.

A second critical dimension of evaluation is the relationship between an individual's values, interests, and goals and his or her use of time. The occupational questionnaire can be used to assess the degree to which people enact their interests and values in daily life. A third dimension of temporal adaptation is the degree to which a person's time use reflects a balance of life roles. A therapist can explore whether or not the individual has sufficient numbers of roles to organize time use, whether there is role conflict (i.e., roles presenting conflicting demands for time use), or whether the individual's time use reflects a failure to meet role demands. A further dimension is the match of a person's time use to the environments within which he or she performs. Each setting has its own requirements for how occupants use time, and competence is reflected in a person's ability to meet those requirements.

Another area to be examined is the relationship of temporal patterns to any pathology or limitations of performance. Here, two issues are involved: adjustments that must be made to disease and its constraints, and the impact of patterns of time use on pathological processes. Some people with psychosocial dysfunction have physical limitations (e.g., cerebral palsy) or emotional or mental limitations (e.g., cognitive problems or low stress tolerance) which necessitate schedules that maximize their strengths while taking into account these limitations. For instance, a man who has cerebral palsy, but who wants to appear neatly dressed may spend a great deal of time each morning in self-care. The value of self-care and appearance to this individual make it important to maintain it as part of his schedule. For someone else, trying to pursue two roles, such as worker and student, might produce more stress than the person can tolerate. In this case, it is important to realize that one role may need to be given up if the person is to cope successfully with the other.

The second issue, the impact of time use on pathology, describes a situation in which a person's time use can be identified as directly contributing to a psychosocial problem. One may identify how the overscheduled day of a workaholic contributes to a sense of helplessness and depression or how the chaotic and unplanned day of a schizophrenic contributes to disorientation and a sense of unreality.

The goals of counseling for temporal adaptation are organized along the same dimensions as evaluation. The therapist and client seek to schedule a balanced daily and weekly routine that allows the client time to pursue work, play, and rest; time to fulfill life roles; and time to enact values and interests while meeting the reasonable demands of the environment. Sometimes, this process involves tasks other than simply planning time. Clarifying values, deciding to drop an unnecessary role, negotiating with others for altered role demands, developing skills for more efficient time use, and identifying interests to guide temporal behavior are examples of strategies that might be pursued as part of establishing a healthy use of time in daily life.

One of the most important aspects of time management counseling is helping people achieve an integration between present time use and future goals. By identifying the tasks needed for a future goal and integrating them into the present, the person may achieve a relationship between present patterns of time use and orientation to the future. This often involves the important process of occupational choice, which, because of its complexity, is treated here as a separate area of occupational therapy counseling.

Occupational Choice Counseling. Occupational choice counseling refers to facilitating a lifelong process of choices for occupational roles that may include work, but that extend to many other occupational behaviors. Further, occupational choice refers to much more than the process of identifying and selecting a job or an area of training for work. It involves the developmental process of anticipating success and satisfaction in life occupations, of developing interests, values, and a personal identity. The occupational therapist intervenes when occupational choice is developmentally delayed and when people demonstrate patterns of having made poor choices for occupational behavior. Occupational choice counseling may culminate in referral of an individual to a vocational or rehabilitation counselor who can help a person select training opportunities, identify resources for training, and so on. Finally, because occupational therapists recognize occupational choice as a process involving a dynamic interplay of action, choice, feedback, and further action, they integrate occupational choice counseling with the prescription and planning of experiences, skill training, values clarification procedures, and other processes that facilitate development of occupational choice.

Paulson[107] and Webster[131] offer schemas of occupational choice and of assessing the developmental level of choice. They also illustrate the various action implications of occupational choice problems that serve as a guide to setting up tasks for clients to pursue as part of a counseling process.

While much of the focus of occupational choice is on the major productive role of the individual (i.e., the worker role), occupational choice is a process involving many decisions about life roles. For example, becoming a volunteer, pursuing an amateur activity, preparing for retirement, and deciding how to replace the homemaker role when children leave home are examples of situations requiring an occupational choice. Therapists can bring the same issues and procedures to these choices as to the choice of the worker role. Additionally, they can enable people to identify what needs are met in other continuing or future roles so as to clarify the main purposes of these occupational choices.

Leisure Counseling. The occupational therapist's role as a leisure counselor extends from concern for people's temporal adaptation and their ability to find meaning in play or leisure. The occupational therapist views leisure as one role within the total occupational life-style of the individual. In leisure counseling, the therapist engages in a collaborative problem-solving endeavor with the goal of enhancing the client's ability to independently plan and use leisure time. The process is more involved than simply exploring or enacting leisure interests—it entails identification of the client's values as they pertain to both work and play and of the client's current and anticipated roles and determination of the presence or absence of skills that will support a leisure role.

Occupational therapists encounter many clients for whom leisure counseling is appropriate. Workaholics, socially isolated individuals such as a mother of five children or a previous drug abuser, or a retiree may be potential candidates.[46] A leisure counseling program can also be part of a transitional discharge planning program for psychiatric patients.

A counseling continuum exists for the development of leisure behavior.[46] In this continuum, optimal leisure behavior is self-chosen and independently enacted; that is, the leisure activity is chosen for its own sake, and the client is intrinsically motivated. At the other end of the spectrum is leisure behavior that is dependent and determined by therapy. In other words, the client does not have the skills or resources to actively and independently pursue leisure, but must learn these skills in the context of therapy.

Kolodner[79] describes a transitional program that meets the needs of clients who fall somewhere between these two ends. The program begins with an initial interview in which the interest checklist is used to help the client ascertain interests and skills. Following this session, the therapist investigates community possibilities for enacting at least two of the client's expressed interests. In a future meeting, the therapist gives the client such information as names of agencies or programs, fees, times and dates for activities, and locations. From this information, a program is selected, and plans are made for the client to attend a session. If the client is hesitant about making the initial contact, either another client or the therapist accompanies the person to the activity. After the client's first attendance at the activity, the therapist and client meet again to evaluate the experience. Thus, the client moves from structure and support to gradual independent leisure in the community.

The following is an example of a leisure planning unit for hospitalized psychiatric patients at an earlier stage of leisure behavior. Referrals to this group were based on an inability to identify interests, poor use of free time in the hospital, difficulty scheduling time, and a lack of awareness of community resources or of how to find out about things to do. Group activities began with an examination of how patients' time was presently structured by the hospital program and how they would ideally like to structure their time after discharge. The next sessions were devoted to values clarification activities in which patients identified activities they enjoyed and characteristics of these activities (such as whether or not they were social, expensive, and so on). To help identify new interests, hobby and sports books were brought to group meetings, and patients were asked to choose an activity from these books to carry out on the ward during the week. The next major activity was typically an outing to the local library, where group members collected information on current community events and planned, in pairs, three possible Saturday outings, one of which would be carried out before the next group meeting. When the group reconvened members reported on their trips and then planned a final activity that would be engaged in by the whole group in the last session. This was a time-limited group that moved from ward uses of free time to planning group and community leisure activities.

Cantor[18] describes preretirement planning for individuals who, because of the changes introduced by retirement, may be unable to reorganize or rebalance their use of time. This program begins with clients completing an activities configuration, to identify their current balance of work, play, and self-care, as well as the source of motivation for these activities, and a self-evaluation of how well they perform them. In the second stage of counseling, the client develops a profile of personal time use and then determines areas to change or maintain. The third stage is a search for alternatives, adaptations, or rearrangements leading to the eventual selection of new options for the client's use of time.

Leisure counseling thus draws on the occupational therapist's skills in helping individuals to define their needs, interests, and ability to satisfy these needs and interests, and to locate community resources where leisure interests can be pursued.[46]

The Therapeutic Use of Self in Occupational Therapy

The importance of the self as a therapeutic agent is a general theme in the training of most mental health workers. It implies that the therapist's personal attributes, actions, and reactions are an essential component of therapy.

The goal of the classical psychoanalytic relationship was to achieve an emotional bond between the therapist and the patient that would result in the unfolding of a series of psychodynamics. The patient would project feelings onto this new relationship and recreate earlier relationships from his or her childhood. The therapist was largely passive and commented only rarely, offering interpretations when he or she felt the patient was "ready" to accept them. Neo-Freudians objected to the classical view of the therapist as a tabula rasa, or blank sheet, upon which the patient replayed the drama of childhood relationships. They argued that the therapist's own behaviors contributed as much to the patient's actions as did such psychodynamic processes as transference. Humanists and existentialists went even further, suggesting that the classical model gave the therapist too much importance and control over the relationship because the therapist ultimately and noncollaboratively set treatment goals for the patient. They advocated a nondirective role for the therapist with the patient being responsible for decisions about his or her life.

The humanistic or client-centered approach to therapy has had a pervasive impact on mental health professionals, including occupational therapists.[45] Dunning[31] described the application of humanism to the role of the occupational therapist, stressing that therapists engage in an "authentic" relationship with their clients, accepting the clients' goals and not imposing their own. In building and consolidating this relationship, activity became "a bridge for the relationship to travel on" (p. 475).[31] This notion of the activity as a bridge, however, represents a crucial dilemma to understanding the therapeutic relationship in occupational therapy. If activity is viewed only as a means to some other end, then the value of occupation as a worthwhile human endeavor is denigrated.

What is required to appreciate the therapeutic use of self in occupational therapy is the recognition that human relations include many types of bonds, mutual expectancies, and responses. The classic therapeutic relationship, with its focus on feelings and unconscious elements in the relationship, is only one of many important ways in which human beings relate to each other. In humans, another entire domain of relations can be recognized, those related to productivity and to recreation, festivity, and ritual. These relationships belong to the general class of occupation and are the relationships associated with work and play. The therapeutic use of self in occupational therapy derives its nature from the genre and ethos of these relationships; thus, when engaging clients in occupations, the therapist assumes the role of teacher, supervisor, coach, player, craftsperson, and so forth. Each of these roles contributes to a therapeutic use of self unique to occupational therapy.

Two sets of relationships characterize the use of self in occupational therapy. One set of relations emerges from the therapist's classic function of engaging patients and clients in productive occupations. When a therapist seeks to induce a person to engage in an art, craft, or other productive occupation, he or she must instruct, coach, and supervise, provide support and encouragement, be a role model, and so on. As is obvious from these behaviors, the therapist's function centers on the patient's performance in the occupation and derives its purpose from their joint efforts to engage in a productive enterprise. In the role of instructor, the therapist becomes someone who must know how to do the activity, who values the occupation enough to want to share this knowledge, and who is able to accept the learner's own motives and values pertaining to the occupation and the process of learning. Also, as an instructor, the therapist must be able to diagnose a person's strengths and weaknesses and the constraints and resources in the environment that will affect learning.

When the therapist serves as a role model, he or she communicates that the endeavor is one that requires correct knowledge of procedure, application of personal energy, perseverance, and willingness of the learner to imitate and take advice from the more knowledgeable person. These communications about the reality of productive enterprise are often those that psychosocially dysfunctional people have not had access to in the course of their life experiences.

Related to such task performance, the therapist often serves as a source of hope to the patient, pointing out the worth of struggle by enumerating the possibilities and criteria of success. The therapist is also an important source of affirmation of success and must honestly praise and rejoice in the success of clients. In the context of productive occupation, the therapeutic interaction is built around enabling people to acquire the emotional and informational resources they need to enter a productive role. An apprentice-like association between therapist and client is the key to this therapeutic relationship.[17]

A second major set of behaviors related to the therapeutic use of self in occupational therapy pertains to the play occupations used as therapy. In play, the goal of participants is the expression of common values; affirmation of common humanity and common circumstance; the discovery of new modes of being and experiencing; the celebration of existence, accomplishment, and survival of hardship; the relief from the efforts of labor; and similar emotions and thoughts. All participants in festivity, celebration, playful competition, and other forms of human play come to a common ground and participate in parallel relationships. Hence, the therapist assumes a commonality with all the players and participates genuinely with them in playing. The therapist must be truly participating or else the spirit and ethos of the activity will not emerge and invite participation.

Certain functions are common to both the productive and playful sets of relationships. The first is that the therapist is consisently a creator of meaning. She or he does this by establishing an external order or dramatic context, within which certain behaviors are expected or relevant and others are out of context or irrelevant.[4,120] Meaning is also created when the therapist believes in the value of the activity and cares deeply about the modality itself.[4] Finally the therapist's ability to understand and manage the environment allows him or her to manipulate the setting to contribute to the creation of meaning.

The second function is that of systems analyst. The therapist becomes a creative problem solver, a hypothesis tester, and a provider of feedback.[57] Finally, the therapist becomes both an advocate for clients, enabling them to locate community resources, and a modulator of the environment, seeking to adjust its demands to match the client's potential for action.[134]

The implications of these modes of therapeutic use of self in occupational therapy is that the therapist must be an expert in the nature of occupations, their requirements, their moods, and their pertinent human relations. Similarly, the therapist must be an expert in analyzing the social and physical contexts for occupations and in identifying both individual and environmental resources and constraints for productive behavior. Without an appreciation of the modes of existence and coexistence represented in the occupational efforts of humans, the occupational therapist cannot make effective therapeutic use of self in the manner that is unique to and important for occupational therapy. This principle was stated very simply in the early literature of the field when writers often noted that the therapist must be a craftsperson and a sportsperson, must have an appreciation of music and dance, and must value the occupations used as therapy for their own sake, for their worthiness to solicit human participation.

The Use of Occupations as Therapy

The oldest and most central role of occupational therapists is that of directly engaging people in occupations as treatment. The history of occupational therapy reveals that a broad spectrum of activities have been considered under the rubric of occupation and used for therapy.[67] The earliest and continuing conceptualization of occupation is that it consists of those behaviors with which people fill the majority of their time. Broadly speaking, all forms of work, play, and self-care are types of occupations.

In the early years of this century, many types of play activities were used. These included art, dance, music, theater and drama, and games and sports. The emphasis of the early leaders of occupational therapy on the playful and creative side of human nature and its role in facilitating healthy adaptation supported this wide use of play activities. However, changes occurred as therapists became embarrassed with their "play lady" image and tended to move away from many playful forms of therapy. Arts and crafts were retained apparently because they had an element of productivity and because they simulated work.

Perhaps the occupation most consistently of concern to psychosocial occupational therapists was self-care. Slagle's early programs of habit training focused on this aspect of occupation, and therapists have continued to develop and use training programs for improved self-care of people with psychosocial dysfunction.

At this point in the history of the field, one might properly ask what occupations are suitable for occupational therapy. The response should come from an examination of what constitutes the occupational behaviors that are currently part of the culture. The changing and varied occupational forms that manifest themselves in the everyday life of society should determine what is useful for therapy. Should arts and crafts lose their place in modern society, their relevance to occupational therapy would diminish. If other behaviors emerge as a form of major occupation (for example, computer based activities), then they should find their way into occupational therapy clinics and programs. The field must be attuned to the occupational life of the culture and adjust its therapeutic media accordingly.

Because many subcultures exist in the United States, occupational therapists must be prepared to offer a wide range of occupations as therapy. What is meaningful to a New York theater director will probably not interest a midwestern farmer. The life occupations of a ghetto youth will differ from the interests and abilities of an elderly middle class lawyer. The common denominator among these people is that they have a human urge to explore and master their worlds, which manifests itself in ways relevant to their socio-cultural environments. To be truly effective, occupational therapists must be prepared to offer this range of occupations. Consequently, the following sections describe a wide range of occupations (dance, arts and crafts, games, play, sport, music, theater, work) as the media of occupational therapy. The most central issue for occupational therapy is the art and science which is the basis for using various media as therapy.[132] Thus, this section begins with a perspective on the art and science of using occupation as a health determinant.

The Art and Science of Occupational Therapy Media. A past approach to psychosocial occupational therapy was the use of media as tools of a psychoanalytic therapy. That is, activities were used as arenas in which patients unconsciously revealed and released feelings through the characteristics of their performances. Thus, therapists designed assessment batteries in which patients created collages, clay objects, and fingerpaintings that were then interpreted by therapists for their symbolic and feeling themes.[2,15,82,83] In parallel fashion, the media were used as cathartic mechanisms whereby patients could express and release pent-up feelings. One hammered out anger, portrayed loneliness in blue watercolors, and enacted a need for affection in psychodrama. Even more classical Freudian approaches were used to help patients gratify immature or blocked needs. Thus, anal fixations were worked out in clay, oral gratification was received through a cooking group, and so on.[35]

This approach to occupational therapy in psychosocial practice is best left to the category of historical curiosity for several reasons. First, it is becoming more recognized that psychoanalytic approaches are best used with the patient who is articulate and who can afford the luxury of a longstanding analytic relationship; however, occupational therapists must be willing to relate methods to patients' needs and problems. The patient population seen by occupational therapists in psychosocial practice is more often the chronic patient whose competence is highly questionable. The majority of these patients suffer primarily from an inability to occupy themselves in a productive and self-satisfying manner. They lack the skills for action, the habits for an organized life-style, and the roles that give them identity and make them acceptable to society. Further, those who have been competent and who now suffer from emotional disturbance often do so from a failure to find meaning in their lives, and the problem is one of bringing their values, goals, and personal view of self into focus and relating them to activity in the real world.

Another reason for giving up the psychoanalytic approach is that occupational therapy should serve as a socializing environment in which patients learn how to construct and organize their actions and identities. This particular orientation is largely incompatible with either an exclusively analytic or combined analytic/competency approach. Reasons for this are found in the communications given when occupations are used as therapy and the context of their presentation to patients. One of the most basic lessons of life is that there is a time and place for everything. Patients in psychiatric care are often heavily engaged in the business of working through pathological or painful feeling states. A great deal of attention is paid to the experience and expression of painful emotions. When such an orientation pervades much of the patient's life, it becomes difficult to discriminate when and where healthy expression of negative feelings should occur.

Of all therapies, occupational therapy should have the most fundamental commitment to the process of doing and to there being a time and a place for performance where negative feelings are tolerated and controlled while the person works toward the positive feelings of accomplishment, satisfaction, control, and self-worth.[37] Such feeling states as anger and self-satisfaction are notoriously incompatible. The importance of occupational therapy as a very special area within the psychosocial treatment arena—one which demands performance and which duly rewards it with recognition—must not be underestimated. The fundamental message of occupational therapy is that positive feelings accrue through the risk-taking, the creativity, and the effort of engaging in work and play. That message should come through clearly in occupational therapy.

Additionally, one should give serious consideration to the possibility that an eclectic approach combining the competency orientation and the expression of unconscious feelings may bear an inherently inconsistent and highly confusing message, because of its potential double-bind communication. In competency-oriented practice, the patient derives satisfaction and feelings of self-worth through completion of some performance or some product that he or she has planned, chosen, and executed. Here the message is that conscious, willful application of effort yielded some worthy outcome. The analytic approach, which views activity as the product or expression of unconscious feeling otherwise not accessible, offers a contradictory message. It suggests the product of performance is shaped by unconscious and negative forces. It appears inconsistent and self-contradictory that a hammered ashtray should be at once an expression of ability and effort as well as the manifestation of latent anger, or that a painting should express insecurity while being an example of competent execution of technique and aesthetic. For patients who are struggling for evidence of their worth and ability, the suggestion that unconscious forces move and direct performances runs too high a risk of undermining a sense of accomplishment or providing conflicting versions of performance. It would do little for one's feelings of competence to be confused about whether the choice of the color red was a manifestation of one's ability to artfully produce or of one's anger.

The fundamental occupational therapy hypothesis is that people can become competent and confident through what they do. Doing enables people to become more fully human as they develop their potential and earn their membership in the culture through their contributions. Operationalization of that hypothesis is a complex enterprise requiring the effort and attention of the field. Dispersing the field's efforts to multiple orientations and techniques does little to fulfill this mandate.

The art and science of occupational therapy underlying the therapeutic use of occupations is based in the understanding of the health-giving nature of occupation and the cultural and personal significance of occupation. As the culture develops and changes or varies among different groups, media will necessarily change and vary. Whereas looms filled the clinics in past generations, computers will likely be important in the future as therapeutic media.[54] For one patient in one part of the country, music may mean a simple hand-wrought instrument, while for another, it is appreciation of the classics. For some people manual labor is demeaning, while for others it signifies the reason and worth of their existence. Recognition of these differences and the flexibility to use a wide range of media as part of the art and science of occupational therapy practice are essential.

Play. The play of childhood is a singularly important contributor to competence in adulthood.[111] Occupational therapists have long acknowledged play to be a critical developmental phenomenon that facilitates adaptation toward adult occupational behavior. In play, children learn symbols or rules that serve as internal maps for acting on the world.[111,113] Play is an important learning medium because it involves the use of musculoskeletal, neurological, and symbolic components of skill;[40] because it incorporates an attitude of curiosity and a state of optimal neurological excitation or arousal;[40,86,113,126] and because it provides a safe context for experimentation. Play facilitates and mirrors the developmental process.[40,125] Early play facilitates sensorimotor development and simple social interaction skills. Later, it develops more complex social behaviors, mastery over tool use, and assumption of roles.

The approaches to using play as therapy are multiple and often complex. To elicit play the environment must have sufficient and suitable objects and people, there should be novelty and opportunities for exploration, repetition, and imitation.[26,40] The approach to eliciting play through environmental manipulation thus includes the use of objects, people, and events. Play activities must also be chosen for the appropriate developmental level of children.

Florey[40] and Michelman[97] offer excellent schemas for identifying the appropriate objects, people, and procedures at different levels of play.

The major rationale underlying the use of play as a therapeutic medium is the identification of skill deficits that can be attributed to a lack or paucity of play experiences. Robinson[113] provides a series of questions to be used to guide judgments about whether a child plays and how well he or she plays. The play history interview also provides data on the quality and quantity of play experiences. Following the identification of children's play deficits, therapists can determine the type of play that would facilitate the development and acquisition of skills. Play is an appropriate arena in which to affect change in all three constituents of skills, because it is a holistic phenomenon.

Games. A subclass of play, games are motivating because they reduce the severity of consequences while still allowing the individual to employ his or her abilities and take risks in situations of competition, uncertainty, and chance. The advent of simulated games has paved the way for a new understanding of gaming technique as a means of encapsulating some complex aspect of reality and allowing one to compete, solve problems, pursue strategies, and receive realistic feedback on consequences.[111]

In adolescent and childhood psychosocial treatment settings, games are routinely used as forms of normal recreation. Here their therapeutic properties are seen largely in the context of providing normal patterns of childhood and adolescent behavior to occupy patients' time. However, games have been used in more specific ways in occupational therapy. For example, Carey[19] explored the utility of games in developing an appreciation of the nature of rules and the reciprocal behavior of following rules in juvenile delinquent youths. According to research and clinical observation, juvenile delinquents exhibit less ability to engage in and enjoy competitive game situations. The program was thus designed to enable delinquent youths to develop a sense of rules through competitive play. A series of game-playing sessions were followed by discussions of what happens when rules are broken, why rules are followed, how rules allow people to play the game together, the implications of cheating, and the nature of competition, winning, and losing.

Hurff[56] created several table games and adapted commercial games to simulate real life situations. These enabled people to try out problem-solving approaches and strategies for social interaction and to learn some concrete skills. This program of games was devised for developmentally disabled adolescents and adults; the program appears to be easily generalizable to all populations of psychosocially disabled people who are experiencing difficulty in daily living skills and judgments. Hurff provides a useful overview of the literature on games as learning situations and a helpful list of properties of games that facilitate the development of skills. These can be used as guidelines for selecting or constructing games.

Hurff observed that her program of games provided patients with the opportunity to experience a variety of simulated situations that arise in community life. One particularly interesting aspect of the games was the simulation of emergency situations. Allowing people to experience and respond to these circumstances in the game facilitated their adaptive response when such situations arose in real life. Overall, simulated games appear to be useful preludes to actual community training and experience.

Sports. Sports are a natural part of everyday life. Many Americans recreate as sport spectators and participants. In early occupational therapy, sports were valued for their ability to teach participants a sense of sportsmanship, which was viewed as an antecedent to citizenship or participation in everyday social reality.[67]

While the use of sports in occupational therapy has been less widespread in recent years, they remain a potentially rich medium for therapeutic application for several reasons. First, their widespread popularity makes them attractive to many people. Second, sports are highly variable and adaptable. They can range from such simple procedures as tag to complex games with many rules and players, such as baseball and basketball. They can be solitary activities such as swimming, fishing, or running, or group activities with highly organized interrelationships. They can involve very simple gross motor movements or quite demanding feats of coordination. The advent of new games[42,43] that have been incorporated into many occupational therapy programs has allowed a creative and noncompetitive use of sporting activities.

While sports have a wide variety of potentially therapeutic properties, three are notable. First, the excitement of competition and/or cooperation tends to attract people, often eliciting performance not otherwise possible.

The second property of sports is their unique ability to teach people role behavior.[69,126] In sports, people assume a variety of roles and have the opportunity to understand how roles determine one's contribution to the team or group and how roles guide reciprocal behavior between participants.

Finally, sports, both in participatory and spectator forms, generate enthusiasm and a sense of belonging to social groups.[126] Everything from the homecoming game to the World Series has a special way of bringing individuals a sense of community and common purpose. No doubt, society needs its games to keep members feeling that they are part of the whole. Games can help overcome feelings of alienation and solidify one's attempts to be a part of a group.

King[72] developed an approach to using sporting activities based on concepts of neurological function and dysfunction in some psychiatric patients. While her primary aim in using games and sports was to facilitate sensory integration, she recognized the importance of mind-body interactions and, thus, the necessity of incorporating desired sensory and motor experiences into sport-like activities. Recognizing that neurological changes could be elicited only when proper mental and conscious experiences are involved, she incorporated "elements of skill, chance surprise, incongruity, and suspense" (p. 535)[72] in the activities in order to make them attractive and meaningful, and to elicit a sense of pleasurable participation on behalf of patients. King's approach is an example of the hierarchical principle that when one wishes to correct a deficit in one constituent of skill, other constituents and their relationships must be recognized.

Kaplan[58] developed a group for low level psychiatric patients of all diagnoses. Her goal was to provide simple adaptations of sports with low demands for both rules and behavior. One example of her adapted sports is a game in which people throw a Nurf ball to other seated members in a circle, while engaging in a parallel verbal behavior such as naming the person to whom the ball is thrown or naming a member of some class of objects (e.g., a type of car) without repeating anything another person has already said. She also employs an adapted form of soccer involving kicking a ball from seated positions and attempting to get it past another person's chair. Kaplan's procedure incorporates simple rules, skills, and roles into an activity that has an element of fun and moderate competition along with cooperation and reality-orientation. The games elicit participation from patients who do not participate in verbal groups or other activities.

Kielhofner and Miyake[69] used sports with mentally retarded adults to elicit a variety of motor, psychosocial, and social behavior changes. These people were unaccustomed to the movements, attitudes, and rules and behaviors of the sport activities. Therapists participated in the sports as peers and as coaches, keeping up the mood and continuity of the game. Over a period of time the program progressed from simple sports such as games of tag to football, frisbee, and baseball, complex games with multiple roles and teams.

Performing Arts. The performing arts include such occupations as drama, dance, film and video, music, magic, puppetry, storytelling, and mime. Many of these media hold a less prominent place in occupational therapy today than in the past. However, their substantial possibilities for therapeutic application are being increasingly recognized. One important reason for the inclusion of such occupations in psychosocial practice is the need for a wide range of media to suit the particular tastes and values of different persons. Not all people are oriented to or find meaning in creative arts that result in the production of an object. They may prefer those that have public performance as their goal. Performing arts also provide opportunities for different kinds of action, emotion, and cognition—as well as a very different social organization—than do creative arts.

Music and drama, for instance, are important agents of socialization in many societies and subcultures. For adolescents, being familiar with the prevailing musical hits and knowing the current dance steps are essential parts of fitting in with one's peers. For certain adults, church singing and piano singalongs are favorite forms of recreation. Drama is closely linked to ritual and in some societies is a means of passing along the traditions and history of the group. In addition, the prescribed role relationships that may exist in drama, folk dancing, music ensembles, and so on provide opportunities to learn and practice different roles in the context of highly coordinated and cooperative behavior. Thus, the expressive arts offer a variety of opportunities for people to learn and practice skills, develop social interaction and role behavior, deepen their appreciation of the cultural meanings of their environments, and experience the success that accrues from personal and mutual application of human effort. Finally, the public nature of expressive arts provides via the intended and actual audience a point of reference and a source of feedback that facilitates self-assessment.

Goldstein and Collins[47] note an additional advantage of film and video as permanent performing media, since they "require integration into the user's environment; that is, one needs to be in a specific environment to take a picture of that environment" (p. 530).[47] They describe a videotape project with hospitalized adolescents that capitalized on the cultural relevance of television to this age group. This project enabled the teenagers to learn how to use equipment, to assume different production roles and levels of responsibility, to achieve some control over their experiences of hospitalization, and to explore issues pertaining to health care and illness in the scripts.

Performing arts also provide opportunities for individuals to recognize, affirm, and appreciate the significant events of a culture. For instance, a Christmas play and talent show allows participants to explore and express the meanings of the holiday. The collective efforts required to execute a play, a circus, a variety show, a musical, or a dance presentation have an unusual organizing effect on patients. Typically, people who have seemed incompetent or withdrawn suddenly muster the ability to perform and maintain a protracted contact with the reality of some purposeful action in the world. The ambience of the performing arts and the way in which they signify the connection between performer and society make them immediately useful as a means of bringing people into the reality of social life. Further, their role as carriers of emotional and symbolic messages such as beauty, hope, courage, joy, triumph over suffering, and so forth makes them especially appropriate as experiences that teach values and meaning to participants.

Arts and Crafts. For a period of time, the utility of arts and crafts in occupational therapy was questioned, in part due to the general devaluation of "handmade" objects in American culture as brought on by mass production and consumerism. Today, there is a resurrection of handcraft represented not only in the increasing number of people engaging in crafts, but in the increased commercial value of handmade items.

Perhaps the single most imporant contribution to the field's understanding of the value of arts and crafts was made by Reilly[109] in her statement that "man, through the use of his hands as they are energized by mind and will, can influence the state of his own health" (p. 2). Though she did not intend the statement to be solely on behalf of the arts and crafts, it served as a reaffirmation of their importance as a therapeutic tool, since crafts bind thought and action. One can view art and craft as a subcategory of play that embodies its freedom, joy, and creativity while resulting in a tangible, useful, and aesthetic object. Thus, while craft is playfully done, it can serve a productive end. As such, it is an important bridge between play and work.

Crafts embody a value system (standards of performance and utility) and procedural rules that make them organizing activities. To engage in the craft, one must correctly apply the rules. One is energized by the possibility of excellence in the craft and the potential for beauty and utility in the product. Crafts can be important simulators of work satisfaction and work conditions.[23]

Crafts lend themselves to both individual and cooperative group processes. The therapist often serves as a kind of master craftsperson who must select tools and materials and demonstrate techniques, serving as an inspiration and a role model to participants. Crafts can be integrated into actual life situations when persons make objects to decorate or to function within their own living spaces or as gifts. Art and craft organized into the individual's life are more meaningful.

A number of therapeutic properties of arts and crafts have been identified.[23,109] They include opportunities for problem solving; learning to deal with materials and people in productive situations; the ability to develop a positive self-image and increased confidence from accomplishment; the potential to productively contribute to society; the development of skills that can carry over into one's life-style; and orientation to the reality of work.

Work. The value of work as therapy has long been recognized, beginning with the efforts of moral treatment practitioners. Occupational therapists have continued to use various forms of work as a part of their therapeutic programs.

Noting that hospitalization often resulted in atrophy of work skills and work roles, Reilly[110] argued that work should be incorporated into all adult therapeutic programs. She also pointed out that for the adult, work is a necessary component of the balance of occupation in daily life. One cannot have true leisure unless it has been earned through work.

Forms of work that are used in therapy vary greatly both in content and in organization. Work may simply be the completion of simple chores on the ward or completion of clerical tasks in a work module organized in occupational therapy. On the other hand, it may involve more serious volunteer work in the institution or the community or even reimbursed labor under the auspices of job training programs. Generally, more serious forms of work are seen as the final phase in a continuum of treatment for people with psychosocial dysfunction. Work is the most demanding of life tasks; it tends to be public, often involves drudgery, and requires substantial ability, commitment, and perseverance.

One approach to providing work for patients with psychosocial problems is to organize simple work modules within the occupational therapy workshop or clinic. In one work program, adolescent inpatients performed different tasks pursuant to making a large table game for the ward. Jobs were posted on the ward, and patients applied and were interviewed by a volunteer who also served as job supervisor. Patients were "hired" for the program to perform such jobs as carpenter, painter, and janitor. Hours were assigned, and patients punched in and out of work. They were paid in the form of tokens that could be used to purchase food and other objects.

Another way that meaningful work roles have been incorporated into a treatment program can be seen in community mental health programs for long-term treatment of psychiatric clients. In a clubhouse program based on Fountain House, members filled needed and important roles related to clubhouse maintenance. They performed jobs such as the clerical tasks of writing, artwork, production, and distribution of member newspapers; food preparation and the associated tasks of menu-planning, money management, serving, and cleanup; and tasks related to special events throughout the year. In addition to these tasks, members were responsible for orienting, touring, and being "buddies" to new members. All jobs were selected for their necessity in developing and maintaining the clubhouse and for their similarity to normal everyday responsibilities and activities. Occasional work projects based on subcontracting from other agencies were also accepted and performed by some members for wages. Finally, volunteer opportunities were made available to interested members. The clubhouse operation depended on the productive participation of its members. Both the maintenance of the organization itself and the services it offered to members and to the community relied on the efforts of members. There were opportunities for members to engage in meaningful work tasks with identifiable purposes, to collaborate with each other, and to contribute toward the maintenance of an organization to which they belonged. The organization of work into a program such as this is probably the most relevant kind of experience that adults with psychosocial dysfunction can have. It serves as a bridge between earlier states of disorganization and the organized labor required for productive community life. However, it does so in the context of a real and functioning institution.

Goodwin[48] describes another, often used approach of placing patients in jobs within the institution. This was once a major function of occupational therapy and was referred to as industrial therapy. The occupational therapist identified supervisors, who then either used patients as volunteers or reimbursed them for work within their departments. The occupational therapist was involved at both ends—consulting with the supervisors and counseling and performing training and mutual problem solving with the person placed on the job.

Another approach is the placement of people in industry in the community. DeMars[25] describes such a program in which she arranged with local industry for retarded people to be placed as janitors in actual job situations. A final level of involvement of the occupational therapist has been in the sheltered workshop. Such programs generally provide reimbursed work that is subcontracted from various groups. Therapists in such settings function in roles from job supervisor and work simplification expert to overall manager of the workshop.

Activities of Daily Living (ADL). Historically, occupational therapists have been concerned with activities of daily living as both a set of skills to be learned or maintained and as providing activities that place demands on clients for normal behavior while in treatment. ADL skills are necessary for adaptive, independent functioning and they reflect the client's self-image. Many of these activities could be considered as hobbies or as work if performed with different intent. Mosey[101] describes ADL as referring to "all those activities one must engage in or accomplish to be able to participate with comfort in other facets of life" (p. 75). The list of ADL areas of concern to occupational therapy includes the following: grooming; personal hygiene; food preparation, shopping, and nutrition; general home maintenance; communications, such as writing notes and using the telephone; money management; ability to arrange for transportation; and time management. The need for and nature of competence in each area varies with the individual's life experiences and the requirements of the setting in which the person lives.[71]

ADL programs have continued as a component of many psychosocial occupational therapy programs, whether in acute or chronic care hospitals, in community day treatment programs, or in transitional programs between the hospital and community. In acute care, the goal is usually to maintain the level of functioning rather than to teach new skills.[21] Community treatment programs frequently have ADL skill training components such as job-seeking skills, cooking, and grooming.[14] A lecture approach has also been used by some therapists to teach the ADL skills of homemaking, cooking, and dress-making, among other topics.[24,59] Yet another approach to increasing independence in the area of ADL is illustrated by a "quarterway house" program developed at a state hospital for a group of predischarge patients.[92] They were given increased responsibility for ADL, and the program included task group meetings in which training in areas of cooking, laundering, transportation, money management, shopping, and medications management were covered.

The benefits of ADL training may extend beyond the immediate skills learned. For instance, an intensive community reorientation training in ADL and leisure skills resulted not only in skill learning, but also in greater social interest among group members, increased social competence, and decreased symptomatology.[88]

The Use of Task-Oriented Groups

Groups have been used in occupational therapy throughout its history in a variety of ways. Although there is an extensive body of knowledge on group dynamics and group processes, the types and structures of groups in occupational therapy should reflect both the profession's unique emphasis on the value of occupation and a client/therapist relationship that directly promotes action and competence. Because the field is concerned with occupational groups, understanding of group process should derive from a sociological, as opposed to a psychodynamic, perspective on groups. In practical terms, this translates into asking, for example, how individuals learn and assume various occupational roles in a group, rather than asking how someone uses the group for multiple transference.

Examples of occupational groups found in everyday life include community task forces, political groups, music ensembles, sports teams, clubs, special interest groups such as weight loss groups, work units, parent-teacher groups, and so on. What these groups share is a task orientation—they exist specifically to accomplish some real and substantial activity, such as developing a program policy, winning a game, putting on a performance, or getting a job done. They differ from the type of group usually found in therapeutic settings in that the latter typically emphasize increasing self-understanding, and rely on talking to accomplish this goal. Self-understanding may well be a product of many occupational groups, but it is neither their explicit nor their only intended function.

The use of groups in psychosocial occupational therapy fills several important roles: It provides a recapitulation of productive and playful normal aspects of life; it allows for the development of social behaviors necessary to participating in occupational roles; and it is an arena for the communication of occupational values.

As a socialization process, occupational therapy communicates the expectations of the larger culture. Groups are an intrinsic part of our society, and people naturally belong to or identify with various groups throughout their lives. Donohue,[29] for instance, discusses a group that she labels an identification group. This is a homogeneous age and sex group to which a person naturally belongs. She uses the term "identification" instead of "reference group," because the latter typically implies a choice of wanting to use the group to define oneself. Many psychosocial patients, however, may not aspire toward membership in the reference group assigned to them by society. The identification group can evolve into a true reference group for the patient, however. In the women's identification group described by Donohue, activities included topic-centered discussions of issues such as birth control, child-rearing, and self-defense; experimentation with new behaviors, such as assertiveness and decision making; exercise and aerobics; and a casual coffee and rap session. These are all activities that would conceivably be engaged in by a group of nonhospitalized women meeting socially.

Similarly, Versluys'[127] role-focused groups are designed around the homemaker's role, maintenance of roles enacted by the patient prior to hospitalization, and family roles. The groups enable patients to discover that "they are capable of being productive within their physical and medical limitations" (p. 612) and to remain somewhat involved in the groups to which they belonged in normal life. In the role maintenance group, for instance, group members help one another to find ways in which they can carry out their family, community, and work obligations while they are hospitalized. This has the effects of minimizing the sick role and of helping the patient to maintain control of his or her life.

Occupational therapy literature is replete with examples of groups that have been used to teach daily living skills, social skills, and work skills. Many behaviors that are encompassed by the role of productive participant are best learned in groups. For instance, cooperation, competition, and consensual decision making can all be natural concomitants to various group activities. Fidler[36] describes the task group as "a shared working experience" where "alternate patterns of functioning can be considered and tested" (p. 45). She highlights the value of task groups as focusing on active and current involvement in a situation that closely simulates real life experience and demands for skilled, responsible, interpersonal behavior.

Skill development groups give patients the opportunity to receive feedback from their peers, to serve as role models for one another, and to experiment with new behaviors in a setting where experimentation is the norm. The therapeutic social club, which uses community resources and settings, enables former mental patients to develop leisure and interpersonal skills in a situation that bridges the gap between hospital and community.[30] Heine[53] described a daily living group that provided didactic and experiential learning in such areas as job hunting and interviewing, leisure planning, using the community, and finding living arrangements, among others. Meacham and Lindemann[95] developed a summer program for adolescents organized around work, social, self-care, and academic skill development in group settings. An assembly project gave teenagers the chance to produce salable products in an assembly-line situation, while the luncheon party unit involved members in learning about nutrition, planning and executive meals, and preparing a formal party for invited guests.

Mosey[100] offered guidelines for structuring task groups that would facilitate different levels of interpersonal skills; these groups range from a parallel level of activity, where individuals work on their own projects, to a mature, co-operative level, where members share responsibility for a completion of a major total group product. The importance of these guidelines lies in the knowledge that many work and leisure occupations are not only conducted in group settings but also require cooperative or team efforts. In addition, most occupational roles are learned and carried out in interpersonal con-texts,[101,127] and even roles that are eventually done somewhat independently, such as homemaker, are initially learned in a social situation (the family).

One example of how patients can assume both cooperative and individual roles can be found in German's[44] avocational interest group. The specific purpose of this group was to enable patients to develop interests in hobbies that could be pursued outside of the hospital. The group was structured with a short workshop period in which patients moved in and out of teaching and learning roles with one another. In addition, the use of written instructions and catalogues encouraged patients to independently pursue their interests outside the group.

In order to successfully communicate relevant occupational values, the group environment must be structured to be consistent with the demands of the group task. If a goal for therapy is to socialize individuals with little or no work history into a worker role, then a work group must embody, through explicit rules, the norms and values that are associated with work by society at large. If a new member perceives that others in the group consider their work to be important and preparatory for moving on to a job in another setting, then he or she will be inclined to adopt this attitude as well. Along with the attitude, the individual will feel group pressure to come on time, to interact in a manner that is appropriate for a work setting, and so forth. Donohue's[29] identification group operationalized this principle by using activities common to women in their daily lives, as well as an organizational format conducive to these activities. Aerobics sessions recreated the atmosphere of an adult education class, while the rap sessions recalled an informal living room or kitchen gathering. The leader acted as a group member, role model, and guide, helping other members to take on these roles as well. This structure, however, would not suffice for a work-skills group. There the emphasis would be on creating an atmosphere similar to what one would encounter in the real work world. Social and personal conversation would be minimal, and the leader would more appropriately function as supervisor or boss, rather than as group member.

THE OCCUPATIONAL THERAPIST AS ENVIRONMENTAL MANAGER

CREATING A CONTEXT FOR TREATMENT:

Occupational therapy influences the attitudes, conscious processes, and recovery of patients by how it organizes the environment.

Therapist's attitudes and indications about the activity and its value all influence how patients experience therapy.

Therapy ultimately has a role in constructing or reconstructing reality for patients via the messages contained in the therapeutic environment.

The environment of therapy is conceptualized as a context that guides and defines behavior and experiences.

These contexts may include exploration, festivity and ritual, sport, craft, work and play as a value, and an educational milieu.

Contexts are communicated by physical and architectural properties of a setting; dress, behavior, values, and ideas of people in a setting; and verbal and nonverbal communication.

Occupational therapy includes a context of competence by structuring the environment to match people's abilities.

MANAGING THE COMMUNITY ENVIRONMENT:

Occupational therapy has a developing role in managing the community environment; there is potential for occupational therapists to assume leadership positions in community mental health programming.

The community is a natural setting for occupational therapy since it provides a meaningful and normal context for learning skills.

Community work in comparison to the hospital is less structured, without physical boundaries, and has more flexible and complex administrative and co-worker relationships, and a relatively nonmedical orientation.

The community therapist must be familiar with community standards; work with a wide range of people and agencies; have a broader understanding of the life situations, culture, history, and environments of clients; and be able to assume roles as program director and consultant.

Community settings include residential programs, halfway houses, clubhouse programs, day treatment, sheltered workshops, quarterway houses, partial hospitalization, and prevention programs for the well elderly.

Models of community programming in which occupational therapists have been involved include aftercare programs to aid adjustment and promote independence, work-oriented day care programs, the clubhouse model (Fountain House), neighborhood extension of activity therapy, and a preventive activity program for elderly people.

THERAPIST AS CO-PROBLEM SOLVER AND CO-PLANNER

Counseling is within the purview of occupational therapy when it focuses on facilitating a person's participation in a pattern of healthy occupation.

Time management planning and problem solving:
- are based on a framework of temporal adaptation;
- focus on balance in daily life behavior; the match of values, interests, and goals to time use; role balance and performance; and temporal adjustments for pathology;
- aim at establishing a schedule of healthy occupation for clients to follow.

Occupational choice counseling:
- occurs when occupational choice is delayed or when a poor choice has been made;
- aims to having people find and operationalize work, play, and other roles consistent with their abilities and desires.

Leisure counseling:
- extends from a concern for overall temporal adaptation and the need for people to find meaning in play or leisure;
- involves identification of clients' values, roles, and skills to support leisure activities;
- applies to people such as workaholics, socially isolated individuals, or retirees with difficulty adjusting to leisure;

- may be part of a discharge planning or transitional program;
- may be part of a preretirement counseling program.

THE THERAPEUTIC USE OF SELF IN OCCUPATIONAL THERAPY

Concepts of the therapeutic use of self have evolved substantially since they originally grew out of psychoanalytic approaches.

In occupational therapy the therapeutic use of self has undergone shifts in emphasis.

Among a variety of human relationships, occupational therapy uses a special class of relationship related to occupation.

The therapeutic relationship in occupational therapy revolves around:
- interactions for accomplishing productive tasks in which people require emotional and information resources to support the struggle to perform competently;
- interactions for accomplishing forms of play such as ritual, celebration, sport, and recreation.

In the therapeutic relationship the occupational therapist influences the creation of the meaning of activities and supports the process of successful performance or participation in an occupation.

In order to enact the therapeutic use of self, the occupational therapist must have expertise in and value the occupations used as therapy.

THE USE OF OCCUPATIONS AS THERAPY

The central role of occupational therapy is providing occupations in which patients and clients participate.

Occupations refer to the broad spectrum of activities in which people engage as part of their routine use of time and include work, play, and self-care.

Emphasis on different types of occupations as therapy has differed over the history of the field.

The criterion for inclusion of occupations as forms of therapy should be their relevance to the culture at large and to the cultural background of people in therapy.

The art and science of occupational therapy media:
- centers on the process of developing competence for performance of work, play, and self-care activities;
- does not include the process of identifying and expressing unconscious feelings;

- is based on the understanding of the health-giving nature of occupation and on understanding the cultural and personal significance of occupation.

Play:
- contributes to the development of competency;
- serves as a therapeutic modality to increase skill and confidence.

Games:
- are a subclass of play that allow people to take risks in controlled and inconsequential contexts;
- may simulate the problems of everyday life and allow practice of problem-solving;
- are part of normal occupational behavior;
- may facilitate the development of moral behavior through appreciation of the functions of rules and their binding nature.

Sports:
- teach participants a sense of sportsmanship;
- evoke motor activity through their motivating properties;
- allow learning of roles, their functions, and reciprocal role relationships.

Performing arts:
- include dance, drama, film and video, music, magic, puppetry, storytelling, and mime;
- can be important forms of socialization and are linked to ritual;
- have a public nature, which means that they provide a point of reference and a source of feedback.

Arts and crafts:
- are enjoying a resurgence of popularity and worth;
- uniquely bind hands and mind to a productive purpose;
- can be integrated into people's life situations;
- can be individual or group activities;
- result in tangible, aesthetic, and useful products.

Work:
- should be a component of all adult therapeutic programs;
- can vary from chores, to work activities in the hospital, to volunteer activities, to actual work training;
- requires integration into a context that gives the work meaning and purpose.

Activities of daily living:
- are both targets and means of therapy;
- include those activities that support participation in other facets of daily life.

THE USE OF TASK-ORIENTED GROUPS

The use of groups in occupational therapy focuses on occupation (i.e., accomplishing tasks).

Groups:
- allow various occupations to take on a real rather than a simulated character;
- facilitate socialization of members into the attitudes and behaviors reflective of similar groups in the culture;
- facilitate social productive role behavior;
- serve as contexts for teaching skills;
- should be structured according to the ethos of groups that are naturally organized to accomplish tasks.

TERMS AND CONCEPTS

closed system	A system that does not interact with its environment and is not alive (e.g., a machine).
competent	Fulfilling the expectations of others.
context	A psychosocial setting that people recognize and that influences how they experience and behave.
custodialism	The process of containing handicapped people in institutions without offering rehabilitation.
cybernetic process	A process of modifying behavior based on feedback.
deinstitutionalization	The placement of people who were formerly in state hospitals into the community along with efforts to reduce the numbers of people sent to state hospitals in the first place.
demoralization	Loss of interest and commitment to one's way of life; a feeling of meaninglessness and hopelessness.
extrinsic motivation	Motivation whose source is not from within the activity itself. Extrinsically motivated behaviors are those done for some underlying motive (e.g., hunger) or motive external to the activity (e.g., payment or social praise) rather than for the activity itself.
fantasy period	A stage in occupational choice when choices are based solely on perceived pleasure in an occupation.

feedback The return of information to a system concerning the process and outcomes of its action.

goals Plans for future accomplishments.

gradation The principle of gradually increasing the complexity and challenge of occupations used as therapy.

habit deterioration The breakdown of routines of everyday life manifest in chaotic and disorganized daily behavior.

habits Internal images that trigger and guide routine performance.

habit training The name for early occupational therapy programs that incorporated full 24-hour schedules of work, play, rest, and sleep. These programs were aimed at restoring healthy patterns of daily occupational behavior.

habituation A process of developing routine behavior patterns. This term is used to describe the subsystem in the Model of Human Occupation which regulates routine behavior. It includes habits and roles as part of its structure.

hierarchy The arrangement of phenomena into levels in which higher ones govern and are constrained by the lower.

intake The importation of information and energy from the environment.

interests Dispositions to find certain objects or activities pleasurable.

internalized expectations Expectations for performance associated with a role that one perceives to pertain to oneself.

internalized role A role and its expectations which one perceives oneself to hold and which one believes others perceive one to hold.

intrinsic motivation	Motivation that emanates from the behavior itself rather than from some extraneous motive. Thus, intrinsically motivated activity is activity done for its own sake and not for some extrinsic reward.
mainstreaming	A policy of placing handicapped people in the types of institutions (e.g., schools) where nonhandicapped people are located.
meaningful activity	Activity which relates to a person's values and interests and which provides a sense of accomplishment and worth when it is performed.
normalization	An ideology that believes in giving handicapped people access to resources and circumstances to which the average (normal) member of the community has access.
occupational behavior	The performace of daily work, play, and self-care tasks.
occupational performance	See *occupational behavior*.
occupations	Activities motivated by the urge to explore and master. They generally include work, play, and activities of daily living.
output	The performance of some action by a system.
perceived role incumbance	The belief that one has the status and obligations of a given role and that others perceive likewise.
personal causation	Images one holds concerning one's effectiveness as an actor in the world.
press	The demands of the environment for certain types of behavior.
realistic period	A stage in occupational choice when the person has made a selection and has begun to operationalize the choice through receiving training and so forth.
role	A recognized position or status in a social group which had defined obligation for performance.

role balance — The healthy integration of roles into a routine of behavior satisfying to self and relevant others.

role dysfunction — Imbalance of roles and/or ability to perform the tasks associated with a role or roles.

sense of efficacy — A feeling that one is able to competently perform necessary and valued tasks.

socialization — The developmental process of acquiring the attitudes, values, and behavioral norms of a particular social group.

temporal adaptation — The organization of daily life behaviors into a satisfying and competent pattern of performance.

tension reduction — The release of pent-up psychic energy.

tentative period — A stage in occupational choice when a person has begun to seriously select an occupation based on interests, values, and an understanding of personal capacity.

throughput — The transformation of energy and information within a system and its incorporation into the function and structure of the system. Throughput often results in a change in the structure of a system.

values — Personal images of what is good, right, or otherwise highly desirable.

volition — The process of willing or choosing. The term is used to describe a subsystem in the Model of Human Occupation which is responsible for making choices. According to this theory, volition begins with the urge to explore and master and incorporates one's personal causation, values, and interests.

REFERENCES

1. Ayres, J. *Sensory integration and learning disorders*. Los Angeles: Western Psychological Services, 1972.
2. Azima, H., & Azima, F. J. Outline of a dynamic theory of occupational therapy. *American Journal of Occupational Therapy*, 1959, *13*, 215–221.
3. Barris, R. Environmental interactions: An extension of the model of

human occupation. *American Journal of Occupational Therapy*, 1982, *36*, 637–644.

4. Bateson, G. Communication in occupational therapy. *American Journal of Occupational Therapy*, 1956, *10*, 188.

5. Beard, H. G., Propst, R. N., & Malamud, T. J. The Fountain House model of psychiatric rehabilitation. *Psychosocial Rehabilitation Journal*, 1982, 5, 47–53.   PSYch. ABSTRACTS

6. Behnke, C. J. *Examining reliability of the play history*. Unpublished master's project, Department of Occupational Therapy, Virginia Commonwealth University, 1982.

7. Black, M. Adolescent role assessment. *American Journal of Occupational Therapy*, 1976, *30*, 73–79.

8. Bledsoe, N., & Shepherd, J. The preschool play scale. *American Journal of Occupational Therapy*, 1983, in press.

9. Bloomer, J., & Williams, S. The Bay Area Functional Performance Evaluation. In B. Hemphill (Ed.), *The evaluative process in psychiatric occupational therapy*. Thoroughfare, N.J.: Charles B. Slack, 1982.

10. Bockoven, J. S. Challenge of the new clinical approaches. *American Journal of Occupational Therapy*, 1968, *22*, 23–25.

11. Bockoven, J. S. *Moral treatment in community mental health*. New York: Springer Publishing, 1972.

12. Borys, S. Implications of interest theory for occupational therapy. *American Journal of Occupational Therapy*, 1974, *28*, 35–38.

13. Brayman, S. J., Kirby, T. F., Misenheimer, A. M., & Short, M. J. Comprehensive occupational therapy evaluation scale. *American Journal of Occupational Therapy*, 1976, *30*, 94–100.

14. Broekema, M. C., Danz, K. H., & Schloemer, C. U. Occupational therapy in a community aftercare program. *American Journal of Occupational Therapy*, 1975, *29*, 22–27.

15. Buck, R. E., & Provancher, M. A. Magazine picture collages as an evaluative technique. *American Journal of Occupational Therapy*, 1972, *26*, 36–39.

16. Burke, J. P. A clinical perspective on motivation: Pawn versus origin. *American Journal of Occupational Therapy*, 1977, *31*, 254–258.

17. Burke, J. P., Miyake, S., Kielhofner, G., & Barris, R. The demystification of health care and demise of the sick role: Implications for occupational therapy. In G. Kielhofner (Ed.), *Health through occupation: Theory and practice in occupational therapy*. Philadelphia: F. A. Davis, 1983.

18. Cantor, S. G. Occupational therapists as members of pre-retirement re-

source teams. *American Journal of Occupational Therapy*, 1981, *35*, 638–643.

19. Carey, C. *Games: An occupational therapy treatment mode for juvenile delinquent boys*. Unpublished master's project, Department of Occupational Therapy, Virginia Commonwealth University, 1981.

20. Casanova, J. S., & Ferber, J. Comprehensive evaluation of basic living skills. *American Journal of Occupational Therapy*, 1976, *30*, 101–105.

21. Corry, S., Sebastian, V., & Mosey, A. C. Acute short-term treatment in psychiatry. *American Journal of Occupational Therapy*, 1974, *28*, 401–406.

22. Cubie, S. H., & Kaplan, K. A case analysis method for the model of human occupation. *American Journal of Occupational Therapy*, 1982, *36*, 645–656.

23. Cynkin, S. *Occupational therapy: Toward health through activities*. Boston: Little, Brown, 1979.

24. Deane, W. N., & Dodd, M. L. Educational techniques for the rehabilitation of chronic schizophrenic patients. *American Journal of Occupational Therapy*, 1960, *14*, 7–12.

25. DeMars, P. K. Training adult retardates for private enterprise. *American Journal of Occupational Therapy*, 1975, *29*, 39–42.

26. deRenne-Stephan, C. Imitation: A mechanism of play behavior. *American Journal of Occupational Therapy*, 1980, *34*, 95–102.

27. Diasio, K. Psychiatric occupational therapy: Search for a conceptual framework in light of psychoanalytic ego psychology and learning theory. *American Journal of Occupational Therapy*, 1968, *22*, 400–414.

28. Dobbins, B. *An investigation of the reliability and validity of the Westphal decision making inventory*. Unpublished master's project, Department of Occupational Therapy, Virginia Commonwealth University, 1980.

29. Donohue, M. V. Designing activities to develop a women's identification group. *Occupational Therapy in Mental Health*, 1982, *2*, 1–19. *women's paper*

30. Dunning, H. Environmental occupational therapy. *American Journal of Occupational Therapy*, 1972, *26*, 292–298.

31. Dunning, R. E. The occupational therapist as counselor. *American Journal of Occupational Therapy*, 1973, *27*, 473–476.

32. Engelhardt, H. T., Jr. Defining occupational therapy: The meaning of therapy and the virtues of occupation. *American Journal of Occupational Therapy*, 1977, *31*, 666–672.

33. Ethridge, D. A. The management view of the future of occupational therapy in mental health. *American Journal of Occupational Therapy*, 1976, *30*, 623–628.

34. Farnham-Diggory, S. Self, future, and time: A developmental study of

the concepts of psychotic, brain-damaged, and normal children. *Monographs of the Society for Research in Child Development*, 1966, *31* (1, Serial No. 103).

35. Fidler, G. Some unique contributions of occupational therapy in the treatment of the schizophrenic. *American Journal of Occupational Therapy*, 1958, *12*, 9–12.

36. Fidler, G. S. The task-oriented group as a context for treatment. *American Journal of Occupational Therapy*, 1969, *23*, 43–48.

37. Fidler, G., & Fidler, J. Doing and becoming: Purposeful action and self-actualization. *American Journal of Occupational Therapy*, 1978, *32*, 305–310.

38. Fidler, G., & Fidler, J. Doing and becoming: The occupational therapy experience. In G. Kielhofner (Ed.), *Health through occupation: Theory and practice in occupational therapy*. Philadelphia: F. A. Davis, 1983.

39. Florey, L. Intrinsic motivation: The dynamics of occupational therapy. *American Journal of Occupational Therapy*, 1969, *23*, 319–322.

40. Florey, L. An approach to play and play development. *American Journal of Occupational Therapy*, 1971, *25*, 275–280.

41. Florey, L., & Michelman, S. Occupational role history: A screening tool for psychiatric occupational therapy. *American Journal of Occupational Therapy*, 1982, *36*, 301–308.

42. Fluegelman, A. (Ed.). *The new games book*. San Francisco: Headlands Press, 1976.

43. Fluegelman, A. *More new games*. Tiburon, Calif.: Headlands Press, 1981.

44. German, S. A. A group approach to rehabilitation occupational therapy in a psychiatric setting. *American Journal of Occupational Therapy*, 1964, *18*, 209–214.

45. Gilfoyle, E. M. Caring: A philosophy for practice. *American Journal of Occupational Therapy*, 1980, *34*, 517–521.

46. Girling, K. L. Leisure counseling. *Canadian Journal of Occupational Therapy*, 1979, *46*, 155–158.

47. Goldstein, N., & Collins, T. Making videotapes: An activity for hospitalized adolescents. *American Journal of Occupational Therapy*, 1982, *36*, 530–533.

48. Goodwin, E. Implementation of the occupational behavior model: A personal account. *Canadian Journal of Occupational Therapy*, 1976, *43*, 14–17.

49. Gray, M. Effects of hospitalization on work-play behavior. *American Journal of Occupational Therapy*, 1972, *26*, 180–185.

50. Gregory, M. *Occupational behavior and life satisfaction among retirees.*

Unpublished master's project, Department of Occupational Therapy, Virginia Commonwealth University, 1981.

51. Hasselkus, B. R. Relocation stress and the elderly. *American Journal of Occupational Therapy*, 1978, *32*, 631–636.

52. Heard, C. Occupational role acquisition: A perspective on the chronically disabled. *American Journal of Occupational Therapy*, 1977, *31*, 243–247.

53. Heine, D. Daily living group: Focus on transition from hospital to community. *American Journal of Occupational Therapy*, 1975, *29*, 628–630.

54. Hofstadter, D. R. *Godel, Escher, Bach: An internal golden braid*. New York: Basic Books, 1979.

55. Howe, M. C., Weaver, C. T., & Dulay, J. The development of a work-oriented day care program. *American Journal of Occupational Therapy*, 1981, *35*, 711–718.

56. Hurff, J. Gaming technique: An assessment and training tool for individuals with learning deficits. *American Journal of Occupational Therapy*, 1981, *35*, 728–735.

57. Kannegieter, R. Environmental interactions in psychiatric occupational therapy—Some inferences. *American Journal of Occupational Therapy*, 1980, *34*, 715–720.

58. Kaplan, K. *Directive group*. Unpublished paper, Department of Occupational Therapy, Virginia Commonwealth University, 1972.

59. Kaseman, B. M. Teaching money management skills to psychiatric outpatients. *Occupational Therapy in Mental Health*, 1980, *1*, 59–71.

60. Kavanaugh, M. *Person-environment interaction: The model of human occupation applied to mentally retarded adults*. Unpublished master's project, Department of Occupational Therapy, Virginia Commonwealth University, 1982.

61. Kielhofner, G. Temporal adaptation: A conceptual framework for occupational therapy. *American Journal of Occupational Therapy*, 1977, *31*, 235–238.

62. Kielhofner, G. A model of human occupation, Part 2. Ontogenesis from the perspective of temporal adaptation. *American Journal of Occupational Therapy*, 1980, *34*, 657–663.

63. Kielhofner, G. A model of human occupation, Part 3. Benign and vicious cycles. *American Journal of Occupational Therapy*, 1980, *34*, 732–737.

64. Kielhofner, G. A paradigm for practice: The hierarchical organization of occupational therapy knowledge. In G. Kielhofner (Ed.), *Health through occupation: Theory and practice in occupational therapy*. Philadelphia: F. A. Davis, 1983.

65. Kielhofner, G., Barris, R., & Watts, J. Habits and habit dysfunction: A

clinical perspective for psychosocial occupational therapy. *Occupational Therapy in Mental Health*, 1982, *2*, 1–22.

66. Kielhofner, G., & Burke, J. P. A model of human occupation, Part 1. Conceptual framework and content. *American Journal of Occupational Therapy*, 1980, *34*, 572–581.

67. Kielhofner, G., & Burke, J. P. The evolution of knowledge and practice in occupational therapy: Past, present and future. In G. Kielhofner (Ed.), *Health through occupation: Theory and practice in occupational therapy.* Philadelphia: F. A. Davis, 1983.

68. Kielhofner, G., Burke, J. P., & Igi, C. H. A model of human occupation, Part 4. Assessment and intervention. *American Journal of Occupational Therapy*, 1980, *34*, 777–788.

69. Kielhofner, G., & Miyake, S. The therapeutic use of games with mentally retarded adults. *American Journal of Occupational Therapy*, 1981, *35*, 375–382.

70. Kielhofner, G., & Miyake, S. Rose-colored lenses for clinical practice: From a deficit to a competence model in assessment and intervention. In G. Kielhofner (Ed.), *Health through occupation: Theory and practice in occupational therapy*. Philadelphia: F. A. Davis, 1983.

71. Kielhofner, G., & Takata, N. A study of mentally retarded persons: Applied research in occupational therapy. *American Journal of Occupational Therapy*, 1980, *34*, 252–258.

72. King, L. J. A sensory-integrative approach to schizophrenia. *American Journal of Occupational Therapy*, 1974, *28*, 529–536.

73. Kirchman, M. M., Reichenbach, V., & Giambalvo, B. Preventive activities and services for the well elderly. *American Journal of Occupational Therapy*, 1982, *36*, 236–242.

74. Klavins, R. Work-play behavior: Cultural influences. *American Journal of Occupational Therapy*, 1972, *26*, 176–179.

75. Kluckholn, F. R., & Strodtbeck, F. L. *Variations in value orientations.* New York: Row, Peterson, 1961.

76. Knox, S. *Observation and assessment of the everyday play behavior of the mentally retarded child.* Unpublished master's thesis, Department of Occupational Therapy, University of Southern California, 1968.

77. Knox, S. A play scale. In M. Reilly (Ed.), *Play as exploratory learning.* Beverly Hills, Calif.: Sage Publications, 1974.

78. Kohler, E. S. The effect of activity/environment on emotionally disturbed children. *American Journal of Occupational Therapy*, 1980, *34*, 446–451.

79. Kolodner, E. L. Neighborhood extension of activity therapy. *American Journal of Occupational Therapy*, 1973, *27*, 381–383.

80. Kuenstler, G. A planning group for psychiatric outpatients. *American Journal of Occupational Therapy*, 1976, *30*, 634–639.

81. Larrington, G. *An exploratory study of the temporal aspects of adaptive functioning*. Unpublished master's thesis, Department of Occupational Therapy, University of Southern California, 1970.

82. Lawn, E. C., & O'Kane, C. P. Psychosocial symbols as communicative media. *American Journal of Occupational Therapy*, 1973, *27*, 30–33.

83. Lerner, C., & Ross, G. The magazine picture collage: Development of an objective scoring system. *American Journal of Occupational Therapy*, 1977, *31*, 156–161.

84. Levin, S. *Test-retest reliability of the Westphal decision making inventory*. Unpublished master's project, Department of Occupational Therapy, Virginia Commonwealth University, 1981.

85. Lillie, M. D., & Armstrong, H. E., Jr. Contributions to the development of psychoeducational approaches to mental health service. *American Journal of Occupational Therapy*, 1982, *36*, 438–443.

86. Lindquist, J., Mack, W., & Parham, D. A synthesis of occupational behavior and sensory integrative concepts in theory and practice, Part 1. Theoretical foundations. *American Journal of Occupational Therapy*, 1982, *36*, 365–374.

87. Lindquist, J., Mack, W., & Parham, D. A synthesis of occupational behavior and sensory integration concepts in theory and practice, Part 2. Clinical applications. *American Journal of Occupational Therapy*, 1982, *36*, 433–437.

88. Linnell, M. W., Caffey, E. M., Klett, C. J., Hogarty, G. E., & Lamb, R. L. Day treatment and psychotropic drugs in the aftercare of schizophrenic patients. *Archives of General Psychiatry*, 1979, *36*, 1055–1066.

89. Linnell, K., Stechman, A., & Watson, C. Resocialization of schizophrenic patients. *American Journal of Occupational Therapy*, 1975, *29*, 288–290.

90. Llorens, L. Facilitating growth and development: The promise of occupational therapy. *American Journal of Occupational Therapy*, 1970, *24*, 93–101.

91. Magill, J., & Vargo, J. Helplessness, hope and the occupational therapist. *Canadian Journal of Occupational Therapy*, 1977, *44*, 65–69.

92. Mann, W. C. A quarterway house for adult psychiatric patients. *American Journal of Occupational Therapy*, 1976, *30*, 646–647.

93. Matsutsuyu, J. S. The interest checklist. *American Journal of Occupational Therapy*, 1969, *23*, 323–328.

94. Matsutsuyu, J. Occupational behavior—A perspective on work and play. *American Journal of Occupational Therapy*, 1971, *25*, 291–294.

95. Meacham, R., & Lindemann, J. E. A summer program for underachiev-

ing adolescents. *American Journal of Occupational Therapy*, 1975, *29*, 280–283.

96. Menarcheck, M. *Examining the validity of the play history.* Unpublished master's project, Department of Occupational Therapy, Virginia Commonwealth University, 1982.

97. Michelman, S. Play and the deficit child. In M. Reilly (Ed.), *Play as exploratory learning.* Beverly Hills, Calif.: Sage Publications, 1974.

98. Moorhead, L. The occupational history. *American Journal of Occupational Therapy*, 1969, *23*, 329–334.

99. Mosey, A. Recapitulation of ontogenesis: A theory for practice of occupational therapy. *American Journal of Occupational Therapy*, 1968, *22*, 426–438.

100. Mosey, A. C. The concept and use of developmental groups. *American Journal of Occupational Therapy*, 1970, *24*, 272–275.

101. Mosey, A. C. *Occupational therapy: Configuration of a profession.* New York: Raven Press, 1981.

102. Neville, A. Temporal adaptation: Application with short-term psychiatric patients. *American Journal of Occupational Therapy*, 1980, *34*, 328–331.

103. Nihara, K., Foster, R., Shellhaas, M., & Leland, H. *AAMD Adaptive Behavior Scale.* Washington, D.C.: American Association on Mental Deficiency, 1974.

104. Nystrom, E. P. Activity patterns and leisure concepts among the elderly. *American Journal of Occupational Therapy*, 1974, *28*, 337–345.

105. Oakley, F. M. *The model of human occupation in psychiatry.* Unpublished master's project, Department of Occupational Therapy, Virginia Commonwelath University, 1982.

106. Parent, L. Effects of a low-stimulus environment on behavior. *American Journal of Occupational Therapy*, 1978, *32*, 19–25.

107. Paulson, C. Juvenile delinquency and occupational choice. *American Journal of Occupational Therapy*, 1980, *34*, 565–571.

108. Potts, L. *Toward a developmental assessment of leisure patterns.* Unpublished master's thesis, Department of Occupational Therapy, University of Southern California, 1969.

109. Reilly, M. Occupational therapy can be one of the great ideas of 20th century medicine. *American Journal of Occupational Therapy*, 1962, *16*, 1–9.

110. Reilly, M. A. A psychiatric occupational therapy program as a teaching model. *American Journal of Occupational Therapy*, 1966, *20*, 61–67.

111. Reilly, M. *Play as exploratory learning.* Beverly Hills, Calif.: Sage Publications, 1974.

112. Riopel, N. J. *An examination of the occupational behavior and life satis-faction of the elderly.* Unpublished master's thesis, Medical College of Virginia, Virginia Commonwealth University, 1982.

113. Robinson, A. Play: The arena for acquisition of rules for competent behavior. *American Journal of Occupational Therapy*, 1977, *31*, 248–253.

114. Rogers, J. Order and disorder in medicine and occupational therapy. *American Journal of Occupational Therapy*, 1982, *36*, 29–35.

115. Rogers, J. C., & Snow, T. An assessment of the behaviors of the institutionalized elderly. *American Journal of Occupational Therapy*, 1982, *36*, 375–380.

116. Rogers, J., Weinstein, J., & Figone, J. An empirical assessment of the interest checklist. *American Journal of Occupational Therapy*, 1978.

117. Roos, P., & Albers, R. Performance of retardates and normals on a measure of temporal orientation. *American Journal of Mental Deficiency*, 1965, *69*, 835–838.

118. Rotter, J. Generalized expectancies for internal versus external control for reinforcement. *Psychological Monographs*, 1966, *80* (1, Whole No. 609).

119. Scaffa, M. *Temporal adaptation and alcoholism.* Unpublished master's project, Department of Occupational Therapy, Virginia Commonwealth University, 1981.

120. Scheflen, A. E. *Body language and social order.* Englewood Cliffs, N. J.: Prentice-Hall, 1972.

121. Shannon, P. Work-play theory and the occupational therapy process. *American Journal of Occupational Therapy*, 1972, *26*, 169–172.

122. Shannon, P. Occupational choice: Decision making play. In M. Reilly (Ed.), *Play as exploratory learning.* Beverly Hills, Calif.: Sage Publications, 1974.

123. Sharrott, G. Occupational therapy's role in the client's creation and affirmation of meaning. In G. Kielhofner (Ed.), *Health through occupation: Theory and practice in occupational therapy.* Philadelphia: F. A. Davis, 1983.

124. Shroeder, C. V., Block, M. P., Trottier, & Stowell, M. S. The adult psychiatric sensory integrative evaluation. In B. Hemphill (Ed.), *The evaluative process in psychiatric occupational therapy.* Thoroughfare, N. J.: Charles B. Slack, 1982.

125. Takata, N. Play as a prescription. In M. Reilly (Ed.), *Play as exploratory learning.* Beverly Hills, Calif.: Sage Publications, 1974.

126. Vandenberg, B., & Kielhofner, G. Play in evolution, culture and in-dividual adaptation: Implications for therapy. *American Journal of Occupational Therapy*, 1982, *36*, 20–28.

127. Versluys, H. P. The remediation of role disorders through focused group work. *American Journal of Occupational Therapy*, 1980, *34*, 609–614.
128. Watts, J., & Barris, R. *Aging: Person-environment interaction and the model of human occupation*. Richmond: Virginia Commonwealth University, 1981. (Audiovisual production)
129. Watanabe, S. Four concepts to the occupational therapy process. *American Journal of Occupational Therapy*, 1968, *22*, 339–444.
130. Webb, L. J. The therapeutic social club. *American Journal of Occupational Therapy*, 1973, *27*, 81–83.
131. Webster, P. Occupational role development in the young adult with mild mental retardation. *American Journal of Occupational Therapy*, 1980, *34*, 13–18.
132. Wiemer, R. Traditional and nontraditional practice arenas. In *Occupational therapy: 2001 A.D.* Rockville, Md.: American Occupational Therapy Association, 1979.
133. Westphal, M. *A study of decision making*. Unpublished master's thesis, Department of Occupational Therapy, University of Southern California, 1967.
134. Yerxa, E. Occupational therapy's role in creating a future climate of caring. *American Journal of Occupational Therapy*, 1980, *34*, 529–534.

16
Criticisms and Limitations

The most obvious limitation of the occupational therapy tradition in psy-chosocial practice is the one that has been emphasized throughout this volume. Occupational therapy practice in the area of psychosocial dysfunction has a very specific and therefore circumscribed purpose and intent: to improve people's capacity for and involvement in healthy occupations. As such, it does not address some of the problems inherent in psychosocial dysfunction. In-terestingly, therapists have not always recognized or agreed to these limits. For example, the whole domain of sexual feelings and unconscious processes are beyond the scope of occupational therapy, yet many therapists have made these issues focal points of their practice.

In addition, since occupational therapy focuses on the maintenance and development of healthy behavior, it has limited relevance to many aspects of psychopathology as conceptualized by the medical model. Reilly[4] suggested that occupational therapy makes no claim to influence pathological states; however, this issue bears further exploration. Occupational therapy has lim-ited impact on pathology in terms of psychiatric diagnostic categories. That is, it is not directed at influencing any psychodynamics underlying such states as anorexia or modifying symptomatic events such as hallucinations. Other contributions in the mental health arena such as psychotherapy and chemo-therapy do make claims to have an influence on such pathological phenomena.

On the other hand, because psychosocial dysfunction frequently involves the interplay of several etiological and syndromatic factors—some of which may be occupational in nature—a program of occupational therapy aimed at influencing healthy occupational behavior could have some impact on path-ological processes. The limitation of occupational therapy is that it does not specifically seek to remediate pathology. For example, occupational therapy, with its concentration on life tasks and concrete performance, may increase the reality-based thinking of the schizophrenic patient. Or because of its emphasis on eliciting feelings of competence and control, it may reduce symptoms of clinical depression or the anxiety level of a psychotic person. But even in such cases, the goal of treatment is not symptom reduction. Thus, while the contribution of occupational therapists to influencing pathology is limited, it nonetheless may exist as an indirect result of therapy.

This is not to suggest that occupational therapy has a more limited contribution than other disciplines to make to those with psychosocial problems. On the contrary, occupational problems are part and parcel of psychosocial disorder, and the occupational therapist is in a special position to address and ameliorate such problems.

The process of setting limits on what one does as a professional is a critical one, lest a field be accused of claiming to be "all things to all people." At times in the past, occupational therapists have come dangerously close to this or have actually made such claims, attempting to use occupational media for any purpose they chose. All fields and their respective views of order and disorder, along with their action implications, offer only partial answers to complex psychosocial problems. Each is limited by its particular focus and expertise.

Another important limitation of occupational therapy is the "state of the art." As a relatively new field that has placed less emphasis on developing a coherent body of knowledge than on refining practical techniques, the field has less sophisticated concepts and fewer connections between theory and practice than fields such as behavioral psychology that have stressed science as much as practical application. The manifestations of this limitation are: (1) the lack of conceptual refinement of theory (especially refinement based on research); (2) the preliminary nature of most clinical assessments (i.e., most lack research claims to reliability and validity); (3) the limited connections between theory and practice (i.e., many theoretical formulations do not have clearly articulated action principles, and many practical programs described in the literature are not firmly based in theory); and (4) the lack of outcome research on practice techniques and programs.

Another limitation of occupational therapy is the degree to which most occupational therapists understand the main tradition and themes of the field. Over the years therapists in a variety of settings have come under pressure to accept and apply the knowledge of traditions other than occupational therapy. For example, one can find occupational therapy programs based primarily on behavioral or psychoanalytic concepts. Such programs not only obscure the uniqueness of occupational therapy, but they limit the contribution that clinical practice could otherwise make to the development of technologies of practice for the field. Because the perspective offered in this volume on occupational therapy practice is not at present universally accepted, disagreement, dialogue, and eventual consensus will have to occur before clear and concentrated development of the knowledge and practice base can take place. In this vein, Bockoven[1,2] has criticized occupational therapy for its lack of recognition of its moral mandate and its inattention to the mental problems of disordered society (i.e., poor conditions of work and play that lead to psychosocial dysfunction). Bockoven is referring to the fact that occupational therapy has often taken the route of existing psychodynamic or other approaches, rather than developing and pursuing its own unique contribution to psychosocial health.

It could be said that occupational therapy's historical mandate is certainly much larger than that which has already been realized in clinical practice. Reilly[3] saw occupational therapy as being one of the great ideas of 20th century medicine, yet its practice does not reflect such importance. This is both discouraging, since it indicates that the field has been slow to operationalize its hypothesis that occupation can influence health, and encouraging, since it points to a great potential for the field if efforts are consolidated to advance theory, research, and practice.

A criticism that occupational therapists in practice will be familiar with is one that comes from other professionals as they view occupational therapy in psychosocial treatment. That is, the practical focus of the field, its concern for playful media and the like, is often misinterpreted by other disciplines as a sign that occupational therapy is not an important therapy or that it is primarily diversional in nature. In other words, it keeps patients busy but doesn't really have any impact on their problems.

In the past it is this criticism that appears to have led therapists to abandon their orientation and their occupational media in favor of assuming roles more like those of others in the setting—for example, running verbal groups with no occupational component. Therapists should recognize that such criticism is not founded in an objective analysis of occupational therapy but in misunderstanding. As Reilly[3] once noted, the vast difference between the complexity of our patient problems and the very simple media we use to address those problems is both our greatest asset and our greatest vulnerability. Therapists should seek ways to translate criticism into a recognition of occupational therapy as an asset. Inservice education and clearly formulated and theoretically based program descriptions are examples of the kinds of tools that therapists can use to explain their therapy, its goals, and how it works.

REFERENCES

1. Bockoven, J. S. Challenge of the new clinical approaches. *American Journal of Occupational Therapy*, 1968, *22*, 23–25.
2. Bockoven, J. S. *Moral treatment in community mental health.* New York: Springer Publishing, 1972.

3. Reilly, M. Occupational therapy can be one of the great ideas of 20th century medicine. *American Journal of Occupational Therapy*, 1983, *16*, 1–9.
4. Reilly, M. A psychiatric occupational therapy program as a teaching model. *American Journal of Occupational Therapy*, 1966, *20*, 61–67.

17
Commentary

Part Two of this book followed the presentation of 11 major bodies of knowledge in psychosocial practice and proposed in detail the occupational therapy approach to psychosocial dysfunction. As we noted in the introduction, the total volume reflects a conviction that occupational therapists must appreciate the perspectives of others in psychosocial practice while having depth and expertise in their own body of knowledge.

In proposing a unique occupational therapy approach to practice, Part Two showed how certain themes and principles have emerged and been enacted by therapists. These themes capture what we perceive to be the longstanding central tradition of the field, and they provide a cohesive framework for delineating the role of occupational therapy in psychosocial practice.

Some will no doubt view our concentration on occupation and occupational dysfunction and our relative exclusion of such concepts and approaches such as psychoanalytically based occupational therapy as unnecessarily confining to both the scholarship and practice of occupational therapy. We are the first to acknowledge that our approach definitively sets limits on the boundaries of occupational therapy's expertise and defines the nature of its practice in a narrower sense than others have proposed.

It is not the intention of this volume to limit occupational therapists' awareness of a wide range of knowledge. For this reason Part One covered major theoretical perspectives in psychosocial practice today. However, we do reject the notion that all this knowledge should be treated equally by occupational therapists. Occupational therapists must evaluate and determine what any knowledge has to offer their practice by selecting judiciously that which is complementary and leaving out that which is not necessary or relevant. To fail to do so perpetuates ambiguity in psychosocial occupational therapy practice and results in the inability of the field to either define its special area of expertise or to admit limitations in the range of competencies of its practitioners. In the past such failure has diluted occupational therapists' grasp of what they should uniquely know how to do and obscured the identity that would make occupational therapists valuable and definable members of a psychosocial health care team.

The dilution of the occupational therapist's knowledge and identity that has resulted from an eclectic, broad-based approach to psychosocial practice can actually be more limiting in the long run. As the introduction to this text suggested, therapists who try to embrace all theories eventually find that their practices reflect the expectations or needs of other professionals, often at the expense of their own beliefs. On the other hand, therapists who identify with a unique theoretical tradition that gives a focus to their role are in a better positon to define what services they have to offer and then to competently provide them. Rather than confining, a unique professional theory allows the practitioner to understand pluralistic viewpoints without losing sight of his or her own perspective.

The focus on occupation that we have identified as central to occupational therapy is far from being a restrictive perspective for the field. Occupation is a complex phenomenon that can take us to a wide range of concerns and studies. Within this general rubric there is ample room for creativity, diversity of thought, and variety of research, theory, and practice. Even more important, the focus on occupation reflects the historical mandate of the field as well as mainstream beliefs and principles of occupational therapists practicing in psychosocial settings today. Belief in the occupational nature of people and a treatment emphasis on work, play, and self-care continues to characterize the practice of many occupational therapists and, in particular, that of therapists who are most likely to think and act as autonomous professionals.[1]

Hence, it is not only *not* confining to set limits on the scope of practice, but it can serve to strengthen and ensure the professional survival of the field. In fact, it is probably unwise to seek survival by trying to fit in and adopt the ideas of others, because the health care system of today is itself in a state of flux.

For instance, such trends as increasing concern over cost-effectiveness, the movement of health care into the private corporate sector, and the growing awareness and power of the consumer who wants to be informed will increasingly make demands on occupational therapy to clearly articulate its service and the benefits of that service. At the same time that such changes in health care will call for a more clearly delineated service, there will be changes that would welcome the kind of occupational therapy service we have articulated in this book. As consumers become more aware that health is a matter of what they do, they will be looking for health care that supports their doing instead of simply repairing their deficits. Health care in general is recognizing that health is a state greatly influenced by the person's daily action and interaction with the environment. A service model which provides opportunity for active involvement and which addresses the process of everyday competence will flourish in such an arena.

While the system is changing, we are well aware that the present health care system has created many impediments to our practice. Issues of reimbursability for our services and gaining recognition from other psychosocial workers can be major obstacles, but they are not insurmountable. In fact, some of the difficulty we currently face in obtaining third-party reimbursement for occupational goals and means has resulted because we did not have a clear sense of our mission in the past and others defined for us what should be reimbursed. Shaping practice to what we can get paid for, rather than to what individuals really need, may allow us to survive in the short run, but in the long run it will fail because we will no longer be maintaining the social contract that initiated the field's existence.

Like all fields, occupational therapy came into existence and initially gained financial and social support from society because it served an identifiable need. This need was for reality-based programs of occupation that could reorient and rehabilitate disabled persons. As we have strayed from this historical mandate, other fields have quickly stepped in to fill the gap, so obviously the need for the type of service we can offer still exists.

Given both the historical reasons for the emergence of occupational therapy and the current changes in the health care system, occupational therapy can hardly afford to remain an ambiguous service, unsure of its unique contribution in health care. While identifying with the knowledge and techniques of other professions or blending into the philosophies of particular settings may be a path of least resistance or a means of gaining acceptance or respect for individual therapists in the short run, it would be professional suicide in the long run.

Having a viable practice in a pluralistic arena requires a unified professional identity. The source of such an identity and practice is already available in the field's tradition of knowledge. This book should be a step toward enhancing the identification and operationalization of a unique and unified occupational therapy service.

REFERENCE

1. Barris, R. *Toward an image of one's own: Sources of variation in the occupational therapist's role.* Unpublished doctoral dissertation, Teacher's College, Columbia University, New York, 1983.